Moxibustion:

The Power of Mugwort Fire

by Lorraine Wilcox, L. Ac.

Published by:
BLUE POPPY PRESS
A Division of Blue Poppy Enterprises, Inc.
1990 North 57th Court, Unit A
Boulder, CO 80301
www.bluepoppy.com

First Edition, May 2008
Second Printing, November 2009
Third Printing, June 2010

ISBN 1-891845-46-2
ISBN 978-1-891845-46-8
LCCN #2008927164

DISCLAIMER: The information in this book is given in good faith. However, the author and the publishers cannot be held responsible for any error or omission. The publishers will not accept liabilities for any injuries or damages caused to the reader that may result from the reader's acting upon or using the content contained in this book. The publishers make this information available to English-language readers for research and scholarly purposes only.

The publishers do not advocate nor endorse self-medication by laypersons.
Chinese and Western medicines are professional medicines.
Laypersons interested in availing themselves of the treatments described in this book should seek out a qualified professional practitioner of Chinese and/or Western medicine.

Cover & page design: Eric J. Brearton & Honora Wolfe

COMP Designation: Original work

10 9 8 7 6 5 4 3

Printed at Edwards Brothers, Ann Arbor, MI, on recycled paper with soy inks.

TABLE OF CONTENTS

PART 3: CONCLUSION

PREFACE

This book investigates the use of moxibustion in treating and preventing disease. Part 1 contains introductory chapters defining moxibustion, describing the various types and techniques, and the history of its practice. Part 2 researches this modality as it was practiced at the end of the Ming dynasty (1368-1644) through the writings of three master physicians. Part 3 is the conclusion. It summarizes and makes recommendations for increasing the scope of moxibustion practice in contemporary clinics of the West.

The heart of this book is Part 2 in which I explore the works of three important authors and physicians through annotated translations and discussions of their relevant writings. These masters are:

- Yang Jizhou (1522-1620), the author of *Great Compendium of Acupuncture and Moxibustion*.[1]
- Zhang Jiebin (1563-1640), also known as Zhang Jingyue, the author of the *Illustrated Supplement to the Categorized Classic* and *[Zhang] Jingyue's Complete Works*.[2]
- Li Shizhen (1518-1593), author of *Great Pharmacopoeia*.[3]

Biographies of the authors and discussions of the source texts can be found in the appendices.

Moxibustion seems to be in a state of decline in the West. In Chinese, "acupuncture and moxibustion" can be said in two syllables: *zhen jiu*. In English, it takes nine syllables. So the word "moxibustion" is often dropped. This tends to de-emphasize its importance.

At the time this book was written, there were few English language books specifically on moxibustion. Textbooks generally focus on acupuncture and give much less space to moxibustion. It is also less emphasized in the average techniques class or teaching clinic. This is a lack that needs to be remedied if

---

[1] 楊繼洲 《針灸大成》 published in 1601, hereafter called *Great Compendium*.
[2] 張介賓, 張景岳 《類經圖翼》, 《景岳全書》 published in 1624 and 1636, respectively. Hereafter called *Illustrated Supplement* and *Zhang's Complete Works*.
[3] 李時珍 《本草綱目》 published (posthumously) in 1596.

moxibustion is to be regarded with equal status to acupuncture (Wilcox, 2007).

This book is intended, in part, to raise the modern practitioner's awareness of and to help restore moxibustion to its honored position. The translations found in Part 2 demonstrate how important moxibustion was in clinical practice during the Ming dynasty. They describe a variety of techniques and a wide range of diseases that were treated with moxibustion. Although some of the treatments are clearly not applicable in the modern Western clinic, many or most are. It is likely that at least some of these techniques can affect a cure when other treatment methods fail.

Since few English language textbooks discuss the use of moxibustion in detail, these translations also allow the modern English-speaking clinician to expand its clinical use. I encourage practitioners to experiment with techniques that are new to them and, in this way, revive some of the "endangered species" techniques of moxibustion. I also hope that more varied moxibustion techniques will be taught in schools of East Asian medicine in the West.

HOW THIS BOOK CAME TO BE

One day as I was flipping through Zhang Jiebin's *Illustrated Supplement*, I came upon a section in Volume 11 on the treatment of disease covering each symptom, pattern, or disease one by one. To my surprise, virtually all of the treatments were moxibustion prescriptions. I found this surprising because Zhang is well-known as a theorist and as an herbalist. I had never heard anyone discuss his use of acupuncture or moxibustion before. In addition, I have been told that most herbalists looked down on acupuncture-moxibustion.

I liked that this section was a complete treatment manual. Further, it was not extremely long, so I began translating it for myself. I still consider this section to be the core of the book.

Later, I was researching the Yuan dynasty doctor, Zhu Danxi. Zhu was also a theorist and an herbalist

and was one of the "four great masters of the Jin-Yuan period." I noticed that, sprinkled throughout his books, were suggestions on using moxibustion and bleeding techniques, although he did not seem to use much acupuncture. It also became apparent that he frequently used moxibustion to treat heat diseases, something that was said to be contraindicated when I was in school.

These discoveries led me to believe that moxibustion was held in high esteem by some of the great physicians of the past and that it was used to treat many more conditions than now. I also noticed that the ancients used a large variety of techniques that I had not been taught; some I had never even heard of.

In order to research moxibustion more thoroughly, I chose it as the topic of my dissertation. This book is a revision of my dissertation, in order to make it more practical and relevant to the modern practitioner.

ACKNOWLEDGEMENTS

Many people contributed to this project. It is impossible to name them all: friends, colleagues, and teachers who have discussed moxibustion, literary Chinese, or the classics of medicine with me in classrooms, cafes, and through e-mail. A few deserve specific mention.

Chen Yongping spent many hours with me pouring over my translations, checking them word for word. This project would have been utterly impossible without her patient help and warm support.

I have a lot of gratitude for the help of Heiner Fruehauf, Jerome Jiang (Jiang Jianyuan), and especially Master Larry Sang of the American Feng Shui Institute.

I would also like to thank Bob Flaws, Peter Deadman, Subhuti Dharmananda, Herman Oving, Jonathan Schell, Frank Popff, Kathryn White, Maya Rosas, and Jose Cornejo.

While many people have contributed tremendously to my work, any errors are mine alone.

PART 1
OVERVIEW OF MOXIBUSTION

CHAPTER 1
MOXIBUSTION

In Chinese, the term for external treatment methods applied mostly to acumoxa points is 針灸 *zhen*1 *jiu*3, which literally means "acupuncture-moxibustion." This term seems to give moxibustion equal status to acupuncture, but this is generally not the case. From the time of the *Yellow Emperor's Inner Canon*[1] until today, moxibustion has received less discussion in the literature, and it has probably been used less frequently in the clinic as well.

The definition of moxibustion is somewhat controversial. According to Wiseman (1998, 402), moxibustion[2] is "a method of applying a heat stimulus to the body by burning the dried and sifted leaf particles from the herb mugwort (*ai*4 *ye*4) on or close to the skin, with the aim of freeing qi and blood, coursing qi, dispersing cold, eliminating dampness and warming yang."

According to Flaws (2003, 1), this definition is too narrow: "Literally, the Chinese word *jiu* only means to cause localized erythema or a burn by means of ei-

ther an external source of heat or the application of a caustic substance when the purpose of causing erythema or a burn is for medical treatment... By itself, the word *jiu* does not imply the method by which such therapeutic erythema or burns are created."

Because the English word "moxibustion" is linguistically linked to mugwort (Wiseman 1998, 402), some prefer to translate *jiu* as cauterization since cauterization does not imply the material used in treatment (Harper 1998, 5n.1; Unschuld 2003).

Artemisia vulgaris (sometimes called mugwort) is the most common material used for moxibustion, but moxibustion can also include sulfur paste, hot wax, the application of various caustic substances to the skin, heat lamps, "liquid moxa," and the burning of Medulla Junci[3] or other medicinals on or near the skin. However, most of the methods mentioned in the texts translated below involve burning mugwort. So there is no need to belabor this point.

---

[1] 《黃帝內經》, hereafter referred to as *Inner Canon*.
[2] 灸法 (jiu3 fa3)
[3] 燈心草 dengxincao

FUNCTIONS

The Chinese edition of *Chinese Acupuncture and Moxibustion* says, "Due to mugwort leaf's warming nature, it is able to rouse and support qi and yang. Also, because of its acrid and strong qi and flavor, it is able to pass through all the channels and regulate qi and blood. The acrid flavor governs scattering cold. The bitter flavor governs drying dampness. Therefore, it is used as the fuel for applying moxibustion."[7]

Zhang Jiebin said in *Illustrated Supplement*, Volume 11, "The functions of moxibustion are to scatter cold evils, eliminate yin toxins, open depression, break stagnation, reinforce qi, and return yang… It expels and scatters wind evils and perfuses the blood vessels" (Zhang 1991, 930).

Historically, moxibustion has been used for a multitude of functions. The functions compiled from two modern Chinese books on moxibustion are listed below (He 2003, 13-14; Liu 1991, 444). These functions will be illustrated and discussed throughout the book.

Of course, point selection and application methods are considered when applying these treatment principles to a particular case.

MOXIBUSTION

- *Warms and scatters cold evils*: The heat of moxibustion and the warming nature of mugwort and other medicinals counteracts coldness.
- *Warms the channels and frees the network vessels*: Cold slows the flow of qi and blood; heat activates qi and blood. Moxibustion penetrates all the channels and removes obstruction.
- *Disperses stasis and scatters bindings*: The heat of moxibustion and the acrid flavor of mugwort move and unblock qi and blood.
- *Quickens the blood and stops pain*: Pain is caused by non-passage. Since moxibustion moves qi and blood, it has an analgesic affect.
- *Eliminates dampness and scatters cold*: Li Shizhen called moxa floss "pure yang" (Li 1996, 435). So it is ideal to treat yin disorders such as cold and dampness.
- *Warms yang and supplements vacuity of qi and yang*: Heat is yang. By adding heat to the proper points, yang is supplemented or restored. The "pure yang" of moxa floss also fortifies qi and yang.
- *Returns yang and stems desertion*: Moxibustion on Guan Yuan (Ren 4) or Shen Que (Ren 8) is prescribed for this type of emergency condition.
- *Upbears yang and lifts the fallen*: Moxibustion on Bai Hui (Du 20) leads sinking qi or yang upward.
- *Supplements the center and boosts qi*: Moxibustion on points such as Zu San Li (ST 36), Qi Hai (Ren 6), and Zhong Wan (Ren 12) boosts center qi.
- *Regulates and contains the thoroughfare and conception vessels*: Moxibustion on Guan Yuan (Ren 4) is often used in gynecology for this purpose.
- *Repositions the fetus*: A well-known treatment for malpositioned fetus is moxibustion on Zhi Yin (UB 67). (continued)

---

[7] 由於艾葉性質的溫暖，所以能振扶氣陽，又因氣味的辛烈，故能通行諸經，調理氣血，辛主散寒，苦主燥濕，故以此作爲施灸的燃料 (Cheng 1964, 420).

MOXIBUSTION, (CONTINUED)

- *Downbears counterflow and descends qi*: Moxibustion on points such as Fei Shu (UB13) or Zhong Wan (Ren 12) descends counterflow qi of the lungs or stomach. In addition, points on the legs can also draw down repletion in the upper body.
- *Calms the liver and subdues yang*: To draw down repletion from the head, apply moxibustion to Yong Quan (KI 1) or similar points.
- *Dispels toxins and discharges heat*: See below on the use of moxibustion in heat conditions. The fire of moxibustion can radiate heat outwards from the body.
- *Prevents disease and safeguards health, strengthens the body, prolongs life and boosts longevity*: This function has been used at least since the Tang dynasty. See the section on preventive moxibustion below.

ADVANTAGES & DISADVANTAGES

Certain factors have brought about an overall decline in the use of moxibustion as well as a more limited range of techniques employed today.

Applying moxibustion is time-consuming. The practitioner must make cones and light them one by one or hold a moxa stick over the body for a period of time. If using isolating substances, the practitioner must keep them in stock and slice or prepare them as needed.

The smoke causes other problems. Some patients may be sensitive to it. Neighbors may complain about the odor (which some say resembles the smell of burning marijuana). Patients may not like the odor clinging to their clothes and hair. The practitioner may also dislike extended exposure to moxa smoke. Smoke alarms may sound. Questions have been raised regarding the toxicity of the fumes when certain powdered medicinals such as Xiong Huang (Realgar) are combined with the mugwort and burned. Realgar has been a common ingredient in moxa sticks (Guo 1991, 15). In addition, the ash from burning moxa can be untidy, and there is the ever-present danger of fire.

There is also the risk of burns. This risk is greater in patients who are diabetic or have loss of sensation, but accidents can occur on any patient. The ancients felt that moxa sores were necessary in order for the treatment to be effective (see below), but ironically, today burns may result in a lawsuit. Some acupuncture malpractice insurance policies do not allow the use of direct moxibustion (private communication with Mary S. Schnuck, 2004).

Patients may be taught to do moxibustion at home on themselves to increase the frequency of treatment. However, teaching the patient takes time. They may have problems with point location or proper technique. They or their family may object to the smoke. If burns result, a lawsuit may ensue.

Moxibustion can cause side effects if used improperly, and there is disagreement about when moxibustion is appropriate. (See below on the use of moxibustion in heat conditions.) Some doctors believe that excessive use of moxibustion, especially on the upper body, may cause or increase yang evils, damage yin, and result in a worsening condition.

Some practitioners feel that the only contribution of moxibustion toward curing illness is the heat of the fire. They feel that the mugwort or other material burned has no additional benefit (Dharmananda 2004, 17). Because of this, some prefer alternate heat sources such as heat lamps or hot packs, believing they are safer and more convenient to use.

Moxibustion also has many advantages (discussed throughout the book): The variety of methods and extensive functions of moxibustion allow for flexible and effective clinical use. It is effective for treating many diseases and in some cases, it is more effective than acupuncture or medicinal formulas. It is also cost-effective and fairly convenient to perform if it is not considered too time-consuming. Moxibustion can be used as a fully-developed system of treatment, as it includes a theoretical foundation, scope of practice, methods for supplementation and draining, contraindications, and a long record of clinical experience.

CHAPTER 2

METHODS OF MOXIBUSTION TREATMENT

Throughout history, many techniques for moxibustion use have been developed. This chapter explains various moxibustion techniques and explores the vast diversity found within the modality of moxibustion. Here are the different types of moxibustion as outlined by He Puren (2003, 29):

Below is an introduction to each type of moxibustion listed in the table. Some of these methods may not be considered appropriate in the modern Western clinic.

MUGWORT MOXIBUSTION

This is the most common type. Mugwort (*Ai Ye*, Folium Artemisiae Argyi) is an ideal material as it is a common plant that is found all over China (and elsewhere). It is processed into "wool" that resembles the texture of cotton balls. The wool is also called moxa floss or moxa punk. Moxa wool can be rolled into cones that hold their shape. It ignites easily, burning smoothly without a flame (O'Connor and Bensky 1981, 438). In addition, many (but not all) doctors feel the medicinal properties of mugwort make it more effective than other substances, although some feel that heat is the only "active ingredient" (for example, Dharmananda 2004, 17).

The specific properties of mugwort are discussed later. However, a few comments regarding the clinical use of mugwort for moxibustion are appropriate here. The best mugwort is from Qizhou[1] because of the climate and soil (Cheng 1987, 339). Historically, it is recommended that mugwort be picked on the third day of the third lunar month (around the vernal equinox) or the fifth day of the fifth lunar month (around the summer solstice). Wang Tao, Sun Simiao (both Tang), and Li Shizhen (Ming) are among many who have stated this. From a practical

---

[1] 蕲州

Mugwort moxibustion 艾灸法	Mugwort cone moxibustion 艾炷灸法	Direct moxibustion 直接灸	Non-scarring moxibustion 無瘢痕灸	
			Blistering moxibustion 發泡灸	
			Scarring moxibustion 瘢痕灸	
		Indirect moxibustion 間接灸		
	Mugwort stick moxibustion 艾條灸	Pure mugwort stick moxibustion 純艾條灸法	Hand-held moxibustion 手持灸	Gentle moxibustion 溫和灸
				Circling moxibustion 回旋灸
				Sparrow-pecking moxibustion 雀啄灸
			Isolating substance moxibustion 隔物灸	Walnut shell moxibustion 胡桃殼灸
				Warm needle moxibustion 溫針灸
		Moxa sticks with other medicinals added 加藥艾條灸	Thunder-fire miraculous needle 雷火神針	
			Taiyi miraculous needle 太乙神針	
			Needle that emits a hundred miracles 百發神針	
	Mugwort cake moxibustion 艾餅灸法	Ironing moxibustion 熨灸		
		Sunbeam moxibustion 日光灸		
	Mugwort-fuming moxibustion 艾熏灸法	Smoke-fuming moxibustion 煙熏灸		
		Steam moxibustion 蒸汽灸		
	Warming device moxibustion 溫灸器灸	Warming cylinder moxibustion 溫筒灸		
		Warming box moxibustion 溫盒灸		
		Reed tube moxibustion 葦管灸		
Moxibustion using other medicinals [non-mugwort moxibustion] 其他藥物灸法	Moxibustion by burning medicinals 藥物火熱灸法			
	Moxibustion without burning medicinals 藥物非火熱灸法	Heavenly moxibustion [blistering] 天灸（藥物發泡療法）		
		Medicinal application moxibustion [non-blistering] 藥物敷灸法		
	Electrical moxibustion 電灸法	Electrical heat moxibustion 電熱灸法		
		Electrical warm needle moxibustion 電溫針灸法		

point of view, this is the time when mugwort leaf is the best quality for use. From a theoretical point of view, since mugwort floss is "pure yang" according to Li Shizhen, it is best picked at the time of the year when yang is increasing (the vernal equinox) or when yang is at its peak (summer solstice).

Mugwort should be harvested after the bottom of the leaf has developed a wooly feeling (Ellis, Wiseman, and Boss 1991, 22). It is then sun-dried, ground or crumbled, and sifted repeatedly until all that is left is a soft fibrous material resembling cotton balls. The more it is sifted and the longer it is aged, the higher the grade. The best moxa wool is very pale tan. The coarser the grade, the greener and darker the color will be. High-grade moxa wool is easily shaped, burns smoothly, and can be made into tiny thread-like cones. It is used in direct moxibustion. Lower grades are used on top of isolating materials, in mugwort sticks, or burned in moxibustion devices (O'Connor and Bensky 1981, 438).

1. Mugwort cone moxibustion

When moxa wool is rolled or shaped between the fingers, it can be made into "cones." There are two words for moxa cones in Chinese. "Cone" is not a literal translation of either word. *Zhuang* 4 is a "number word" and is used only to state the number of cones. It literally means "strong, able-bodied, or healthy" (Mathews 1943, 205). To say "three cones" of moxibustion (三壯) is actually to say "three strengthenings" or "three invigorations."

The form of the cone is denoted by *zhu*4 , which also means the wick of an oil lamp or candle, or a stick of incense (Mathews 1943, 189). Although the shape is often cone-like, sometimes a moxa "cone" resembles a short thread or piece of string.

The old Chinese texts often specified the size of a cone by comparing it to a common object

rather than using a unit of measurement. Cones vary from the size of a grain of millet to as large as the top of the thumb. Chen Yanzhi (Southern and Northern dynasties) stated that the base of a moxa cone should be three fen in diameter. This was quoted by many later doctors, including Sun Simiao (Tang) and Gong Yanxian (Ming). Generally, direct moxibustion requires smaller cones that are made of higher grade mugwort than indirect moxibustion.

The number of cones is also variable, depending on the condition of the patient, the location on the body where treatment is applied, and the philosophy of the doctor. Recommendations range from one to one thousand cones. In surveying the literature, larger numbers of cones are generally used for urgent conditions, on the back and abdomen, and for supplementation. Fewer cones are used in non-urgent situations (especially due to repletion), on the head and limbs, and when the patient has a heat condition. Doctors who favor warm supplementation tend to use more cones.

Occasionally powdered medicinals are added to the moxa wool before it is made into cones. An example of this is found in [Zhu] Danxi's *Heart Methods [of Treatment]*.[2]

➤ **Direct moxibustion:** For direct moxibustion, burn cones directly on the skin. There are different degrees of stimulation:

 • **Non-scarring moxibustion:** Remove the mugwort cones before they burn close to the skin. The patient feels warmth and the area becomes red, but the flesh is not damaged. Use non-scarring moxibustion for vacuity cold patterns (He 2003, 33).

 • **Blistering moxibustion:** Burn small thread-like cones to the flesh, but do not allow deep

---

[2] 《丹溪心法·卷二·咳嗽》 Yuan dynasty (Zhu 2000, 186).

damage. A blister will form although no scar remains after it heals. Apply blistering moxibustion for chronic vacuity cold patterns, such as asthma, dizziness, diarrhea, and warts (He 2003, 33).

• **Scarring moxibustion:** This is also called suppurating moxibustion and is the most intense type. Larger cones are burned down to the flesh, although these cones are not as large as those used in indirect moxibustion. This leaves a larger blister, and pus may form before the sore heals. Scarring moxibustion is used to treat asthma, scrofula, consumption, lumps and accumulations, epilepsy, open sores, and chronic gastrointestinal diseases. It is applied to prevent wind stroke in patients with high blood pressure. It is also used to prevent disease and promote longevity in healthy people (He 2003, 33-4).

Traditionally, most doctors believed that without blistering or scarring, the treatment would not be effective. Today, few in the West dare to use this type of treatment.

➤ **Indirect moxibustion:** In indirect moxibustion, an isolating substance is placed between the cone and the skin. This is generally less painful and a blister or scar is less likely, although it is not impossible. A variety of substances are used, such as ginger, garlic, Fu Zi (Radix Lateralis Aconiti) slices, or salt. Powdered substances are sometimes made into a cake to isolate the moxa cone from the skin. The cake or slice is usually the thickness of a coin. Small holes are punched into the isolating substance to help the smoke, heat, and mugwort qi penetrate into the skin. The cake or slice is changed every few cones when it dries up or becomes charred.

The properties of the isolating substance are thought to affect the treatment, although in some cases an isolating substance is used simply to moderate the amount of heat stimulation. Today, it is common to find self-adhesive moxa on a neutral isolating base. You can also buy "skin shields" to further isolate the self-adhesive moxa cones (Lhasa OMS catalogue 2003-4, 33).

The uses of indirect moxibustion are extensive and depend, in part, on the properties of the isolating substance. For example, moxibustion on garlic is used for abscesses, sores that have not ulcerated, toxic swellings, consumption, abdominal lumps and accumulations, and snake bites. Salt is used as an isolating substance to return yang, stem counterflow or desertion, and to treat acute abdominal pain, vomiting and diarrhea, dysentery, reversal cold of the limbs, and strangury (He 2003, 37-40).

2. Mugwort stick moxibustion

Mugwort wool is packed and rolled up in paper to make a stick that resembles a cigar or a large cigarette. The moxa wool is often mixed with other medicinals. The stick is lit and held near the skin or is sometimes used with an isolating substance (He 2003, 60, 62, 64).

➤ **Pure mugwort stick moxibustion:** In this case, mugwort alone is rolled into a stick.

• **Hand-held moxibustion:** This is the most common method of moxibustion used in the clinic today (Ellis, Wiseman, and Boss 1991, 24). Moxa rolls are convenient. They can be bought ready-made, so there is no need to roll cones or sticks or prepare isolating substances. There is less chance of burns because the amount of heat is fairly easy to control. Patients can easily be taught to use moxa sticks at home (He 2003, 60).

• **Gentle moxibustion:** Hold the moxa stick over an area or point to gently warm it. Redness will appear but there should be no blister or scarring (Cheng 1987, 343). Use this method to warm and unblock the channels and vessels, scatter cold and eliminate evils. It is more frequently used in chronic diseases (He 2003, 61).

Circling moxibustion: Move the stick in circles over the area to be warmed. Use this method to warm an area rather than a point. Apply it for wind damp impediment, paralysis, and skin diseases (He 2003, 61).

Sparrow-pecking moxibustion: Raise the stick up and down over the point or area to be warmed. Focus on a point or small area so that the heat penetrates more easily (O'Connor and Bensky 1981, 442). It is used more often in acute diseases, clouding reversal, malposition of the fetus, insufficient lactation, etc. (He 2003, 61).

• **Isolating substance moxibustion**: Even with moxa rolls, sometimes isolating substances are used.

➤ **Walnut shell moxibustion:** A walnut shell is cracked in two and the meat is removed. Three to five small holes are drilled into each half of the shell. The inside is filled with chicken manure.[3] It is placed upside down on the affected site. A mugwort stick is lit and applied over the holes in the shell. This method is said to resolve toxins, disperse swelling, and check pain (He 2003, 61-2).

Since the 1970s, walnut shells with holes are dipped in Ju Hua (Flos Chrysanthemi) water and then joined to eyeglass frames. Pieces of moxa sticks are attached to the outside and burned. Chrysanthemum has an affinity for the eyes. The walnut shells suggest the brain. The qi of walnut and chrysanthemum is thought to enter the body through the eyes and benefit the brain and the eyes (Unschuld 2000, 86). This method is used to treat various eye problems and paralysis of the eye muscles (He 2003, 61-2).

• **Warm needle moxibustion:** Moxibustion can be applied to the handle of an acupuncture needle. There are many ways to do this. Slice a moxa stick and place the slices on the handle of a needle that has been inserted into a point. The needle must be relatively thick and inserted deeply in order to hold the additional weight on the handle. The handle must be metal and not plastic. The heat of the moxibustion travels through the needle into the point (He 2003, 63-4).

Others simply hold a moxa stick and warm the area of the needle insertion.

Some doctors pack mugwort wool on the handle of the needle and ignite it. You can also buy metal caps that hold the moxa wool. These caps sit on the handle of the needle and protect the skin from falling ash (Lhasa OMS catalogue 2003-4, 36).

The warm needle is used to treat many types of disease, including wind, cold, and damp impediment, menstrual block, lumbar pain, impotence, prolapse of the rectum, and facial paralysis (He 2003, 64).

➤ **Moxa sticks with other medicinals added:** Doctors design recipes of powdered medicinals to add to the mugwort roll. Different formulas are prescribed to treat various types of illness. Examples of the names of these sticks are "thunder-fire miraculous needle," "*taiyi* miraculous needle," and "needle that emits a

---

[3] Chicken manure has been used as a medicinal for millennia. It was used in a formula in *Elementary Questions*, Chapter 40, for example (Wu and Wu 1997, 196).

hundred miracles" (He 2003, 64-7). Later, a few types will be discussed in detail.

If the sticks are handmade, they can be formulated for the condition of a patient. This was common in the Ming and Qing dynasties. Moxa sticks were highly regarded at that time, as is evident by their names, almost all including the word *shen*: "miraculous, spiritual, godlike." Today, moxa sticks are commercially manufactured and seem to be used more for convenience than because they are highly regarded.

At the present, one can buy pure moxa sticks, a few types of sticks with other medicinals added, and also what is called "smokeless moxa sticks" (Lhasa OMS catalogue 2003-4, 35). These are sticks of charcoal that have been infused with mugwort and sometimes other medicinals. They emit less smoke and odor (Dharmananda 2004, 15-16).

3. Mugwort cake moxibustion
Mugwort wool is shaped and packed until it has the appearance of a cake. The cakes of mugwort are applied to a site in conjunction with an external heat source. The heat penetrates through the mugwort wool and permeates into the flesh (He 2003, 68). There are two types of mugwort cake moxibustion:

➤ **Ironing moxibustion:** Here, the mugwort cake is placed on a point or an area such as the abdomen. The cake is covered with a few layers of cloth. Then it is ironed or a hot-water bottle is placed on top. The patient should feel an appropriate amount of heat. This method is suitable for wind, cold, or damp impediment, wilting, abdominal pain due to cold, diarrhea, etc. (He 2003, 68).

Since the heat source is often a hot iron, this method is also considered an aspect of the heat treatment called ironing[4] (He 2003, 68).

➤ **Sunbeam moxibustion:** This is similar to the previous method, but the external heat source is the sun. Usually, the treatment lasts 10-20 minutes. You must be careful to avoid overexposure, such as sunburn, heat stroke, or sun stroke. You can also use a heat lamp. This method is suitable for wind, cold, or damp impediment, the five types of slow development in children, and chronic diseases with vacuity and weakness (He 2003, 68).

4. Mugwort-fuming moxibustion
This is the application of smoke from burning or steam from boiling mugwort wool to treat a point or affected area. The steam or smoke must be below the area to be treated (He 2003, 68).

➤ **Smoke-fuming moxibustion:** Place the mugwort wool in a fireproof container and light it. The smoke treats the affected site or point. This method is also called "warm cup moxibustion." It is used to treat wind, cold, or damp impediment or wilting (He 2003, 69).

➤ **Steam moxibustion:** Boil mugwort wool or a leaf in a container with water. Place the affected site or point in the rising steam. This treats wind, cold, or damp impediment, abdominal pain due to vacuity cold, distention, fullness, and diarrhea (He 2003, 69).

5. Warming device moxibustion
Various devices are manufactured to hold burning moxa wool, sticks, or cones:

➤ **Warming cylinder moxibustion:** This is a metal can or cylinder with small holes to let air in and smoke out. The cylinder may have a flat or a pointed bottom. Use the flat-bottom cylinder for larger areas and the pointed-

---

[4] Ironing was discussed in the Mawangdui text, *Formulas for Fifty-two Diseases*, and in the *Yellow Emperor's Inner Canon*.

bottom cylinder to direct the treatment to specific points or angular locations. The device often has a handle to make it easier to hold or move over the affected site or targeted point (O'Connor and Bensky 1981, 442). Warming cylinder moxibustion treats wind, cold, and damp impediment, abdominal pain or distention, diarrhea, wilting, etc. (He 2003, 70).

➤ **Warming box moxibustion:** Use a metal box with a screen across the bottom. Burn the moxa inside. This device is used to warm a larger area of the body (O'Connor and Bensky 1981, 442). Cover the skin with a cloth to prevent burns from the hot metal box. Then place the box on the affected area. The warming box is used for menstrual pain, lumbar pain, epigastric pain, enuresis, seminal emission, impotence, and diarrhea (He 2003, 70-1).

➤ **Reed tube moxibustion:** A reed (or bamboo) tube is used to apply moxibustion in the ear. This technique was first described in the early Tang dynasty by Sun Simiao in Volume 26 of *Supplement to Prescriptions Worth a Thousand Pieces of Gold*[5] (He 2003, 71). Tube moxibustion is the forerunner of the warming cylinder (O'Connor and Bensky 1981, 400).

At the present, there are two types of tube moxibustion. In one, the diameter of the tube's opening is about a half centimeter, and the tube is five or six centimeters long. One end is cut into the shape of half a duck's bill. Adhesive is applied to the other end to seal it when it is inserted into the external auditory meatus (He 2003, 71).

The second type of device consists of two sections of reed. One section is relatively larger in diameter, about 0.8-1.0 centimeter, and is four centimeters long. One end is cut into a "duck

bill." The other section is smaller, with a diameter of about 0.5-0.6 centimeters, and is about three centimeters long. One end is inserted into the external auditory meatus and the other end goes into the larger tube. Again, adhesive is used to seal it (He 2003, 71).

In either type, a pinch of mugwort the size of a half of a peanut is placed in the "duck bill" and lit. Three to nine cones are applied until the ear feels warm. This method is used to treat facial paralysis, dizziness, tinnitus, etc. (He 2003, 71).

MOXIBUSTION USING OTHER MEDICINALS (NON-MUGWORT MOXIBUSTION)

Although mugwort is the most common material used for moxibustion, other materials have been used historically and in clinical practice today.

1. Moxibustion by burning medicinals

Many substances have been burned for moxibustion, including sulfur, hot wax, incense, Deng Xin Cao (Medulla Junci), and peach or mulberry twigs (He 2003, 72-80).

For example, a chunk of sulfur can be burned on a fistula or boil (Wang 1984, 5).

Juncus moxibustion is usually used on children. A stalk is dipped in oil and lit. Then the burning end is applied to a point or area (Wang 1984, 5). Juncus moxibustion is still used in clinics of China. *Chinese Acupuncture and Moxibustion* recommends it in the treatment of mumps (Cheng 1987, 472).

Mulberry or peach twigs can be lit and then blown out so that the end of the twig becomes a burning ember. The twig is then touched to carbuncles, sores, or ulcers (Wang 1984, 6).

---

[5] 孫思邈《千金翼方》

2. Moxibustion without burning medicinals

This is the application of a medicinal paste to the skin without any use of fire or mugwort. The medicinals may be applied to an acupuncture point or locally to the affected site. Generally, acrid, warm or hot medicinals that contain irritating volatile oils are used (Flaws 2003, 2). The effect depends on the nature of the medicinal that is employed.

➤ **Heavenly moxibustion (blistering):** Heavenly moxibustion is the application of medicinals to irritate the skin enough to cause blistering. These medicinals include Bai Jie Zi (Semen Sinapis), Da Suan (Bulbus Allii Sativi, garlic), Wei Ling Xian (Radix Cleamtidis), Cong Bai (Bulbus Allii Fistulosi, scallion white), Ba Dou (Semen Crotonis), Ban Mao (Mylabirs), Mao Gen Ye (Folium Ranunculi Japinici), and Ban Xia (Rhizoma Pinelliae) (He 2003, p.81-84).

➤ **Medicinal application moxibustion (non-blistering):** This is the application of less irritating medicinals to the skin; so no blisters erupt. This category includes Ma Qian Zi (Semen Strychnotis), Tian Nan Xing (Rhizoma Arisaematis), Gan Sui (Radix Euphobiae Kansui), Wu Zhu Yu (Fructus Evodiae), Fu Zi (Radix Lateralis Aconiti), Xi Xin (Herba Asari), Bo He (Herba Menthae Haplocalycis), Ya Dan Zi (Fructus Bruceae Javanicae), Wu Bei Zi (Gallus Rhois), Bi Ma Zi (Semen Rici Communis), and Tao Ren (Semen Persciae) (He 2003, 84-87). "Liquid moxa," a solution with mugwort and possibly other medicinals can be purchased. It is applied to a point or area, often in combination with electric heat treatment (Flaws 2003, 2-3).

3. Electrical moxibustion

These techniques are, of course, a modern invention.

➤ **Electrical heat moxibustion:** Heat lamps or other sources of electric heat are applied to the surface of the body. In the earliest stage of its development, doctors used an external heat source with an electric fan aimed at the point, but the strength of the heat was insufficient to penetrate. Today, people use specially made electrical moxibustion devices. Some are similar to a regular lamp, but are designed to emit particular types of radiation, such as infra-red. The amount of heat is relatively focused, the area that directly receives the heat is relatively small, and the strength of the heat is sufficient to penetrate into the flesh. A treatment usually lasts about 10-15 minutes (He 2003, 88).

➤ **Electrical warm needle moxibustion:** Electrical heat combined with acupuncture mimics the warming needle. The difference between this and electro-acupuncture is that heat, not electrical current, is the goal. Points are selected based on the disease or pattern. The points are needled and after qi sensation is obtained, the electrical warm needle moxibustion equipment is applied for 15-30 minutes. This is appropriate for many patterns, including impediment, wind stroke, asthma, abdominal pain, and infertility (He 2003, 88).

➤ **Other types of electrical moxibustion:** Today, some use experimental techniques to apply moxibustion using various types of waves, such as light, laser, and ultrasound.

CHAPTER 3
THE HISTORY OF MOXIBUSTION

Moxibustion is an age-old part of indigenous Chinese medicine, developing over a long period of time. Here, the history is discussed chronologically and then certain aspects are explored in more detail.

PRE-HISTORY

Moxibustion must have developed gradually, sometime after humans began to use fire, about 1.7 million years ago. The ability to work with fire allowed great changes to occur in human diet and lifestyle. People found that the heat of fire dispelled the cold and relieved fatigue. Perhaps because its warmth eases the suffering of many illnesses and painful conditions, people began to use fire to treat disease. This is the likely origin of moxibustion (He 2003, 1; O'Conner and Bensky 1981, 398).

The early materials for moxibustion were probably burning twigs and branches. Even as late as the Ming dynasty, Li Shizhen discussed moxibustion using peach or mulberry twigs. At some point, people found that mugwort burns easily and that it possesses medicinal qualities, such as warming the channels and scattering cold. Eventually, people developed theories about the nature and actions of the materials used in moxibustion and integrated this knowledge with the channel system (He 2003, 1; O'Conner and Bensky 1981, 400).

PRE-HAN

The character for moxibustion, 灸 *jiu*3, is defined in the Eastern Han *Analytical Dictionary of Chinese Characters*: "Moxibustion means burning [or cautery]."[1] This word, *jiu*, may have been used in very early times as the verb for applying a red-hot poker to a tortoise shell to make it crack (Harper 1998, 96). The cracks would be interpreted in divination. The *Analytical Dictionary* says, "Divination means to burn the shell of the tortoise. The image has the form of *applying moxibustion [jiu]* to the tortoise."[2] Here, "applying moxibustion," does not mean applying a medical treatment to the tortoise. It signifies applying the burning stick to the tortoise shell to make it crack.

In 1973, an early Han tomb was opened at the site called Mawangdui[3] in Changsha, Hunan province. In it, archeologists found a number of books written on silk. These books date to sometime before 168 BCE. They are generally said to be pre-Qin. In these silk books, moxibustion was written simply as 久 *jiu*3 (Harper 1998, 194). The fire radical 火 must have been added later.

Two of the Mawangdui silk books are the earliest recorded medical literature on moxibustion. Indeed, they are also the earliest extant Chinese medical texts (Unschuld 1985, 93-4). These two are titled: *Moxibustion Canon of the Eleven Yin and Yang Vessels* and *Moxibustion Canon of the Eleven Vessels of the Foot and Forearm.*[4] They discuss the pathway of the vessels (channels), their symptoms when diseased, and their treatment using moxibustion. Neither text tells us the specific location for the moxibustion treat-

ment nor exactly how the treatment was performed. For example, after giving the pathway for a vessel and the diseases that might affect it, *Eleven Yin and Yang Vessels* simply says to apply moxibustion to the vessel (Harper 1998, 91).

The Mawangdui texts tell us that the 11 vessels contain qi. Six were on the legs and five were on the arms. They were named somewhat differently than today. The vessel that we now call the pericardium channel is missing. In these two silk books, moxibustion was the only treatment method specifically discussed for affecting the vessels (Harper 1998, 23; Unschuld 1985, 94).

Another book from the Mawangdui tombs, called *Formulas for Fifty-two Diseases,*[5] discussed many treatment modalities, but never mentioned acupuncture with the fine needle. This book also prescribed moxibustion as one of five types of heat treatment[6] (Harper 1998, 95). Several materials besides mugwort were specified to be used for moxibustion. For example, *Fifty-two Diseases* says to treat warts, "Take a worn-out cattail mat or the soft leaves of a cattail bedmat and make them into a cord. Then ignite the tip and cauterize the tip of the wart with it. When it becomes hot, pluck off the wart and discard it."[7] Another entry says, "Take hemp refuse and wrap in *ai* (mugwort). Use this to cauterize the center of the crown of the head of the person with inguinal swelling. Let it blister and no more."[8] Clause 135 contains the only mention of applying moxibustion according to channel theory. It says, for "inguinal swelling... cauterize the great yin and the great yang."[9] Mugwort was burned as a fumigant for hemorrhoids in Clause 155 (Harper 1998, 275).

---

[1] 灸，灼也。《說文解字》 (Around 100 CE) (Xu S. 1997, 1381)
[2] 卜，灼剝龜也，象灸龜之形。《說文解字》(Xu S. 1997, 452)
[3] 馬王堆
[4] 《陰陽十一脈灸經》,《足臂十一脈灸經》
[5] 《五十二病方》
[6] The others were roasting (by applying herbs then heating the affected part near a fire), ironing (hot-pressing), fumigating with steam or smoke, and medicinal soaks or baths.
[7] Clause 64, translated by Harper (1998, 244).
[8] Clause 127, translated by Harper (1998, 263).
[9] Translated by Harper (1998, 267).

While these early works were lost for 2,000 years, the *Yellow Emperor's Inner Cannon* was passed down through the generations. It is the earliest Chinese book on medical theory that has been transmitted in some form continuously until today.

There is debate over when the *Inner Canon* was written. It is most likely that its language and ideas were developed between 400 BCE and 260 CE (Unschuld 2003, 3). This estimate places the *Inner Canon* as mostly pre-Han and Han. During this period of more than 600 years, its essays were gathered together and lost, edited and annotated, reordered and recopied many times.

The *Inner Canon* gives a description of the origin of moxibustion in *Elementary Questions*, Chapter 12:[10] "The north is the region where heaven and earth close up and store. The land is high and the people dwell in mounds. There is wind, cold, and crystal-clear ice. The people enjoy the wilderness and drink milk. Their viscera are cold, which engenders the disease of fullness. The appropriate treatment is to burn moxibustion. Thus, burning moxibustion also came from the north." While moxibustion may have originated in the north, by the time this passage was written, the therapies from all five regions[11] were in general use.

The *Inner Canon* discusses moxibustion in many places. It is recommended or warned against in more than 10 chapters of *Elementary Questions*.[12] Chapter 60 gives a detailed account of the use of moxibustion. Chapter 24 states, "When disease is generated in the vessels, treat it using moxibustion and pricking."[13]

Moxibustion is also recommended in the *Magic Pivot*: Chapter 73 states, "Moxibustion is suitable for what the needle does not do."[14] Chapter 10 says, "Apply moxibustion to what is sunken."[15] Chapter 51 gives directions for using moxibustion on the back transport points as well as for dispersing and supplementation techniques using moxibustion.

There are also descriptions of moxibustion in some of the non-medical literature of the time. For example, *Zuo's Commentary on the Spring and Autumn Annals* recounts that in 518 BCE, Doctor Huan said of Prince Jing of Jin, "His illness cannot be handled. The disease is located above the *huang* and below the *gao*.[16] It cannot be attacked. Penetrating cannot reach it. Medicinals cannot treat it."[17] It is generally agreed that "penetrating" indicates the needle stone and "attacking" means moxibustion (He 2003, 2; Duan 1984, 4; Wang 1984, 2).

Mengzi, known in the west as Mencius, said, "A disease of seven years requires three-year-old mugwort."[18] Mugwort and moxibustion are also mentioned a few times in *Zhuangzi*[19] (Wang 1984, 2).

Even the *Book of Songs*, already old by the time of Confucius, had a number of poems that refer to

---

[10] 《素問·異法方宜論篇第十二》北方者，天地所閉藏之域也。其地高陵居，風寒冰冽，其民樂野處而乳食，臟寒生滿病，其治宜灸焫。故灸焫者，亦從北方來。(Wu and Wu 1997, 71-72)

[11] The therapies from the five regions are: the healing *bian* stone from the east, medicinals from the west, the nine needles from the south, *dao yin* (basically ancient qigong) and massage from the central region, and moxibustion from the north (Wu and Wu 1997, 71-2).

[12] Including Chapters 12, 19, 24, 28, 36, 40, 47, 60, 76, and 77.

[13] 病生於脈，治之以灸刺。《素問·血氣形志》(Wu and Wu 1997, 133)

[14] 針所不為，灸之所宜。《靈樞·官能》(Wu and Wu 1997, 781)

[15] 陷下者灸之。《靈樞·經脈》(Wu and Wu 1997, 556)

[16] The *gao huang* is "the region below the heart and above the diaphragm. When a disease is said to have entered the *gao huang*, it is difficult to cure" (Wiseman 1998, 239). The *gao* is the region below the heart. The *huang* is the region above the diaphragm.

[17] 醫緩，晉景公。疾不可為也，病在肓之上，膏之下，攻之不可，達之不及，藥不治焉。《左傳》(Duan 1984, 4)

[18] 七年之病求三年之艾。《孟子·離婁》(Mengzi 1997, 124)

[19] 《莊子》

mugwort. It is the earliest reference we have to this plant (Wang 1984, 4). For example, Song 76 says:

> Picking kudzu, one day not seeing him is like three months!
> Picking southernwood, one day not seeing him is like three autumns!
> Picking mugwort, one day not seeing him is like three years![20]

Sima Qian's biography of Bian Que in *Historical Records* says, "Zhong Dafu from Qi suffered tooth decay. Chen Yi applied moxibustion to the left great yang brightness vessel[21] and made a decoction of flavescent sophora (Ku Shen Tang). Every day he rinsed his mouth with three *sheng* of the decoction. Five or six days came and went and the disease was already eliminated."[22] While written early in the Western Han dynasty, this story refers to pre-Han times, as Bian Que was said to have lived during the Warring States period.

It seems evident from these non-medical writings that moxibustion was already common enough during the Spring and Autumn and Warring States periods that authors could expect their readers to understand these passages.

HAN DYNASTY (206 BCE–220 CE)

The *Treatise on Cold Damage* and *Essential Prescriptions of the Golden Cabinet* were written in the Eastern Han dynasty by Zhang Zhongjing.[23] Between these two books, more than 20 sections mention moxibustion. Zhang's views can be summarized as "Acupuncture is appropriate for yang patterns and moxibustion is appropriate for yin patterns" (He 2003, 2).

Moxibustion was not mentioned in the *Classic of Difficulties*.[24]

The earliest moxibustion treatise, *Master Cao's Moxibustion Classic*, was written by Cao Weng who was the son of Cao Cao,[25] the Three Kingdoms period ruler of the state of Wei. This book has been lost, although later authors such as Sun Simiao[26] included much of its contents in their books (He 2003, 2-3).

JIN, SOUTHERN AND NORTHERN & SUI DYNASTIES (265 - 618)

During the Jin dynasty, Huangfu Mi compiled the *Systematic Classic of Acupuncture and Moxibustion*.[27] It is the earliest treatise on acupuncture and moxibustion that is still available in its original form. The *Systematic Classic* is based on the contents of three books: *Elementary Questions*, *Magic Pivot*, and *Acupuncture and Moxibustion Treatment Essentials from the Bright Hall of Points*.[28] The last book has not survived to the present, but the *Systematic Classic* preserved much of it (He 2003, 3). Huangfu compiled and rearranged these three books in a logical, easy to use order.

The *Systematic Classic* does not discuss the techniques of moxibustion much beyond quoting from the *Inner Canon*. However, in Volume 3, a section compiled from *Essentials of the Bright Hall*, Huangfu

---

[20] 彼采葛兮，一日不見，如三月兮！彼采蕭兮，一日不見，如三秋兮！彼采艾兮，一日不見，如三歲兮！《詩經》 (Anonymous 1999, 180-183)
[21] Probably large intestine, hand yang brightness channel.
[22] 齊中大夫病齲齒，臣意灸其左大陽明脈，即為苦參湯，日嗽三升，出入五六日，病已。司馬遷 《史記·扁鵲倉公列傳》 (Duan 1984, 28)
[23] 《傷寒論》，《金匱要略》 張仲景
[24] 《難經》
[25] 曹翁, 曹操 《曹氏灸經》
[26] 孫思邈
[27] 皇甫謐《針灸甲乙經》, hereafter called the *Systematic Classic*.
[28] 《明堂孔穴針灸治要》, hereafter called the *Essentials of the Bright Hall*.

outlined the acu-moxa points one by one. He listed the number of cones to be used on each point (between 1-10 cones, with 3-5 being most common) and also noted points that were contraindicated for moxibustion. Twenty were explicitly contraindicated,[29] while six more did not have a reference to the number of cones.[30] Later doctors also generally prohibited these same points for moxibustion.

The *Pulse Classic* was written by Wang Shuhe,[31] who lived around the same time as Huangfu Mi. In the *Pulse Classic*, Wang said little about moxibustion, except to summarize Zhang Zhongjing's works regarding when moxibustion is appropriate and when it is prohibited. This summary was sometimes quoted by later doctors, such as Zhu Danxi (Zhu 2000, 350).

Eastern Jin doctor Ge Hong wrote *Emergency Prescriptions to Keep Up Your Sleeve*.[32] Ge strongly advocated the use of moxibustion for urgent and critical patterns and wrote many moxibustion prescriptions for treating them, for example:

- "To rescue a patient with sudden death, gaping eyes, and bound-up tongue, apply 14 cones of moxibustion behind the nails of both the hands and feet."
- "Make your nail enter into the patient's Ren Zhong (Du 26), aiming to wake him up. Roll up his hand and apply moxibustion at the end of the lower crease [probably Hou Xi, SI 3], following the years [of age for the number of cones]."[33]

- "For someone who suddenly gets cholera [sudden turmoil] with abdominal pain, first apply 14 cones of moxibustion to the umbilicus. The point named Tai Cang (Ren 12), four *cun* below heart meeting[34] has a higher degree of success."[35]

Ge Hong was the first to record the use of moxibustion on isolating substances (He 2003, 3). He wrote, "I have tried it [moxibustion on garlic] on great swellings below the patient's small abdomen and there was a prompt cure. Every time it is used, it has a great effect."[36] He used moxibustion on dough, "For all unendurable toxic swelling and pain, seek a piece of flour dough the size of a coin for the head of the swelling. Fill the center with pepper. Use this flour cake to cover the head of the swelling. Apply moxibustion to make penetrating pain. This promptly stops it."[37] Ge also recorded the use of salt as an isolating substance. For example, one of his recommendations for sudden turmoil (*i.e.*, cholera) says, "Use salt inside the umbilicus. Apply 27 cones of moxibustion on top."[38]

Ge Hong frequently recommended the application of moxibustion locally to the affected site and to any place on the exterior of the body that reflected a sign of internal imbalance (He 2003, 3).

Ge Hong's wife, Baogu,[39] was also famous as a moxibustion specialist. She became well-known for treating tumors and warts. She is one of the few female

---

29   Tou Wei (ST 8), Nao Hu (Du 17), Feng Su (Du 16), Cheng Guang (UB 6), Yin Men (Du 15), Ji Zhong (Du 6), Xin Shu (UB 15), Bai Huan Shu (UB 30), Si Zhu Kong (SJ 23), Cheng Qi (ST 1), Ren Ying (ST 9), Ru Zhong (ST 17), Yuan Ye (GB 22), Jiu Wei (Ren 15), Jing Qu (LU 8), Tian Fu (LU 3), Yin Shi (ST 33), Fu Tu (ST 32), Di Wu Hui (GB 42), and Yang Guan (GB 33)

30   Quan Liao (SI 18), Su Liao (Du 25), Ying Xiang (LI 20), Ju Liao (ST 3), He Liao (LI 19), and Di Cang (ST 4)

31   《脈經》王叔和   Wang also collated and edited Zhang Zhongjing's *Treatise on Cold Damage* and *Essential Prescriptions of the Golden Cabinet*.

32   救卒死而張目結舌者，灸手足兩爪後十四壯。葛洪 《肘後備急方》, hereafter called *Emergency Prescriptions*. Volume 1 (Ge 1996, 3).

33   令爪其病入人中，取醒，捲其手灸下紋頭隨年。 Volume 1 (Ge 1996, 2). Using the age as the number of cones originated in *Elementary Questions*, Chapter 60 (Wu and Wu 1997, 277).

34   This seems to refer to the lower angle where the seventh rib joins the sternum.

35   卒得霍亂，先腹痛者，灸臍上，十四壯，名太倉，在心厭下四寸，更度之。 Volume 2 (Ge 1996, 27).

36   余嘗小腹下患大腫，灸即差。每用之則可大姣也。 Volume 5 (Ge 1996, 146).

37   一切毒腫疼痛不可忍者，搜麵團腫頭如錢大，滿中安椒，以麵餅子蓋頭上，灸令徹痛，即立止。 Volume 5 (Ge 1996, 146-7).

38   以鹽內臍中上灸二七壯。 Volume 2 (Ge 1996, 28).

39   鮑姑

doctors that was written about in ancient China (He 2003, 3).

In the Southern and Northern dynasties, Chen Yanzhi also wrote about moxibustion. His *Short Sketches of Formulas*[40] was lost, but large portions of it were quoted in later works, such as the Japanese medical classic *Medical Heart Formulas*[41] (He 2003, 3). In addition to recommending it as treatment for different diseases, Chen wrote about practical issues regarding moxibustion, for example, forbidden points, how to light the fire, and which kinds of wood should not be used for fire.

Chen felt that people could use moxibustion as a home remedy; it wasn't necessary to be treated by a doctor: "You must have a teacher before practicing the techniques of acupuncture, but even the ordinary person can apply moxibustion. If a teacher has explained the *Classic* [*Inner Canon*], you can readily practice acupuncture-moxibustion, but if a teacher has not explained this text, you can apply moxibustion according to diagrams and explanatory texts. However, in the uncultivated places without diagrams or anyone to explain the texts, you can expel disease from a site by applying moxibustion to it. All these are good methods. However, avoid applying moxibustion to exposed places on the face and four limbs, leaving damage such as scars."[42]

During the Southern and Northern dynasties, moxibustion was quite popular in southern China. The *Southern History* recorded that both "The eminent and the humble people contended to get it. Many found it effective."[43]

TANG DYNASTY (618 - 907)

During the Tang dynasty, medical schools were established. Professors taught acupuncture and moxibustion as an academic branch of knowledge. Moxibustion was officially an independent subject of study and "moxibustion master" was a title for this specialty (He 2003, 4).

The famous doctor Sun Simiao wrote *Essential Prescriptions Worth a Thousand Pieces of Gold* and *Supplement to Prescriptions Worth a Thousand Pieces of Gold*.[44] He wrote comprehensively about medicine, including specialties such as gynecology, pediatrics, and diseases of the sense organs. Sun often included prescriptions for moxibustion, for example:

- "In bloody stool, apply moxibustion at the twentieth vertebra. Follow the years of age for the number of cones."[45]
- "For someone with intermittent episodes of mania evil, with disheveled hair, great arousal, desire to kill people, and who does not avoid fire or water: Apply moxibustion to Jian Shi (PC 5) on the left for males, on the right for females. Follow the years of age for the number of cones."[46]
- "Formula to treat a child of four or five years who does not speak: apply three cones of moxibustion to both of the ankle bones."[47]

Sun usually advised using large amounts of moxibustion often exceeding 100 cones. He also recommended that moxibustion be used preventively in people without disease or in the early stages. (See the section on preventive moxibustion, below.)

---

[40] 陳延之 《小品方》
[41] 《醫心方》
[42] 夫針術，須師乃行，其灸則凡人便施。為師解經者，針灸隨手而行，非師所解文者，但依圖，詳文則可灸。野間無圖，
不解文者，但逐病所在便灸之，皆良法。但避其面目，四肢顯露處，以創瘢為害耳。《醫心方·卷二·灸例法》
(Tamba 1993, 69)
[43] 貴賤爭取之，多得其驗。《南史》 (He 2003, 3)
[44] 孫思邈 《千金要方》，《千金翼方》，hereafter called *Prescriptions* and *Supplement*, respectively.
[45] 大便下血，灸第二十椎，隨年壯。《千金翼方·卷二十七·脾病》 *Supplement*, Volume 27 (Sun 1997a, 274).
[46] 狂邪發無常，披頭大喚欲殺人，不避水火者，灸間使，男左女右，隨年壯《千金翼方·卷二十七·小腸病》。 *Supplement*,
Volume 27 (Sun 1997a, 273).
[47] 治小兒四五 不語方：灸足兩踝各三壯。《千金要方·卷五·孫兒雜方》 *Prescriptions*, Volume 5 (Sun 1996, 146).

Sun prescribed moxibustion using isolating substances such as garlic, fermented bean cakes, Fu Zi (Radix Lateralis Aconiti), and salt. He also recognized that mugwort is not the only material used in moxibustion. For example, to treat swellings he suggested, "Scrape a bamboo arrow and use the shavings to make cones. Apply two times seven cones of moxibustion on it. It will promptly disperse."[48]

Sun thought a good doctor should prescribe medicinals, acupuncture, and moxibustion as appropriate. Although he gave higher status to medicinal decoctions, all treatment modalities should cooperate and be coordinated. Sun said, "When medicinal decoctions attack the interior and acupuncture and moxibustion attack the exterior, the disease has no place to escape. If you know how to attack with acupuncture and moxibustion, it is more than half compared to medicinal decoctions."[49] Sun also advocated the use of the warming needle: "A great method is to settle the needle, then apply moxibustion to it. This is a good formula."[50]

Wang Tao included extensive and varied prescriptions for moxibustion in his book, *Secret Necessities of a Frontier Official*. He held an extreme view on the benefits of moxibustion and the dangers of acupuncture. In Volume 39, Wang said, "Since ancient times, acupuncture has been taken as profound but, in the end, people cannot understand it."[51] Wang cited *Magic Pivot*, Chapter 60,[52] "The *Classic* says, 'Acupuncture is able to kill living people,' but it is unable to

raise dead people. If you want to employ it, I fear it will damage life. Today, do not employ acupuncture on the channels; only apply moxibustion."[53]

In Volume 14 of *Secret Necessities*, Wang quoted Sun Simiao:[54] "Burning mugwort especially has extraordinary abilities. Although it is said acupuncture, decoctions, and powders all have something they can reach, moxibustion is the most important… It is the most essential of all the essentials. Nothing exceeds this technique."[55] These quotations illustrate how Wang emphasized moxibustion and belittled acupuncture.

Even poets wrote about moxibustion. Han Yu wrote a poem called "Dispelling the Malarial Ghost." One line says, "Moxibustion masters apply mugwort cones cruelly like hunting with encircling fires"[56] (Han 2002; Wang 1984, 3).

In the late 19th century, a collection of Sui and Tang dynasty manuscripts were found behind a wall in a cave in Dunhuang, in northwest China. Dunhuang was located on the "silk road." These caves had been made into Buddhist temples. When word spread that documents were discovered, European explorers, including Auriel Stein, came to take what they could. Stein (and other explorers) bribed the monk in charge of the temple and was given a number of documents which he sent to England (Wright and Twitchett 1973, 122). Two of these books or scrolls include *Moxibustion Diagrams* and the *Moxibustion Classic of the Bright Hall*[57] (Wei 1987, 15). Other

---

[48] 刮竹簡上取茹作炷灸上二七壯，即消矣。《千金翼方·卷二十四·癭瘤》 *Supplement*, Volume 24 (Sun 1997a, 241).

[49] 湯藥攻其內，針灸攻其外，則病無所逃矣。方知針灸之功，過半于湯藥矣。《千金要方·卷二十九·明堂三人圖》 *Prescriptions*, Volume 29 (Sun 1996, 514).

[50] 大法得針訖乃灸，此為良方。《千金要方·卷三十·孔穴主對法》 *Prescriptions*, Volume 30 (Sun 1996, 549).

[51] 其針法古來以爲深奧，令人卒不可解。王燾《外台秘要·卷三十九·明堂序》, hereafter called *Secret Necessities*. (Wang 1979, 1077).

[52] 《靈樞·玉版第六十》 (Wu and Wu 1997, 736)

[53] 經曰：針能殺生人，不能起死人，若欲錄之，恐傷性命，今不錄針經，唯取灸法。《外台秘要·卷三十九·明堂序》 (Wang 1979, 1077)

[54] 《千金翼方·卷十七·中風》 *Supplement*, Volume 17 (Sun 1997a, 164).

[55] 至於火艾，特有奇能，雖曰針湯散皆所不及，灸為其最要。。。要中之要，無過此術。《外台秘要·卷十四·中風及諸風方》 (Wang 1979, 375)

[56] 韓愈《昌黎先生集》灸師施艾炷，酷若獵火圍。

[57] 《灸圖》，《灸經明堂》

documents ended up in Paris, Berlin, Leningrad, Kyoto, and Beijing (Wright and Twitchett 1973, 122).

The first emperor of the Later Liang dynasty, Tai Zu,[58] personally applied moxibustion to his ailing heir (Wang 1984, 3).

SONG DYNASTY (960 - 1279) & JIN DYNASTY (1115 - 1234)

Song dynasty doctor Wang Weiyi wrote the *Illustrated Classic of Acupuncture Points as Found on the Bronze Man*.[59] This book was influential because it standardized acu-moxa point locations (He 2003, 5).Wang listed the number of cones to be burned on each point and sometimes the size of the cone or whether the point was contraindicated for moxibustion. This book was the most comprehensive update on points since the *Systematic Classic* by Huangfu Mi.

There are quite a few Song dynasty publications that described and prescribed moxibustion extensively. *General Record of Sage-like Benefit*[60] contains a large collection of moxibustion formulas. It covered more than 50 categories of disease that could be treated by moxibustion, such as wind stroke, water swelling, steaming bones, eye diseases, abscesses, sores and swellings, gynecology, and pediatrics. *Sage-like Prescriptions of the Taiping Era* by Wang Huaiyin[61] and *Prescriptions of Universal Benefit from My Own Practice* by Xu Shuwei[62] also recorded a great number of moxibustion prescriptions (He 2003, 5).

Moxibustion on Gao Huang Shu [UB 43] was written by Zhuang Chuo[63] during the Southern Song dynasty. He discussed the treatment of consumption with moxibustion. His book contained a number of diagrams along with the text. Zhuang compiled past writings, adding his own comments on the location and treatment methods for Gao Huang (UB 43) (He 2003, 6).

The Book of Bian Que's Heart was written by Dou Cai. Even today, it is considered an important work on moxibustion. The first volume includes theory, stories, and treatment protocols regarding moxibustion. The other two volumes cover the patterns of internal and external medicine, gynecology, pediatrics, etc. Although Dou prescribed many medicinal formulas, he suggested moxibustion treatments for more than 60 types of illnesses. He attached more than 40 case studies, about 90% of them using moxibustion (Wei 1987, 16). An example of Dou's treatment recommendations is, "A postpartum woman with a fever that does not abate is likely to gradually develop consumption. Quickly apply 300 cones of moxibustion below the umbilicus."[64]

Dou felt that moxibustion was essential for treating disease: "A doctor's use of moxibustion to treat disease is like the use of fuel to cook a meal."[65] Dou was also a strong supporter of moxibustion as a preventive measure. He advocated moxibustion to promote longevity even when there was no illness. (For details, see the section on preventive moxibustion, below.)

Other distinguishing features of Dou Cai's use of moxibustion are:

• The large number of cones: 100 or more cones on each point. If the case was severe, he would even suggest 500 or 600 cones. Dou said, "It is a common custom to use no more than 30 or 50

---

[58] 太祖 (reigned from 907-910)

[59] 王惟一《銅人腧穴針灸圖經》, hereafter called the *Bronze Man*.

[60] 《聖濟　錄》

[61] 《太平聖惠方》王懷隱

[62] 《普濟本事方》許叔微

[63] 《灸膏肓拡穴法》莊綽

[64] 婦人產後，熱不退，恐漸成勞瘵，急灸臍下三百壯。《扁鵲心書·卷上·黃帝灸法》 (Dou 2000, 18)

[65] 醫之治病用灸，如做飯用薪。竇材《扁鵲心書·卷上·大病宜灸》 (Dou 2000, 9)

cones of moxibustion. They still do not know how to eliminate minor disease and bring about recovery. So retaining the root of life is then difficult. That is why the *Illustrated Classic of Acupuncture and Moxibustion as Found on the Bronze Man* said, 'Generally in major disease, it is appropriate to apply 500 cones of moxibustion below the umbilicus to supplement and receive true qi,' meaning this method. But when eliminating minor disease, such as wind evil in the four limbs, you should use only three, five, or seven cones."[66]

- Warm supplementation of the spleen and kidneys: Dou's application of moxibustion was mostly limited to treating these organs. He said that "The spleen is the mother of the five viscera and the kidneys are the root of the whole body."[67] Dou favored Ming Guan (SP 17) to supplement spleen yang and Guan Yuan (Ren 4) to supplement kidney yang.

Besides Dou Cai, many doctors developed the use of moxibustion for warm supplementation. Xu Shuwei, the author of *Prescriptions of Universal Benefit from My Own Practice*,[68] used moxibustion to supplement kidney yang and developed a theory of dual supplementation of the spleen and kidneys, similar to Dou Cai. Luo Tianyi (see p. 25) also promoted the use of moxibustion to supplement the spleen and stomach. These doctors laid the foundation for the school of warm supplementation that was developed by doctors like Zhang Jingyue and Zhao Xianke during the Ming dynasty (Wei 1987, 16).

Wang Zhizhong wrote the *Classic of Nourishing Life with Acupuncture and Moxibustion*. He chose moxibustion as the treatment method for more than a 100 types of diseases. Wang summarized the writings of earlier doctors and discussed his own viewpoint (He 2003, 5-6).

Wang discussed the number of moxa cones recommended by a few earlier authors. Each had a different set of guidelines, leading him to conclude, "All should observe the degree of seriousness of the disease and use this [to determine the number of cones]. You cannot be tied down by one theory without also knowing that surely there is another theory."[69]

Wang's point selection was simple, often using only one or two points, for example, "In diarrhea, it is appropriate to first apply moxibustion to the umbilicus, then apply moxibustion to points like Guan Yuan (Ren 4)."[70] Wang applied few cones, generally in the range of three to seven. He advocated using many methods together to treat disease, saying, "Modern people only know acupuncture and not moxibustion, moxibustion and not acupuncture, or only use medicinals and do not know acupuncture and moxibustion. All these offend True Person Sun's admonishments."[71]

Ming dynasty authors such as Xu Feng, Gao Wu and Yang Jizhou frequently quoted Wang's *Classic of Nourishing Life* when discussing moxibustion.

Moxibustion Equipped for Emergencies was written in the Southern Song dynasty and is generally attributed to Wenren Qi'nian (Knowledgeable Aged Person).[72] This book specializes in moxibustion, describing protocols for more than 20 types of disease, including abscesses, sores, abdominal pain,

66 世俗用灸，不過三五十壯，殊不知去小疾則愈，駐命根則難，故《銅人針灸圖經》云：「凡大病宜灸臍下五百壯，補接真氣。」即此法也。若去風邪四肢小疾，不過三，五，七壯而已。《扁鵲心書·卷上·大病宜灸》(Dou 2000, 9)
67 脾為五臟之母，腎為一身之根。《扁鵲心書·卷上·五等虛實》(Dou 2000, 16)
68 《普濟本事方》許叔微
69 皆視其病之輕重而用之，不可泥一說，而又不知其有一說也。王執中《針灸資生經·論壯數多少》(Huang 1996, 268)
70 泄瀉宜先灸臍中，次灸関元等穴。《針灸資生經·泄瀉》(Huang 1996, 280)
71 今人或但知針而不灸，灸而不針，或唯用藥不知針灸者，皆犯孫真人之所戒也。《針灸資生經·針灸須藥》(Huang 1996, 266). 'True Person Sun' refers to Sun Simiao, who said, "When medicinal decoctions attack the interior and acupuncture and moxibustion attack the exterior, disease has no place to escape" (see above).
72 《備急灸法》聞人耆年

vomiting, and diarrhea. The author praises moxibustion as the treatment of choice for acute disease and records successful cases (He 2003, 6).

Zhang Congzheng[73] was one of the "four great doctors of the Jin-Yuan period." He advised caution in using moxibustion. "Burning 100,000 cones of moxibustion is completely without any effect. On the contrary, it makes the patient suffer this misfortune. How is it not painful!"[74] Zhang stressed that the practitioner of moxibustion should pay attention to the season to prevent violation of the prohibition against "replenishing repletion and evacuating vacuity."[75] "The application of moxibustion is greatly prohibited distal to the wrists and ankles in the hot summer months because the hands and feet both are the exterior of yang, which arises on the outside of the five fingers and toes."[76]

Moxibustion was popular enough that the famous Song artist, Li Tang,[77] painted a moxibustion scene.

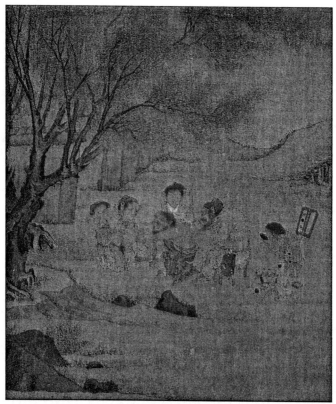

李唐灸艾图

Moxibustion with Mugwort by Li Tang (Song) with permission from Palace Museum in Taiwan

---

[73] 張從正, also known as Zhang Zihe 張子和
[74] 燔灸千百壯者，全無一效，使病者反受其殃，豈不痛哉！《儒門事親·卷十一·論火熱》 (Zhang 1996, 260)
[75] This prohibition is stated in *Elementary Questions*, Chapter 70 (Wu and Wu 1997, 372), as well as in the *Classic of Difficulties* and *Essential Prescriptions of the Golden Cabinet*.
[76] 大忌暑月于手腕足踝上著灸，以其手足者，諸陽之表，起于五指之外。《儒門事親·卷十一·風門》 (Zhang 1996, 265)
[77] 李唐 This painting is in the National Palace Museum, Taiwan.

YUAN DYNASTY (1271 - 1368)

In the *Precious Mirror of Protecting Life*, Luo Tianyi advocated using moxibustion for warm supplementation of the spleen and stomach and for prevention of wind stroke. For example, he wrote, "Usually in a person with wind, you must pay special attention to this moxibustion. You can safeguard without worry. This method of moxibustion can be applied to sudden death."[78] Luo also advocated using moxibustion to regulate the spleen and stomach and bank up original qi. He recorded case studies of this sort, "The patient had fever, emaciated flesh, fatigued and cumbersome limbs, somnolence, night sweating, and sloppy diarrhea… I applied moxibustion to Zhong Wan (Ren 12), Qi Hai (Ren 6), and Zu San Li (ST 36)"[79] (Liu 1991, 172-3).

Wei Yilin wrote *Effective Formulas Obtained from Generations of Doctors*, an encyclopedic treatment manual. He collected numerous moxibustion formulas, for example:

- "Running piglet rushing to the heart with inability to catch the breath: Apply 50 cones of moxibustion to Zhong Ji (Ren 3)."[80]
- "To treat extreme vacuity: Apply moxibustion to Gao Huang (UB 43) and Qi Hai (Ren 6), the more cones, the more wonderful the results."[81]
- "Lip disease: To treat tight lips that are unable to open and close, apply moxibustion to Hu Kou (LI 4), on the left on males and on the right on females."[82]

MING DYNASTY (1368 - 1644)

During the Ming dynasty, moxibustion was frequently discussed in the many voluminous books that were published. The comprehensive medical book, *Prescriptions of Universal Benefit*,[83] described a large number of moxibustion protocols. Xu Feng's *Great Completion of Acupuncture and Moxibustion*[84] and Wang Ji's *Questions and Answers on Acupuncture and Moxibustion*[85] both included an enormous amount of material on moxibustion (He 2003, 8).

Miraculous Formulas from Longevity Land by Zhu Quan[86] was the first book to record the use of the moxa roll (He 2003, 7; Wei 1987, 17). Although Zhu's moxa roll only used mugwort, many types of moxa rolls developed afterwards. (See discussion of moxa rolls, below.)

Moxibustion using Deng Xin Cao (Medulla Junci) was first mentioned in Volume 6 of Li Shizhen's *Great Pharmacopeia*.[87] Sang Zhi (Ramulus Mori, mulberry twig) moxibustion was described in the same volume. Brass mirror moxibustion[88] also appeared during this period. It uses a special brass mirror placed in the sun to generate focused heat onto the intended site on the body. In a similar way, some use a lens to gather sunlight as a means of moxibustion in modern times (He 2003, 7).

Even though the use of acupuncture, moxibustion, or medicinals alone could be relatively effective, quite a few doctors at this time felt that their

---

[78] 如素有風人，尤須留意此灸法，可保無虞。此法能灸卒死。羅天益《衛生寶鑑·卷八·中風灸法》
[79] 病發熱，肌肉消瘦，四肢困倦，嗜臥盜汗，大便溏多。。。經灸中脘，氣海，足三里。《衛生寶鑑·卷五·胃中有熱治驗》
[80] 奔豚搶心不得息：灸中極五十壯。危亦林《世醫得效方·卷四·五積·腎積·灸法》(Wei 1964, 168-9)
[81] 諸虛極：灸膏肓腧，氣海穴，壯數愈多愈妙。《世醫得效方·卷八·痼冷·灸法》(Wei 1964, 400)
[82] 唇病：治緊唇不能開合，灸虎口，男左女右。《世醫得效方·卷十七·唇病·灸法》(Wei 1964, 874)
[83] 《普濟方》
[84] 徐鳳 《針灸大全》
[85] 汪機 《針灸問對》
[86] 《壽域神方》朱權
[87] 《本草綱目·卷六·燈火》 (Li 1996, 203-4)
[88] 陽燧灸

combined use was synergistic. Many Ming dynasty doctors advocated this integration, including Gao Wu, Wu Kun, and Yang Jizhou (He 2003, 7). For example, in the introduction to *Six Collections of Acupuncture Formulas*, Wu Kun tersely stated, "No acupuncture: no miracle. No moxibustion: no good."[89] In the same section, he stressed that medicinals were also necessary.

Gao Wu pointed out in *Gatherings from Eminent Acupuncturists*, "Someone who acts according to the disease in applying acupuncture, moxibustion, and medicinals is a good doctor."[90] Gao Wu recorded moxibustion formulas for many types of diseases. He also included memorization songs on internal and external medicine, gynecology, pediatrics, etc. *Gatherings* was a frequent source of material for Yang Jizhou's *Great Compendium of Acupuncture and Moxibustion.*

In the *Great Compendium*, Yang Jizhou analyzed and explained the use of acupuncture, moxibustion, and medicinals. He felt that these three modalities were all of equal importance. Yang wrote, "If you do not take medicinals for illness in the intestines and stomach, you cannot be helped. If you do not use acupuncture for illness in the blood vessels, it cannot be reached. If you do not use iron-burning for illness in the interstices, it cannot be penetrated. These needles, moxibustion, and medicinals: a medical doctor cannot lack any of them"[91] (He 2003, 7).

In Volume 11 of Zhang Jiebin's *Illustrated Supplement to the Categorized Classic*, there is a chapter called *Important Points for Moxibustion for the Various Patterns*. It recorded numerous moxibustion formulas for wind stroke, reversal counterflow (*jue ni*), cold dam-

age, etc. For scrofula, Zhang said, "Use a slice of single-clove garlic. First, begin moxibustion on the most recently erupted nucleus. When you reach the mother nucleus of the initial eruption, stop. A lot of moxibustion is spontaneously effective."[92]

Zhang also gave an overview on the use of moxibustion. For example, he wrote: "If using moxibustion on both the upper and the lower body, you must first apply it above and then below. You cannot first apply it below and then above."[93]

QING DYNASTY (1644 - 1911)

The *Organized Supplement of Gathering Mugwort*[94] is an anonymous treatise on moxibustion. Volume 2 recorded treatment principles and moxibustion formulas for each medical specialty such as adult medicine, pediatrics, external medicine, and emergency medicine (He 2003, 8).

Wu Qian *et al.* wrote the 90 volumes of the *Golden Mirror of Medicine*. The chapter called "Essential Poems of the Heart Method of Pricking and Moxibustion"[95] used acupuncture and moxibustion memorization songs to convey information. It included 22 moxibustion memorization songs regarding treatment of nineteen types of diseases (He 2003, 8).

Chen Yanquan's *Collection of Missing Writings*[96] discussed the application of moxibustion to extraordinary points, such as Yin Tang, Yao Yan, Zhou Jian, the Four Flowers, and the Riding the Bamboo Horse points (Liu 1991, 321-328; He 2003, 8).

Li Xuechuan was the author of *Meeting the Source of*

---

[89] 不針不神，不灸不良。吳崑《針方六集·針方六集序》(Huang 1996, 1027)
[90] 針灸藥因病而施者，醫之良也。高武《針灸聚英·針灸聚英引》(Gao 1999, 1)
[91] 疾在腸胃，非藥餌不能以濟；在血脈，非針刺不能以及；在腠理，非熨焫不能以達。是針灸藥者，醫家之不可缺一者也。楊繼洲《針灸大成·諸家得失策》(Huang 1996, 844)
[92] 用獨蒜片，先從後發核上灸起，至初發母核而止，多灸自效。張介賓《類經圖翼·諸症灸法要穴》(Zhang 1991, 931)
[93] 若上下俱灸，必須先上而後下，不可先下後上也。《類經圖翼·諸症灸法要穴》(Zhang 1991, 931)
[94] 《采艾編翼》
[95] 吳謙《醫宗金鑒·刺灸心法要訣》
[96] 陳延銓《羅遺篇》

Acupuncture and Moxibustion. He discussed many treatment protocols using moxibustion, for example, "Someone grew a tumor on his arm that gradually got as big as a Long Yan Rou (Arillus Longanae). The person used seven small cones of mugwort moxibustion on the tumor. He finished and it gradually dispersed and did not grow back."[97]

Wu Yiding compiled *Principles of Miraculous Moxibustion.* This book is a treatise of about 200,000 characters summarizing the writings on moxibustion up through the Qing dynasty (Wei 1987, 88). Wu favored moxibustion in urgent patterns: "Sudden strike of wind and cold can become critical in an instant. Using medicinals will not reach it. Moxibustion obtains the essential. Life can immediately return. For a medical doctor, nothing surpasses applying effective treatment and seeing results."[98] Wu also explained various aspects of the practice of moxibustion, such as the use of aged mugwort, the appropriate size of cones, contraindications, and the importance of moxa sores (Liu 1991, 335-7).

BRIEF SUMMARY OF MODERN HISTORY

During the Qing dynasty, the influence of Western medicine grew tremendously. Due to this and other factors, acupuncture and moxibustion lost status. Among the various forms of indigenous medicine, the herbal tradition retained more influence than acupuncture and moxibustion. The intellectuals of the 20th century (and even up to the present) have tended to favor Western science and many scorn indigenous medicine (Fruehauf 1999, 7; Unschuld 1985, 251).

However, due to political and social concerns, Chinese medicine could not be totally abandoned. Therefore, the government of the People's Republic of China decided to "tame the beast." Chinese medicine was systematized, standardized, and integrated with Western medicine. Many techniques and theo-

ries of the past lost favor. In addition, Western-style clinical or laboratory research became the most accepted way to validate a treatment (Fruehauf 1999, 9-10; Unschuld 1985, 252).

This trend necessarily affected moxibustion. New moxibustion techniques, such as "electrical moxibustion," liquid moxa, smokeless moxa, self-heating moxa pads, and stick-on cones, were developed (He 2003, 88; Flaws 2003, 2; Dharmananda 2004, 15-6). While these new techniques may expand the scope of moxibustion, there seems to be a concurrent reduction in the view of how, why, and when this modality should be used.

Do modern doctors still prefer mugwort picked on the fifth day of the fifth month? Do they still use an odd number of cones, or the same number of cones as the age of the patient? Are there still many who feel that moxibustion can be used in heat conditions? Is the heat of burning mugwort the only active ingredient? Who still applies moxibustion to the left on males and the right on females? Even more important, who still sees the patient as a small *tai ji*, a mini heaven and earth? Or is all of this just a vestige of a time when superstition ruled?

Perhaps some of the past may be viewed with an archeologist's eye, but before we discard the ideas of classical Chinese medicine, we had better examine them. Otherwise, we may know less than our predecessors, rather than more.

Below, the history of a few specific aspects of moxibustion are discussed.

MOXIBUSTION AS AN INTEGRATED PART OF CHINESE MEDICINE

It is a common myth that, in ancient times, doctors only practiced acupuncture-moxibustion or internal

---

[97] 一人于臂上生一瘤漸大如龍眼肉，其人用小艾于瘤上灸七壯，竟而漸消不長。李學川《針灸逢源》 (He 2003, 9)
[98] 風寒卒中危在須臾，用藥有所不及，灸得其要，立可回生，醫家取效見功莫過於此。吳亦鼎 《神灸經綸·卷一·說原》

medicine using medicinals, but not both types of modalities. This has never been true. Many or most famous herbalists included acupuncture and/or moxibustion in their treatments, although to a lesser degree than their use of internal medicine.

The *Inner Canon*, while focused on acupuncture and moxibustion, contained 13 herbal formulas and extensive discussion of the theories of herbal medicine. Zhang Zhongjing focused on herbal formulas but recommended acupuncture or moxibustion a number of times. Ge Hong used all these modalities. Sun Simiao said, "When medicinal decoctions attack the interior and acupuncture and moxibustion attack the exterior, the disease has no place to escape" (Sun 1996, 514). All of the four great masters of the Jin-Yuan period (Liu Wansu, Zhang Zihe, Li Dongyuan, and Zhu Danxi), while famous for their use of medicinals, also applied acupuncture and/or moxibustion. Zhu Danxi (1281-1358, Yuan dynasty), the last of these four masters, was no exception. In fact, he had his own unique theories about how and why acupuncture and moxibustion should be used. Li Shizhen and Zhang Jiebin were considered herbalists, yet the use of acupuncture and especially moxibustion is evident in their writings. Ye Tianshi also included formulas for many types of moxa rolls.

Many doctors who were primarily herbalists favored moxibustion over acupuncture when they used these external modalities, including Chen Yanzhi, Ge Hong, Wang Tao, Zhu Danxi, and Zhang Jiebin. Perhaps this is because moxibustion is performed using medicinal substances.

Styles of usage were quite varied: for example, whether or not moxibustion could be used against hot diseases, the necessity of using suppurating moxibustion, and the advisability of using moxibustion preventively or to expand lifespan. These ideas are discussed below. Another issue was the number of cones used in a treatment. Some doctors liked to

use hundreds, even a thousand cones (Sun Simiao, Dou Cai). Others used moxibustion often, but usually burned less than 10 cones (Zhu Danxi). It is clear from perusing the pre-modern books that moxibustion was used widely. Because of this, many techniques developed throughout the ages.

In ancient Chinese medical books, there is a spectrum ranging from no mention to extreme reliance on moxibustion. Examples:

- No moxibustion: *Classic of Difficulties*. Mugwort and moxibustion were never mentioned in the text, although acupuncture is discussed frequently.
- Moxibustion less than acupuncture: Many books, including the *Inner Canon*.
- Moxibustion and acupuncture more or less equally important: This is hard to judge, but perhaps Sun Simiao's *Supplement to Prescriptions Worth a Thousand Pieces of Gold* or Yang Jizhou's *Great Compendium of Acupuncture and Moxibustion*.
- Moxibustion more than acupuncture: Many books including those by Ge Hong, Zhu Danxi, and Zhang Jiebin.
- Moxibustion but no acupuncture: Books by Wang Tao and Dou Cai.

A HISTORY OF PREVENTIVE MOXIBUSTION

Preventive moxibustion is a technique in the Chinese tradition of "nourishing life." It is the application of moxibustion to guard against disease, strengthen the body, and slow the aging process.

The use of moxibustion to prevent disease has a long history. Although the *Yellow Emperor's Inner Canon* did not explicitly describe preventive moxibustion, it laid the groundwork for it in two ways:

- The *Inner Canon* emphasized preventive treatment. For example, *Elementary Questions*, Chapter 2 says, "The sages did not treat what was

---

[99] 聖人不治已病，治未病。《素問·四氣調神大論篇》 (Wu and Wu 1997, 16)

already ill. They treated what was not yet ill."[99]
- The *Inner Canon* identified one of the functions of moxibustion as supplementing vacuity. For example, *Magic Pivot*, Chapter 73 states, "Fire is naturally appropriate when yin and yang are both vacuous."[100] Chapter 51 describes supplementation technique for moxibustion.

Later doctors developed the theory and practice of preventive moxibustion from this.

The earliest recorded use of moxibustion to guard against disease progression was from the Jin dynasty writings of Fan Wang (Gu and Zhao 1994, 1). He said, "Whenever someone has sudden turmoil [or cholera], apply moxibustion. Although sometimes they do not recover, in the end they will be without the worry of death."[101] He called this type of treatment "counter-moxibustion."[102]

During the Sui dynasty, Chao Yuanfang expressed disapproval of a popular custom in certain areas of China—using moxibustion to guard against pediatric fright wind. He wrote, "In healthy newborns, be careful not to use counter-acupuncture and moxibustion. When counter-acupuncture and moxibustion are applied, the child endures pain and it stirs up the five pulses,[103] causing susceptibility to epilepsy. It is very cold in the region between the Yellow River and the Luo River. Children are susceptible to tetany. Their custom is to use counter-moxi-

bustion on three day old infants to guard against it. They also apply moxibustion to the cheek to guard against clenched jaw."[104] Chao opposed this type of practice because the child suffered pain and possible side effects.

At the beginning of the Tang dynasty, the concepts of nourishing life and prevention were prevalent and the clinical use of moxibustion was widespread. Therefore, the use of preventive moxibustion expanded (Gu and Zhao 1994, 1). Sun Simiao was a strong advocate of prevention. He warned, "Do not take health as if it were constant. You must constantly secure it, and never forget danger. Guard against all disease."[105]

Sun taught that healthy people should regularly apply moxibustion to prevent illness. He explained, "Generally when entering the lands of Wu and Shu, traveling officials must constantly apply moxibustion to two or three sites on their body. If the moxa sores are not allowed to heal even for a short while, miasmic pestilence, warm malaria, and toxin qi are unable to touch the person. That is why people traveling to Wu and Shu frequently apply moxibustion."[106] This is the origin of the practice of making long-term moxa sores to prevent disease.

Sun also was the first to discuss moxibustion on Gao Huang (UB 43) in detail. He stated, "There is nothing Gao Huang Shu does not treat... When this

---

[100] 《靈樞·官能》陰陽皆虛，火自當之。(Wu and Wu 1997, 781)
[101] 凡得霍亂，灸之或時雖未瘥，終無死憂。範汪 (晉代). He was the author of *Fan Dongyang's Assorted Herbal Formulas* 《範東陽雜藥方》. This book of 170 volumes has been lost (Li 1995, 877). However, the quotation was cited in *Medical Heart Formulas*, Volume 11 《醫心方·卷十一·治霍亂方第一》(Tamba 1993, 235).
[102] 逆灸《醫心方·卷十一·治霍亂方第一》 (Tamba 1993, 235)
[103] Probably referring to the pulses of the five viscera. *Elementary Questions*, Chapter 23 says, "The corresponding image of the five pulses: The liver's is string-like. The heart's is hook-like. The spleen's is [regularly] interrupted. The lungs' is hair-like. The kidneys' is stone-like. These name the pulses of the five viscera." 五脈應象：肝脈弦、心脈鉤、脾脈代、肺脈毛、腎脈石。是謂五臟之脈。《素問·宣明五氣篇第二十三》(Wu and Wu 1997, 131)
[104] 新生兒疾，慎不可逆針灸。逆針灸則忍痛動其五脈因喜成癇。河洛間土地多寒，兒喜病痓。其俗生兒三日，喜逆灸以防之，又灸頰以防噤。巢元方《諸病源候論·卷四十五·養小兒候》 Volume 45 of *Discussion on the Origins of Symptoms in Illness* (Chao 1992, 1280).
[105] 勿以健康便為常然，常須安不忘危，預防諸疾也。孫思邈《千金要方·卷二十七·居處法》 Volume 27 of *Prescriptions* (Sun 1997b, 933)
[106] 凡入吳蜀地遊宦，體上常須兩三處灸之，勿令瘡暫差，則瘴癘，溫瘧毒氣不能著人也，故吳蜀多行灸法。《千金要方·卷二十九·灸例》 *Prescriptions*, Volume 29 (Sun 1997b, 1027-8)

moxibustion is completed, it makes a person's yang qi healthy and vigorous."[107] Moxibustion on Gao Huang has been used since that time to treat vacuity taxation and emaciation.

Sun Simiao also wrote, "Generally, at the onset of leg qi, there is weakness of the legs. Quickly apply moxibustion to it."[108] He then suggested applying moxibustion to various points on the legs. In this case, Sun advocated treating a mild condition to prevent it from worsening.

Later in the Tang dynasty, Wang Tao proposed that constant application of moxibustion on Zu San Li (ST 36) had anti-aging effects. He said, "Whenever people over the age of 30 do not apply moxibustion to Zu San Li, qi is allowed to ascend, dimming their eyes. San Li is used to descend qi."[109] Wang was actually misquoting from Sun Simiao's *Supplement*,[110] leaving out a phrase. Sun said the problem of excessive ascent of qi to the eyes occurs *when moxibustion is applied to the head* without also applying it to Zu San Li. Sun considered these eye problems a side effect of improper use of moxibustion. Wang Tao, whether by misquoting or by rephrasing Sun's statement, gave impetus to the idea that frequent moxibustion on Zu San Li can prevent some of the effects of aging.

The Tang dynasty treatise called the *Yellow Emperor's Moxibustion Classic of the Bright Hall*[111] expanded the scope of preventive moxibustion on Zu San Li by prescribing it to guard against the occurrence of wind stroke: "Generally two months before, maybe three or five months before someone has wind stroke, not at any particular time, he will suddenly develop an aching, heavy, insensitive impediment on his shins... This is a predromal symptom of wind stroke. You must quickly apply moxibustion to San Li and Jue Gu [GB 39]: three cones to each of these four places. Afterwards, decoct the four flavors of Cong [Bulbus Allii Fistulosi], Bo He [Herba Menthae Haplocalycis], peach and willow leaves. Wash the moxibustion sores with the decoction. This treatment expels wind qi from the opening of the moxa sores and moves it out"[112] (Gu and Zhao 1994, 2).

Volume 165 of the *Old Tang [History] Book* recorded a case of moxibustion used for longevity and health: Liu Gongquan[113] was over 80 years old and still walked lightly. Someone asked him his technique for nourishing life. He said, "I have not used original qi to aid joy and anger and I constantly warm Qi Hai (Ren 6). That's all"[114] (Gu and Zhao 1994, 2).

This shows that during the Tang dynasty, moxibustion was not only used to guard against the occurrence of disease, but it also had begun to be used to enhance the constitution, delay aging, and lengthen life.

In the Song dynasty, medical doctors and specialists in nourishing life continued to apply preventive moxibustion; its use for this purpose increased and theories explaining its effects were developed. Dou Cai wrote copiously about the importance of moxi-

107 膏肓抦無所不治。。。此灸訖，令人陽氣康盛。《千金要方·卷三十·雜病》*Prescriptions*, Volume 30 (Sun 1997b, 1088)
108 凡腳氣初得腳弱，速灸之。《千金要方·卷七·論風毒狀·論灸法》*Prescriptions*, Volume 7 (Sun 1997b, 272)
109 凡人年三十以上，若不灸足三里，令人氣上眼闇，所以三里下氣。《外台秘要·卷三十九·不宜灸禁穴及老少加減法》(Wang 1979, 1078)
110 《千金翼方·卷第二十八針灸下·雜法》*Supplement*, Volume 28 (Sun 1997a, 282)
111 《黃帝明堂灸經》*The Yellow Emperor's Moxibustion Classic of the Bright Hall* was written at the end of Northern Song. The name of its author is lost. During the Yuan dynasty it was made part of the *Four Books of Acupuncture and Moxibustion* (Li 1995, 1351).
112 凡人未中風時，兩月前，或三五個月前，非時，足脛上忽發酸重頑痹。。。此乃中風之候也。便須急灸三里穴與絕骨穴，四處各三壯。後用葱，薄荷，桃，柳葉四味煎湯，淋洗灸瘡，令驅逐風氣于瘡口中出也。《針灸四書·黃帝明堂灸經·正人形第四》
113 柳公權 (778-865), statesman and calligrapher (Liu 1999, 166).
114 未嘗以元氣佐喜怒，氣海常溫耳。《舊唐書·卷一百六十五》

bustion in the *Book of Bian Que's Heart*. He said, "In the method of preserving life, burning mugwort is first, elixir medicinals are second, and Fu Zi [Radix Lateralis Aconiti] is third."[115]

Dou elaborated on the theory and principles of preventive moxibustion. He believed that yang was the key to life: "If yang essence is vigorous, you will have a lifespan of a thousand years. If yin qi is strong, it will bring death and damage. It is also said, if yin qi is never dispersed, the end is death. If yang essence exists, it will bring long life."[116] Dou also stated, "When yang qi has not expired, life is firm and fast."[117] He felt that treatment to conserve life and guard against illness must focus on "preserving and supporting yang qi as the root."[118] Moxibustion was an ideal means for this.

Dou described a protocol for preserving life: "When people reach their later years, yang qi is debilitated. That is why their hands and feet are not warm, the lower origin is vacuous and worn out, and movement is difficult. Now, as long as people have qi remaining, they will not die. Qi is yang, which is life. This is why you must die when yang qi is exhausted. When people are without disease, they should frequently apply moxibustion to Guan Yuan [Ren 4], Qi Hai [Ren 6], Ming Guan [SP 17], and Zhong Wan [Ren 12]. In addition, take Bao Yuan Dan [Elixir to Preserve the Origin] or Bao Ming Yan Shou Dan [Elixir to Preserve Life & Longevity]. Although you may not obtain [an extremely] long life, you can still maintain a lifespan of 100 years."[119]

Dou theorized that a person who was old and feeble gradually reached exhaustion of original yang. Fre-

quent moxibustion on points like Guan Yuan could strengthen original yang, delay decline and aging, and lengthen the lifespan. Application of moxibustion to Guan Yuan in healthy people could strengthen and fortify their body, while in those who were already ill, applying moxibustion could also prevent disease progression. Based on this, Dou recommended that preventive moxibustion on Guan Yuan should keep pace with the age, increasing the number of cones as years go by, in order to delay aging and decline.

Dou related his personal experience with preventive moxibustion, "At the time I was 50, I frequently applied 500 cones of moxibustion to Guan Yuan… I gradually achieved a light and fortified body, and had a good appetite. When I was 63, because of anxiety and anger, I suddenly found a death pulse in my left *cun* position — 19 beats and one rest. I then applied 500 cones of moxibustion each to Guan Yuan and Ming Men [Du 4]. Fifty days later the death pulse had not returned. Each year I constantly add to this moxibustion, pursuing and obtaining health in my old age."[120]

Dou Cai expanded the point selection for moxibustion to nourish life and recognized that healthy people who often used moxibustion on these points were more likely to resist disease and live longer.

Southern Song author and doctor Wang Zhizhong wrote the *Classic of Nourishing Life with Acupuncture and Moxibustion*. He stated, "Qi Hai [Ren 6] is the sea of original qi. Man uses original qi as his root. If original qi is not damaged, disease will not harm him. Once original qi is damaged, he dies even without disease. It

---

[115] 保命之法，灼艾第一，丹藥第二，附子第三。《扁鵲心書·卷上·住世之法》(Dou 2000, 9)
[116] 陽精若壯千年壽，陰氣如強必斃傷。又云陰氣未消終是死，陽精若在必長生。《扁鵲心書·卷上·須識扶陽》(Dou 2000, 8)
[117] 陽氣不絕，性命堅牢。《扁鵲心書·卷上·大病宜灸》(Dou 2000, 9)
[118] 保扶陽氣為本。《扁鵲心書·卷上·須識扶陽》(Dou 2000, 8)
[119] 人至晚年，陽氣衰，故手足不煖，下元虛憊，動作艱難。蓋人有一息氣在則不死，氣者陽所生也。故陽氣盡必死。
   人于無病時，常灸關元，氣海，命關，中脘，更服保元丹，保命延壽丹，雖未得長生，亦可保百年長壽矣。
   《扁鵲心書·卷上·須識扶陽》(Dou 2000, 8)
[120] 余五十時，常灸關元五百壯。。。漸至身體輕健，羨進飲食。六十三時，因憂怒，忽見死脈于左手寸部，
   十九動而一止，乃灸關元，命門各五百壯，五十日後死脈不復見矣。每年常加此灸，遂得老年健康。
   《扁鵲心書·卷上·住世之法》(Dou 2000, 9)

is appropriate to frequently apply moxibustion to this point in order to invigorate original yang. If you wait for disease before applying moxibustion, I am afraid the opportunity will be lost until it is too late."[121]

Southern Song medical doctor Zhang Gao used suppurating moxibustion on Zu San Li (ST 36) to guard against wind stroke. He wrote the often quoted statement that "If you desire to be secure, San Li must not be dry."[122] Zhang explained his reasoning: "San Li is the irrigation canal of the five viscera and six bowels. You need to constantly circulate and unblock it so that there is no wind disease"[123] (Gu and Zhao 1994, 3).

During the Ming and Qing period, preventive moxibustion continued to develop, for example, in the prevention of wind stroke, Zhu Quan[124] prescribed moxibustion on Bai Hui (Du 20), Da Zhui (Du 14), Feng Chi (GB 20), Jian Jing (GB 21), Qu Chi (LI 11), Zu San Li (ST 36), and Jian Shi (PC 5) for the initial signs of wind stroke with symptoms of wind evils entering the viscera. He also indicated, "If you have a wind condition in general, constantly apply moxibustion to these seven points every spring and autumn in order to discharge wind qi. Especially watch out for people who have had long-term wind conditions."[125]

Li Chan recorded an interesting type of preventive moxibustion in *Entering the Gate of Medicine*: "Smelting the umbilicus method" was suggested for curing vacuity taxation and for prevention. Li claimed that when someone uses this technique four times a year, once in each season, "original qi is firm and secure, and the hundred diseases are not engendered."[126] Yang Jizhou described a similar "method of steaming the umbilicus to treat disease" in Volume 9 of the *Great Compendium of Acupuncture and Moxibustion*. It is roughly the same technique as Li Chan's "smelting the umbilicus method" but the medicinals in the prescription are different. Both make a ring around the navel with dough, fill it with powdered medicinals, and then burn moxa cones on top. Yang advocated applying this type of moxibustion at specific times:[127]

DATE		TIME	
SEASONAL MARKER	APPROXIMATE DATE	BRANCH	DOUBLE HOUR
Spring establishment	February 4th	*si*	9-11 am
Spring equinox	March 21st	*wei*	1-3 pm
Summer establishment	May 5th	*chen*	7-9 am
Summer solstice	June 22nd	*you*	5-7 pm
Autumn establishment	August 8th	*xu*	7-9 pm
Autumnal equinox	September 22nd	*wu*	11am-1 pm
Winter establishment	November 7th	*hai*	9-11 pm
Winter solstice	December 22nd	*yin*	3-5 am

---

[121] 氣海者，元氣之海也。人以元氣為本，元氣不傷，雖疾不害，一傷元氣，無疾而死矣。宜頻灸此穴，以壯元陽，若必待疾作而後灸，恐失之晚矣。王執中《針灸資生經·第三·虛損》(Huang 1996, 270)

[122] 若要安，三里莫要干。張杲。《醫說·卷二》 Volume 2 of *Medical Explanations*. *Medical Explanations* has 10 Volumes, and was published in 1224 (Li 1995, 835).

[123] 三里者五臟六腑之溝渠也，常欲宣通即無風疾。《醫說·卷二》

[124] 朱權《乾坤生意》 *Vitality of Qian and Kun*

[125] 如風勢略可，凡遇春，秋二時，常灸此七穴以泄風氣；若素有風人尤當留意。According to 《針灸大成·卷八·中風癱瘓針灸秘訣》 *Great Compendium of Acupuncture and Moxibustion*, Secret Formula for Acupuncture and Moxibustion [to treat] Wind Stroke Paralysis (Huang 1996, 972).

[126] 一年四季各熏一次，元氣堅固，百疾不生。《醫學入門·卷之一·針灸·煉臍法》(Li Y 1999, 283)

[127] The reasoning behind this will be discussed in Part 2 of this book. It is based on the eight astronomical landmarks of the solar year, and the six unities 六合 relationship between the earthly branches.

Yang explained that using this timing "Unites with the right qi of the four seasons, and completes the creation and transformation of heaven and earth. This moxibustion is never ineffective."[128]

Famous author and doctor Zhang Jiebin discussed the application of preventive moxibustion on various points in the *Illustrated Supplement to the Categorized Classic*. He recommended Feng Men (UB 12) to guard against certain skin ailments: "This point is able to drain hot qi from the whole body. Someone who constantly applies moxibustion to it will never suffer abscesses, sores, and scabs."[129] He also discussed salt moxibustion on Shen Que (Ren 8): "If three or five hundred cones of moxibustion are applied to it, not only will illness be cured, but it will also prolong life."[130] Zhang also warned, "Avoid applying moxibustion on San Li (ST 36) in children. Those beyond 30 years can apply moxibustion. Otherwise, it will generally produce illness."[131] Apparently, according to Zhang, although Zu San Li can delay some of the effects of aging, it may have adverse effects in the very young.

In summary, preventive moxibustion arose during the Jin dynasty (265-419 CE) and developed over the next 1,500 years, in step with preventive medicine in general and the concept of nourishing life. Clinical observation seemed to support its use. Over the centuries, moxibustion expanded from a modality to treat disease into a method of prevention and nourishing life.

CAN MOXIBUSTION BE APPLIED IN HEAT PATTERNS?

Historically there have been two opposing schools of thought on this question: The larger school is op-posed to the use of moxibustion in heat patterns, but others say its use is appropriate.

An early representative of the school that prohibits moxibustion in heat patterns is Zhang Zhongjing (Han dynasty), the author of the *Treatise on Cold Damage*.[132] Analysis of his works shows that Zhang felt moxibustion should only be used in yin patterns — repletion cold or vacuity cold — and was inappropriate for yang exuberance and yin vacuity.

Zhang's ideas, including those about moxibustion, had great influence throughout the ages. Xu Hong (Song dynasty) wrote the *Overall Discussion Guidebook* as an appendix to the famous *Professional and Popular Prescriptions from the Taiping Era*. He stated, "In cold damage which has caused chest and rib-side pain and abdominal fullness, one cannot rashly use mugwort moxibustion. You see this pattern in the villages. If they are without medicinals, it is convenient to use mugwort moxibustion. Often, this results in toxin qi along with fire becoming exuberant. This leads to drum distention, panting, and then death. They do not know that chest and rib-side pain belong to lesser yang, and abdominal distention and fullness belong to greater yin. Besides this, moxibustion can only be applied in yin patterns."[133] While the case that Xu discusses was caused by cold damage, by the time it had entered into the chest and abdomen, it had transformed into heat. He felt that an error in moxibustion could result in death. Thus, he advocated using moxibustion only in yin patterns.

The *Classic of the Central Viscera* is attributed to Hua Tuo who lived near the end of the Han dynasty, although it was probably written much later. Chapter 47 of this book states, "Moxibustion arouses yin and

---

[128] 立春巳時，春分未時，立夏辰時，夏至酉時，立秋戌時，秋分午時，立冬亥時，冬至寅時。此乃合四時之正氣，全天地之造化，灸無不驗。《針灸大成·卷九·蒸臍治病法》(Huang 1996, 990)
[129] 此穴能瀉一身熱氣，常灸之，永無癰疽瘡疥等患。張介賓《類經圖翼·卷七·經絡五》(Zhang 1991, 851)
[130] 若灸之三五百壯，不惟愈疾，亦具延年。《類經圖翼·卷八·經絡六》(Zhang 1991, 899)
[131] 小兒忌灸三里，三十外方可灸，不爾凡生疾。《類經圖翼·卷六·經絡四》(Zhang 1991, 832)
[132] 張仲景《傷寒論》
[133] 傷寒胸脅痛及腹滿，不可妄用艾灸。覺見村落間有此証，無藥便用艾灸，多致毒氣隨火而盛，鼓脹發喘而死。不知胸脅痛自屬小陽，腹脹滿自屬太陰，此外惟陰証可灸。許洪《太平惠民和劑局方·指南總論·傷寒十勸》(Xu H. 1997, 129)

frees yang… If moxibustion is applied when it is inappropriate, it causes serious damage to the channels and network vessels and internal amassment of flaming toxins. Contrary [to the intention of the treatment], it injures the harmony of the center, until the patient cannot be saved… If yin qi is not exuberant or yang qi is not debilitated, do not apply moxibustion."[134]

Zhang Jiebin (Ming dynasty) wrote in *Jingyue's Complete Book*, "Using the method of fire is only appropriate for yang vacuity, lots of cold, or congealed and stagnant channels and vessels. If there are symptoms such as exuberant fire, debilitated metal, depleted water, lots of dryness, rapid pulse, fever, dry throat, red face, thirst, hot bowel movement or urination, one cannot rashly add mugwort fire. If one mistakenly uses it, the result will be that the blood becomes dryer and the heat becomes more severe. This, on the contrary, quickens the peril."[135]

Wang Mengying[136] (Qing) strongly opposed the use of moxibustion in yin vacuity. He felt that moxibustion plunders yin, and regarded the use of moxibustion in heat patterns as the "dreaded path" (Wei 1987, 16).

However, historically, there were also a number of doctors who held the view that moxibustion could be effective in treating heat patterns. Sun Simiao (Tang dynasty) said, "When the head and body are hot, apply 100 cones of moxibustion to Wei Guan [Ren 13]. Do not apply acupuncture,"[137] and, "When the body has heat vexation, needle Zhong Fu [LU 1].

Also apply 50 cones of moxibustion to Jue Gu [GB 39]."[138]

Wang Tao (Tang dynasty) had a chapter on using moxibustion to treat steaming bone syndrome in Volume 13 of *Secret Necessities*.[139] Liu Wansu and Li Dongyuan,[140] (both Jin dynasty) supported the use of moxibustion for repletion and heat patterns. For example, Liu, who began the school of cold and cooling treatment, used moxibustion to treat sores caused by heat in order to "discharge the evil qi."[141] He also used moxibustion to "lead heat to move downward"[142] when the body is hot but the feet are cold. In addition, Liu wrote, "A person with thirst that leads them to drink has heat above the diaphragm… In this pattern, you should apply three times five cones of moxibustion to Da Zhui [Du 14]. The patient will immediately recover. This treatment drains the governing vessel."[143]

It is said that Zhu Danxi (Yuan dynasty) perfected the theory that moxibustion can be used in heat patterns (Wei 1987, 67). Zhu's writings clearly show that he used moxibustion to drain fire as well as to supplement yin vacuity. His views about the use of moxibustion in heat conditions can be summarized as follows:

- Moxibustion "drains and leads heat downward." In *The Heart and Essence of Danxi's Methods of Treatment*, Zhu wrote, "Sometimes leg qi surges into the heart. This is blood vacuity with ascending fire qi… Use Fu Zi [Radix Lateralis Aconiti] powder mixed with spittle to make a

---

[134] 灸則起陰通陽。。。不當灸而灸，則使人重傷經絡，內蓄炎毒，反害中和，至於不可救。。。陰氣不盛，陽氣不衰，勿灸。華佗《中藏經·論諸病治療交錯致于死候》 (Huang 1973, 524)
[135] 用火之法，惟陽虛多寒，經絡凝滯者爲宜。若火盛金衰，水虧多燥，脈數發熱，咽乾面赤，口渴便熱等證，則不可妄加艾火。若誤用之，必致血愈燥而熱愈甚，是反速其危矣。張介賓《景岳全書·非風·灸法》 (Zhang J.Y. 1995, 233)
[136] 王孟英 also known as Wang Shixiong 王士雄 (1808-1866).
[137] 頭身熱，灸胃管百壯，勿針。《千金翼方·卷二十七》 (Sun 1997a, 271)
[138] 身體煩熱，針中府。又，灸絕骨五十壯。《千金翼方·卷二十七》 (Sun 1997a, 271)
[139] 王燾《外台秘要·卷十三·灸骨蒸方》 (Wang 1979, 351-3)
[140] 劉完素，李束垣
[141] 以泄邪氣。《素問病機宜氣保命集·瘡瘍論》 (Liu 1998, 170)
[142] 引熱下行。《素問病機宜氣保命集·心痛論》 (Liu 1998, 144)
[143] 假令渴引飲者，是熱在膈上。。。此証當灸大椎三五壯，立已，乃瀉督也。《素問病機宜氣保命集·瀉痢論》

cake the size of a small coin. Apply it to Yong Quan [KI 1]. Use mugwort fire moxibustion on it. This will drain and lead the heat downward."[144]

Zhu also wrote, in *Pulse Factors, Patterns and Treatment*: "Great heat of the two hands is bone reversal [jue]. It feels as if the hands were placed in fire. You can apply five cones of moxibustion to Yong Quan [KI 1]. There will be immediate recovery."[145]

• Moxibustion "scatters fire and dispels phlegm." *Additional Categorized Cases of Famous Doctors*,[146] records that Zhu treated a runny nose with foul-smelling snivel. He diagnosed it as "a pattern of phlegm, depressed fire, and heat." Zhu applied moxibustion to Shang Xing (Du 23), San Li (ST 36), and He Gu (LI 4), and added a formula to clear heat and dispel phlegm. The patient recovered.

In the same set of cases, another patient had a runny nose with yellow snivel and "brain pain." Zhu applied seven cones of moxibustion each on Xin Hui (GB 22) and Tong Tian (UB 7). The patient then eliminated a lump of "foul-smelling flesh" and recovered.

Moxibustion can be used for heat in the lungs. Zhu said to treat cough with phlegm, apply moxibustion to Tian Tu (Ren 22) and Fei Shu (UB 13) because this "can discharge fire and heat, and greatly drain qi."[147]

• Zhu rationalized the use of moxibustion in repletion heat patterns as: "Fire uses uninhibited radiation to transfer and lead fire toxins out. This is a type of following or paradoxical treatment."[148]

• Moxibustion can even "nourish yin and clear heat." In *Classified Case Histories of Famous Physicians*,[149] there is a record of a patient with fever attributed to yin vacuity heat who was coughing up blood. Zhu applied five cones of moxibustion on Fei Shu (UB 13), and the patient recovered (Wei 1987, 67).

The theory behind Zhu's use of moxibustion for nourishing yin is to supplement yang so it can generate yin. He said, "Great disease vacuity desertion is rooted in yin vacuity. Use mugwort moxibustion on the *dan tian* [cinnabar field]. This is to supplement yang, because when yang is generated, yin is also generated."[150] This is a reasonable explanation for the use of moxibustion in vacuity heat conditions, firmly based in yin-yang theory.

A number of later doctors followed Zhu's lead in using moxibustion for heat conditions. Gong Juzhong (Ming dynasty) indicated in *A Spot of Snow on a Red [Hot] Stove*[151] that moxibustion can be used in all patterns: cold and heat, vacuity and repletion. He claimed that moxibustion is suitable in every case (Wei 1987, 16).

In *Questions and Answers on Acupuncture and Moxibus-*

---

[144] 有腳氣沖心者，乃血虛而有火氣上行。。。再于湧泉穴用附子為末，津拌如小錢大，貼之，以艾火灸，泄引其熱。朱丹溪《丹溪治法心要·腳氣》(Zhu 2000, 646)
[145] 兩手大熱為骨厥，如在火中，可灸湧泉五壯，立愈。《脈因証治·熱》(Zhu 2000, 499)
[146] 《續名醫類案·卷二十二·鼻》(Lu 1996, 4116) *Additional Categorized Cases of Famous Doctors* by 魏之琇 Wei Zhixiu (Qing). This book contained a number of cases where moxibustion was used in heat conditions (He 2003, 8).
[147] 能泄火熱，大瀉氣。《丹溪治法心要·咳嗽》(Zhu 2000, 593)
[148] 火以暢達，撥引熱毒，此從治之意。(Wei 1987, 67)
[149] 江瓘《名醫類案》by Jiang Guan, 1549 (Ming)
[150] 大病虛脫，本是陰虛，用艾丹田者，所以補陽，陽生則陰生故也。《金匱鈎玄·腳氣》*Probing into the Subtleties of the Golden Cabinet* (Zhu 2000, 114). The idea that 'when yang is generated, yin is [also] generated' comes from *Elementary Questions*, Chapter 5 《陰陽應象大論》(Wu and Wu 1997, 31).
[151] 龔居中《紅爐點雪》

tion, Wang Ji (Ming dynasty) explained this theory, "Apply moxibustion in vacuity conditions to make fire qi reinforce original qi. Apply moxibustion in repletion conditions to make the repletion evil follow the fire qi and scatter. Apply moxibustion in cold conditions to make qi return and warm the patient. Apply moxibustion in heat conditions to lead depressed hot qi to discharge outwardly"[152] (Wei 1987, 16).

Besides the cases of Zhu Danxi, mentioned above, *Additional Categorized Cases of Famous Doctors* recorded a number of medical cases where moxibustion was used to treat hot diseases, for example, "A 14-year-old child had lumbar and back pain after having the pox. He was unable to bend forward and backward and had afternoon tidal fevers. This was desiccated and diminished bone marrow, water unable to overcome fire, and hot kidney qi. Three cones of moxibustion were applied on each Kun Lun [UB 60] and Shen Mai [UB 62]."[153] The child was also given a formula, and recovered.

Li Xuechuan (Qing dynasty), the author of *Meeting the Source of Acupuncture and Moxibustion*, wrote, "Generally abscesses and malign sores are all due to toxins from lingering heart fire. When moxibustion is applied, the heart fire circulates and the toxins spontaneously scatter"[154] (He 2003, 9).

The use of moxibustion in heat conditions sounds counter-intuitive to many. However, no one recommends taking a medicinal decoction cold, even when treating patients with heat conditions. Decoctions are usually taken warm at the very least. Perhaps the use of heat in moxibustion is similar to the use of fire in cooking the medicinals. Even though mugwort is classified as warm-natured, we are not using it inter-

nally. Its effects when burned externally are not the same as its effects when used in a decoction.

Modern contraindications of moxibustion in heat conditions are not absolute and are mainly intended for those with less knowledge and experience.

BLISTERING OR SUPPURATIVE MOXIBUSTION

Suppurative moxibustion and its close cousins, scarring and blistering moxibustion, are types of direct moxibustion, allowing the cone to burn down to the skin. A blister forms, sometimes it fills with pus, and after it heals, a scar may be left.

Moxa sores (sores from scarring, suppurative, or blistering moxibustion) were sometimes called moxa flowers, for example in the *Collected Works of Acupuncture and Moxibustion*, by Liao Runhong (Qing).[155]

Doctors have discussed moxa sores for untold years. Zhang Zhongjing's *Essential Prescriptions of the Golden Cabinet* (Han dynasty) mentions moxa sores, but in this case, they are part of the problem, not part of the cure. Zhang says in chapter two, "It is difficult to treat tetany in a patient with moxa sores."[156]

Huangfu Mi's *Systematic Classic* (Jin dynasty) is the first extant book that implies that moxa sores are desirable (Wei 1987, 16). At the end of Volume 3, he wrote, "If you want to make moxa eruptions, heat the sole of a shoe and use it to iron [the site of the moxibustion treatment]. In three days the sores will erupt."[157] This section of the *Systematic Classic* is derived from the lost *Essentials of the Bright Hall for*

[152] 虛者灸之，使火氣以助元氣也；實者灸之，使實邪隨火氣而發散也；寒者灸之，使其氣復溫也；熱者灸之，引鬱熱之氣外發。汪機《針灸問對·卷之下》
[153] 一兒年十四，痘後腰背痛，不能俯仰，午後潮熱，此骨髓枯少，水不勝火，腎氣熱也。灸昆侖穴，申脈穴各三壯。《續名醫類案·卷四十·痘腰痛》(Lu 1996, 4280)
[154] 凡癰疽惡瘡皆心火留滯之毒，則以心火流通而毒自散也。李學川《針灸逢源》
[155] 灸花: 廖潤鴻《針灸集成·卷一·灸後治法》(Liao 1986, unpaginated)
[156] 痓病有灸瘡，難治。張仲景《金匱要略·痓濕暍病脈證治》(Zhang Z.J. 1992, 17)
[157] 欲令灸發者，灸履〔革+扁〕熨之，三日即發。皇甫謐《針灸甲乙經》(Huang 1996, 53)

Points and Acupuncture Moxibustion Treatment;[158] it is unclear if this particular sentence is a comment of Huangfu's or if it is also from that source. As late as the Ming dynasty, doctors such as Gong Yanxian[159] continued to recommend this method.

Suppurative moxibustion flourished over time. In the 6th century, Wei Shou wrote the biography of Li Hongzhi in the *Wei Book*. He said that Li Hongzhi "endured a lot. He received moxibustion to treat a disease with rash. The mugwort was put around the rash at a distance of two *cun* on more than ten places from his hands to his feet. In a short while, moxibustion was applied on all, but he calmly spoke and laughed."[160] We can guess that the treatment involved blistering moxibustion from the phrase "he endured a lot" (Wei 1987, 16).

The *Song Book* recorded in the biography of Qian Ruoshui, "Moxibustion was applied to both feet because of his disease. The wounds ulcerated and bled a few *dou*"[161] (Wei 1987, 16-7).

Although these last two references are not in medical works, they seem to describe blistering moxibustion. This shows that contemporary readers were probably familiar with blistering moxibustion.

Yang Xuancao[162] lived at the beginning of the Tang dynasty and advocated suppurative moxibustion. Volume 2 of *Medical Heart Formulas* cites him as saying, "If moxibustion sores suppurate and decay, the disease will be expelled. If there is no decay, the disease is not eliminated."[163]

Wang Huaiyin, *et al.,* edited *Sage-like Prescriptions of the Taiping Era*. This 100 volume book was ordered by the Song Emperor Taizong. The last volume said, "Even if the number of moxibustion cones is sufficient, sores must erupt with suppuration and decay for the patient to promptly heal. If there is no eruption of sores with suppuration and decay, the disease will not recover"[164] (Wei 1987, 17).

Wenren Qi'nian (Knowledgeable Aged Person), who wrote *Moxibustion for Emergencies*[165] during the Southern Song dynasty, also elaborated on the relationship between moxa sores and the treatment of illness (Wei 1987, 17).

Li Shouxian (Qing dynasty) thought treatment would not be effective without moxa sores. In *Easy Studies in Acupuncture and Moxibustion*, he said, "Moxa sores must erupt; they eliminate disease as if plucking it out"[166] (Wei 1987, 17).

Although today most in the West think this type of treatment is too drastic to use, we should note that historically, many doctors have indicated that moxa sores were necessary for an effective treatment. In addition to the above, Song dynasty Wang Zhizhong and Dou Cai; Yuan dynasty Dou Hanqing; and Ming dynasty Xu Chunfu, Xu Feng, Gong Yanxian, and Li Chan[167] all supported this viewpoint and developed methods for making moxa sores erupt. These methods include the external application of heat; the external application of acrid warm medicinals that engender flesh, unblock, and scatter (as in heavenly moxibustion, see below); or internally taking enriching and supplementing formulas or foods (such as

158 《明堂孔穴針灸治要》
159 龔延賢《壽世保元》, in *Long Life and Protecting the Origin,* Volume 10 (Gong 2001, 446).
160 洪之志性慷慨，多所堪忍，疹疾灸療，艾炷圓將二寸，手足十餘處，一時俱下，而言笑自若。魏收
   《魏書·列傳酷史第七十七·李洪之》
161 因疾灸兩足，創潰出血數斗。《宋書·列傳第二十五·錢若水》
162 楊玄操
163 灸瘡得膿壞，其病乃出；不壞，則病不除。《醫心方》 (Tamba 1993, 70)
164 灸炷雖然數足，得瘡發膿壞，所患即差；如不得瘡發膿壞，其疾不愈。王懷隱《太平聖惠方》
165 聞人耆年《備急灸法》
166 灸瘡必發，去病如把抓。李守先《針灸易學》
167 王執中,竇材,竇漢卿,徐春甫,徐鳳,龔延賢,李梴

fish) to help the body make more pus (Wei 1987, 17).

Some modern doctors concur. For example, Xie Xiliang (born 1926), explains that "The suppuration under the moxibustion scar is quite different to other inflammatory symptoms of boils, sores, or wounds, because it does not lead to any bad results... In general, pustulation after the direct moxibustion belongs to a benign stimulation which may improve body constitution and strengthen the body resistance in order to prevent or treat a disease... The wound after the direct moxibustion usually does not need to be treated, and it will spontaneously recover within 30 days." Later in this passage, Dr. Xie described the warning signs of a secondary infection (Chen and Deng 1989, 593).

Yan Dingliang (born 1924) recommends suppurating moxibustion for asthma and chronic diarrhea. He believes that one cone of suppurating moxibustion is the equivalent of ten cones without suppuration. Therefore, it is only necessary to use it on a few points each year (Chen and Deng 1989, 202-3).

A number of methods were developed to ease the pain of burns. Sun Simiao (Tang dynasty) discussed the use of moxibustion to treat fistulas in Volume 24 of *Prescriptions*. He burned a mixture of Ma Hua (Flos Cannabis, hemp flower) and mugwort floss on the sore, probably a way of numbing the area.[168]

In the *Book of Bian Que's Heart*, Dou Cai suggested an internal formula called *Sleeping Sage Powder*[169] as a way to lessen the patient's suffering during the application of moxibustion. This formula consists of Man Tuo Luo Hua (Flos Daturae) and Huo Ma Hua (Flos Cannabis). It made the patient sleep so that

treatment could be applied painlessly. This is the earliest record of the use of an anesthetic to apply moxibustion (He 2003, 5).

During the Ming dynasty, Gong Xin suggested in Volume 13 of *Ancient and Modern Mirror of Medicine* that before moxibustion, "paper impregnated with medicinals applied to the site, making the skin and flesh numb"[170] should be used in order to partially anesthetize the area. The formula included powdered wasp nest that came from a flowering pepper tree, soaked in wax, powdered again, and mixed with sesame oil.

Gong Xin's son, Gong Yanxian, said in Volume 10 of *Long Life and Protecting the Origin*, "If the pain is unendurable when applying mugwort fire, use a finger to firmly cover the site of the point in advance. Even better, use something made of iron to press it, and the pain will promptly stop."[171] The pressure partially anesthetizes the site of moxibustion.

MOXIBUSTION ON ISOLATING SUBSTANCES

The idea of moxibustion on isolating substances, often called 'indirect moxibustion,' was pioneered by Ge Hong in *Emergency Prescriptions*.[172] He used many types of isolating substances and was the first to record moxibustion on garlic, salt, Sichuan pepper, flour dough, etc. From his time to the present, many doctors, including Sun Simiao and Zhang Jiebin, have commonly used this technique.

During the Yuan dynasty, Zhu Danxi[173] used both direct and indirect moxibustion. He wrote about a variety of prescriptions using isolating substances; he used garlic, salt, Zao Jiao (Fructus Gleditsiae), ginger,

---

[168] 孫思邈 《千金要方·卷第二十四·九漏方》 (Sun 1996, 385)
[169] 睡聖散 《扁鵲心書·卷一·附竇材灸法》 (Dou 2000, 23)
[170] 用藥制過紙擦之，使皮肉麻木。龔信 《古今醫鑒·卷十三·癬疾》 (Gong 1999, 1347)
[171] 著艾火，痛不可忍，預先以手指緊罩其穴處，更以鐵物壓之，即止。龔延賢 《壽世保元》 (Gong 2001, 446)
[172] 葛洪 (c. 283-243, Eastern Jin) 《肘後備急方》
[173] 朱丹溪

cakes made of Fu Zi (Radix Lateralis Aconiti) powder mixed with spittle, and even dandruff (Zhu 2000).

During the Ming dynasty, Xue Ji wrote *External Medicine Formulas from Experience*[174] He recommended moxibustion on garlic to disperse toxins and reduce swelling; moxibustion on bean cake for swellings and hardenings that have not ulcerated or those that have ulcerated but do not close; moxibustion on Fu Zi (Radix Lateralis Aconiti) cake for sores with clear thin pus; and moxibustion on Xiang Fu (Rhizoma Cyperi) and Mu Xiang (Radix Auklandiae) cake to treat liver qi depression patterns (Wei 1987, 17).

Experimentation with isolating substances has continued. Many types can be found in Chinese medical literature. He Puren (2003, 37-60) lists 53 types of isolating moxibustion, including scallion, Chinese chive, Chen Pi (Pericarpium Citri Reticulatae), Hou Pom (Cortex Magnoliae Officinalis), peach leaf, Chuan Jiao (Fructus Zanthoxyli, Sichuan pepper), walnut, flour cake, paper, toad, egg, yellow earth, bowls, etc. The list includes plant and animal products, minerals, and household items.

However, there were some who saw the use of isolating substances as unnecessary. Ming dynasty Monk Zhuhong, author of *Jottings from the Bamboo Window* disparaged this method, saying "There is pain, but there is no useful function"[175] (Wei 1987, 17).

MOXA ROLLS

The most recent major development in moxibustion is the moxa roll or moxa stick. This technology quickly became popular during the Ming dynasty.

Zhu Quan was the first to discuss the moxa roll in *Miraculous Formulas from Longevity Land* at the beginning of the Ming dynasty. In Volume 3, he said, "Use paper to firmly roll up mugwort. Use paper to isolate the point. Use firm force to press the roll into the isolating paper. Wait for the abdomen to feel hot. When the patient sweats, he will promptly recover"[176] (Wei 1987, 17).

This earliest roll was pure mugwort. Moxa rolls with powdered medicinals mixed in seem to have first appeared in Volume 6 of Li Shizhen's *Great Pharmacopeia*[177] and shortly after in Yang Jizhou's *Great Compendium of Acupuncture and Moxibustion*[178] (Wei 1987, 17). These doctors added various medicinal powders, which included substances such as She Xiang (Secretio Mochi), Chuan Shan Jia (Squama Manitis), or Ru Xiang (Olibanum) into the mugwort wool. Li called his formula "thunder-fire miraculous needle"[179] while Yang named his "thunder-fire needle moxibustion."[180]

During the Qing dynasty, doctors such as Fan Yuqi, Li Xuechuan, and Chen Xiuyuan[181] added different types of medicinals to the mugwort roll. Each new formula received a new name, such as "*tai yi* needle" or "*tai yi* miraculous needle"[182] (Wei 1987, 17).

In Ye Tianshi's *Collectively Selected Good Formulas from the Hall of Planting Happiness*, there are moxa rolls with names like "needle for combined three qi impediment," "needle that emits 100 miracles," "miraculous fire needle that disperses aggregation," and "needle to scatter toxins in yin patterns."[183] All of these use different medicinal powders mixed with the mugwort.

[174] 薛己《外科經驗方》
[175] 有痛苦而無功能。沙門株宏《竹窗隨筆》
[176] 用紙實卷艾，以紙隔之點穴，于隔紙上用力實按之，待腹內覺熱，汗出即差。朱權《壽域神方·灸陰証 》
[177] 李時珍《本草綱目》
[178] 楊繼洲《針灸大成》
[179] 雷火神針 (Li 1996, 203)
[180] 雷火針灸 (Huang 1996, 990)
[181] 範毓奇，李學川，陳修園
[182] 太乙針，太乙神針
[183] 三氣合痹針,百發神針,消癖神火針,陰証散毒針葉天士《种福堂公選良方·針灸》(Ye 1999, 388-9)

Qing dynasty writers frequently praised the curative effects of the moxa roll. For example, Qiu Shimin, the author of the introduction to *Taiyi Miraculous Needle Heart Method* (written by Han Yifeng),[184] said that he himself suffered an aching pain of the right arm and numbness of the thumb. Over 16 days he applied moxibustion to himself seven times and then recovered. He also said moxibustion treats "repeated meetings with difficult illnesses. No one does not achieve the effect"[185] (Wei 1987, 17).

Another example is in Guo Yingao's introduction to *Miraculous Needle Appended Formulas* (written by Zhou Yonghe):[186] He told the story of how he himself suffered numbness of the feet. He applied moxibustion to himself and recovered. Guo used this method on four other patients, and all of them recovered (Wei 1987, 17).

In *Tai Yi Miraculous Needle Collection and Explanation*, the author, Kong Guangpei,[187] reported that his concubine suffered from *shan* disorder. He used a moxa roll and in less than a month she recovered (Wei 1987, 17-18).

Other Qing treatises recording this method include Lei Shaoyi's *Thunder Fire Needle Method* and Chen Huichou's *Tai Yi Miraculous Needle Formulas*[188] (Wei 1987, 17).

In contemporary times, moxa rolls are often used because of their convenience.

HEAVENLY MOXIBUSTION

Heavenly moxibustion[189] is the application of medicinals to the skin, most often on a point, to cause irritation or blistering. For example, garlic, Mao Gen Ye (Foilum Ranunculi Japonici) or Ban Mao (Mylabirs) may be used. No fire is involved. He Puren (2003, 81-7) lists nine medicinals that are used to cause blisters and 11 others that are only irritants.

Heavenly moxibustion was first recorded in the Mawangdui manuscript, *Formulas for Fifty-two Diseases*, Clause 52, which says to "mince Lan [Herba Eupatorii]. Pour liquor over it. Drink the liquid and seal the wound with the dregs. Change it continually."[190] This was a treatment for the bite of a certain kind of lizard or poisonous snake[191] (Harper 1998, 240). The same plant is still used today for heavenly moxibustion (He 2003, 83).

Heavenly moxibustion was not mentioned again in works that we have received until *Emergency Prescriptions*. In Volume 5, Ge Hong recommended application of a paste of Ban Xia (Rhizoma Pinelliae) and egg white to abscesses on the back.[192] When applied externally, pinellia makes a blister and is used to treat various sores, abscesses, and nodules (He 2003, 84).

During the Song dynasty, Wang Zhizhong, in the *Classic of Nourishing Life with Acupuncture and Moxibustion*, cited one of Sun Simiao's treatments for malaria: The application of Han Lian Cao (Herba Ecliptae) to a point. Wang added, "Use an ancient coin to press it. Bind it with old silk. After a short

[184] 邱時敏《太乙神針心法》，韓貽丰
[185] 復迂沉疴，無不奏效。
[186] 《太乙神針附方》郭寅皋, 周雍和
[187] 孔廣培《太乙神針集解》
[188] 雷少逸《雷火針法》, 陳惠疇《太乙神針方》
[189] 天灸法
[190] Translation by Harper (1998).
[191] 虺
[192] 葛洪《肘後備急方》 (Ge 1996, 137)

time, a small blister will promptly arise. This is called 'heavenly moxibustion.' It is even able to cure malaria."[193] This was the first use of the term "heavenly moxibustion" (Zhang Q.W. 1992, 61-2; Li 1995, 168).

During the Yuan dynasty, Zhu Danxi[194] recommended heavenly moxibustion for mouth sores.

After applying some medicinals topically to the sores, he said to apply Nan Xing (Rhizoma Arisaematis) powder mixed with vinegar to Yong Quan (KI 1) (Zhu 2000, 459).

Throughout history, many other doctors also discussed heavenly moxibustion and it is still used today (He 2003, 80).

---

[193]以古文錢壓之，係之以故帛，未久即起小泡，謂之天灸，尚能愈瘧。王執中《針灸資生經·第三·瘧》(Huang 1996, 288)
[194]朱丹溪《丹溪手鏡》

MOXIBUSTION IN THE MING DYNASTY

CHAPTER 4

INTRODUCTION TO THE TRANSLATIONS

In Part 2, we explore the works of three important authors and physicians through annotated translations and discussions of their relevant writings. These masters are:

- Li Shizhen (1518-1593), author of the *Great Pharmacopoeia*[1]
- Yang Jizhou (1522-1620), the author of *Great Compendium of Acupuncture and Moxibustion*[2]
- Zhang Jiebin (1563-1640), also known as Zhang Jingyue, the author of the *Illustrated Supplement to the Categorized Classic* and *[Zhang] Jingyue's Complete Works*[3]

The end of the Ming dynasty was a fertile time for Chinese medicine, and these books were all published within a period of 40 years. They are still considered masterpieces today, yet most of them have not been translated into English.

These three authors were elite scholar-practitioners.

So their writings document the views of Ming dynasty medical literati on moxibustion. Although these voluminous books did not focus on this modality, each contains detailed information about its theory and practice.

Yang Jizhou and Zhang Jiebin wrote comprehensively on moxibustion. Yang focused on its techniques and clinical use, while Zhang gave a formulary covering many diseases and patterns. Li Shizhen did not write a section on moxibustion, but he discussed the materials used in its practice.

WHY THE MING DYNASTY?

It can be argued that the peak of Chinese medicine occurred during the Ming dynasty (1368-1644). At this time, doctors were able to study many schools of medical thought, from the *Inner Canon* (*Nei Jing*) and the *Treatise on Cold Damage* (*Shang Han Lun*) to the works of the Four Great Masters of the Jin-Yuan

---

[1] 李時珍《本草綱目》published (posthumously) in 1596.
[2] 楊繼洲《針灸大成》 published in 1601, hereafter called the *Great Compendium*.
[3] 張介賓, 張景岳《類經圖翼》, 《景岳全書》 published in 1624 and 1636, respectively. Hereafter called the *Illustrated Supplement* and *Zhang's Complete Works*.

period.[4] The Ming preceded the decline of Chinese medicine during the Qing dynasty when the influence of Western biomedicine took root.

The Ming dynasty was the last period of imperial sovereignty by the Chinese. It was sandwiched between the Yuan (ruled by the Mongols) and the Qing (ruled by the Manchurians). During the Ming, Neo-Confucianism became political and social orthodoxy. People from all levels of society were able to sit for the imperial exams (Unschuld 1985, 191).

The Ming was also a time when China was exposed to foreign thought. China's imperial fleets traveled to South Asia and Africa.[5] There was also constant commerce through over-land trade routes, commonly called the "silk roads." Father Mateo Ricci arrived in Beijing in 1601, the year the *Great Compendium* was published. Ricci and others like him translated or wrote works on Western medicine for the Chinese. These books were kept only for the Emperor, as the knowledge was considered dangerous for the common people. Because of this, Western influence had not yet penetrated into Chinese medicine (Huard and Wong 1968, 47, 49). The seed (or weed, depending on your point of view) of Western medicine that was sown in the Ming did not really flower until the Qing dynasty. In addition, the state of publishing was technologically advanced. Therefore, voluminous books could be printed and distributed. Both movable type and block printing were at a high level of development (Liu 1985, 72, 80).

The Ming emperors supported acupuncture-moxibustion. They ordered a new casting of the bronze man[6] and the renewal of the stone tablets of its accompanying book so that medical students could make rubbings of the tablets. In this way, they could

have accurate guides for the points (Yang and Liu 1994, viii).

Yang Shouzhong stated, "Towards the late Ming dynasty, acupuncture and moxibustion developed to such a height that each and every branch of the study, from its theories of the channels and connecting vessels to its needling manipulations, had become mature and had reached a consummate level. From this point of view, the flourishing of acupuncture and moxibustion during this period was but the fruition and harvesting of many centuries of slow growth and development" (Yang and Liu 1994, viii).

In this period of great achievement, Li Shizhen, Yang Jizhou, and Zhang Jiebin were three of the most influential medical writers. Therefore, this study on moxibustion focuses on the works of these brilliant men who lived in a period of brightness called the Ming dynasty.

It should be noted, however, that Li, Yang, and Zhang were not the only influential authors during the Ming dynasty. Xu Feng, Wang Ji, Gao Wu, Wu Kun, Li Chan, Gong Juzhong, Gong Xin, and Xue Ji also wrote works that were important in the field of acupuncture-moxibustion. However, Li, Yang, and Zhang came at the end of the Ming dynasty and so were able to incorporate the research of many earlier doctors. Each of them wrote extensively and tried to summarize and incorporate the essence of all the important writings that came before. It is not an exaggeration to say that their writings are the culmination of the medical works of the previous 1,600 years.

Unfortunately, the atmosphere of the Ming did not last. Unschuld wrote that during the Qing dynasty:

---

[4]   Liu Wansu, Zhang Zihe, Li Dongyuan, and Zhu Danxi.
[5]   Some say further. See *1421: The Year China Discovered America* (Menzies 2002).
[6]   Based on the Song dynasty work of Wang Weiyi, the author of the *Illustrated Classic of Acupuncture Points as Found on the Bronze Man*.

The widespread belief in the inadequacy of traditional healing influenced some authors to reject vehemently all post-Sung [Song] innovations in medical thought and to seek instead a 'true' understanding of the ancient sources. The broad influx of Western therapeutic practices beginning in the mid-nineteenth century, in particular anatomical knowledge and the minor surgical skills of Western physicians, as well as the introduction of Western scientific methods, caused a number of Chinese practitioners to lose all faith in their own system (Unschuld 1985, 195).

By the end of the Ming dynasty, the government had become relatively ineffective. Many natural catastrophes appeared in various provinces. Taxes were quite high. Because of this, uprisings began to occur. The Northern "barbarians" were a continuous threat. Ming rule eventually disintegrated and lost power (Unschuld 1985, 192). The Ming collapsed in 1644, four years after Zhang Jiebin's death, the last of the three authors featured in this section.

Identification of the Passages Translated

Since the passages translated below are excerpts from larger texts and since the ability to cross-reference is important, I have adopted the following system of identification for the passages:

The specific passage will be identified as follows:

- The volume number will follow the identification of the book.
- A number representing a heading within that volume will follow although original authors did not give numbers to these headings. They were added based on the sequence found in the primary source.
- If there are subheadings, a third number is added.

For the *Great Pharmacopeia* (**BCGM**), I retained the numbering system used in the English translation from Foreign Languages Press (Li, 2004).

Examples:

- **ZJDC: 9-7** is the seventh heading in Volume Nine of Yang Jizhou's *Great Compendium of Acupuncture and Moxibustion*.
- **ZJDC: 4-31-8** is the eighth subheading under the thirty-first heading of Volume Nine of Yang Jizhou's *Great Compendium of Acupuncture and Moxibustion*.

An index of the passages is also found in the appendices.

Annotation & discussion

These three authors often covered the same topics. Therefore, the passages are arranged into chapters of related entries by different authors. Annotations and discussions are added as necessary to explain a topic.

ABBREVIATION	A PASSAGE FROM:	
ZJDC	楊繼洲 《針灸大成》 *Zhen Jiu Da Cheng*	Yang Jizhou's *Great Compendium of Acupuncture and Moxibustion*
LJTY	張介賓 《類經圖翼》 *Lei Jing Tu Yi*	Zhang Jiebin's *Illustrated Supplement to the Categorized Classic*
JYQS	張介賓 《景岳全書》 *Jing Yue Quan Shu*	Zhang Jiebin's *Jingyue's Complete Works*
BCGM	李時珍 《本草綱目》 *Ben Cao Gang Mu*	Li Shizhen's *Great Pharmacopeia*

Parentheses ( ) are the original author's words, usually written in small print in the original. Brackets [ ]
are used when additional words are needed to clarify
the translation.

Division of the Topics

The translations are divided into 10 chapters as follows:

- *General Guidelines and Techniques for Moxibustion*:
  Basic skills and practical information for
  treatment with moxibustion. This includes
  supplementation and draining techniques, the
  size and number of cones, lighting the cones,
  making and taking care of moxa sores, etc.
- *Points Used for Moxibustion*: Points of the 14
  channels, extraordinary points, and special
  points commonly used for moxibustion.
- *Points Contraindicated for Moxibustion*.
- *The Materials of Moxibustion*: Discussion of the
  materials, such as mugwort, ginger, garlic, and
  aconite.
- *Special Methods and Formulas*: Moxa sticks,
  steaming the umbilicus, etc.
- *Treatment, Part 1*: This section contains Zhang
  Jiebin's treatment formulary from the *Illustrated
  Supplement*. This is Zhang's comprehensive
  manual for treatment of various diseases using
  moxibustion.
- *Treatment, Part 2*: Other treatments for various
  conditions from all three authors.
- *Case Studies Using Moxibustion*.
- *Timing of Treatment*: Including day selection for
  treatment, the best time of day to apply
  moxibustion, and when to pick mugwort.
- *Magical Moxibustion*: This chapter is a discussion
  of the magical or supernatural aspects of
  moxibustion mentioned by Zhang, Li, and Yang.

COMMENTS ON YANG JIZHOU'S USE OF MOXIBUSTION

Yang Jizhou's Sources

In this section of the *Great Compendium*, Yang
seemed to have used three main sources:

1. His own family tradition: Some sections are drawn
   from prior literary sources, but edited by Yang according to his own experience, or an annotation is
   attached to the end. Only a few passages in the section on moxibustion seem to be original to the *Great
   Compendium*. These include **ZJDC: 9-18** *Thunder-Fire
   Needle Method*, **ZJDC: 9-35** *Nursing Health after Moxibustion*, and **ZJDC: 9-36** *Appended Case Studies of Master Yang*. The heading for **ZJDC: 9-9** states that its
   source is the Yang family, but it is quite similar to
   the corresponding passage in *Gatherings*.

2. Gao Wu's *Gatherings from Eminent Acupuncturists*:[7]
   Zhang adapted the following passages from *Gatherings*: **ZJDC: 9-7, 9-9** through **9-11, 9-20** through
   9-32, and **9-34**. He acknowledges this in many of
   the section headings, and a comparison of the
   texts verifies it in the rest.

   Gatherings does not give attribution for its sources
   but most of these quotations are almost identical
   to both Wang Zhizhong's *Classic of Nourishing Life
   with Acupuncture and Moxibustion*[8] and Xu Feng's
   Great Completion of Acupuncture and Moxibustion.[9]
   Editors (Huang 1996, 600; Gao 1999, 5) seem to
   attribute the sections in *Gatherings* directly to
   Nourishing Life. It is possible that *Gatherings* and
   the *Great Completion* are siblings, both having
   Nourishing Life as their parent, rather than in a direct chain of transmission.

3. Li Chan's *Entering the Gate of Medicine*:[10] **ZJDC: 9-6,**

---

[7] 高武 (Ming, 16th c.), 《針灸聚英》, published in 1537. Hereafter known as *Gatherings*.
[8] 王執中 (Song, dates unknown), 《針灸資生經》, published in 1220. Hereafter known as *Nourishing Life*.
[9] 徐鳳 (Ming, 14th c.), 《針灸大全》, published c.1439. Hereafter known as the *Great Completion*.
[10] 李梴 (Ming, 16th c.), 《醫學入門》, published in 1575. Hereafter known as *Entering the Gate*.

9-8, 4-31-4, 4-31-8, 4-31-13, 4-27. *Entering the Gate* does not give its sources for individual sections. However, based on a comparison of the two texts, it seems that one of Li Chan's sources was Wei Yilin's *Effective Formulas Obtained from Generations of Doctors*. (Wei 1964)[11]

All of these sources quote from books such as:

- Sun Simiao's *Essential Prescriptions Worth a Thousand Pieces of Gold*.[12]
- Luo Tianyi's *Precious Mirror of Protecting Life*.[13]
- Wang Weiyi's *Illustrated Classic of Acupuncture Points as Found on the Bronze Man*.[14]
- The *Yellow Emperor's Inner Canon*.
- Other books, which will be mentioned as they occur.

It is difficult to trace a passage back to its earliest source. Every so often, when perusing an ancient book on acupuncture-moxibustion, an earlier source is uncovered. I have found earlier sources than modern books (both in Chinese and English) claim for some of the passages. There is always the possibility that a passage originated in another obscure earlier book. In addition, many early books have been lost. Therefore, all suggested sources are tentative.

The Contents of Yang Jizhou's Section on Moxibustion

ZJDC: 9-6 through **9-11** discusses special points for moxibustion, and gives the location, indications, and specific treatment methods for these points. Most, but not all, of these are non-channel points.

ZJDC: 9-12 through **9-17** give the instructions for treating certain conditions, such as hemorrhoids, *shan* [mounting] qi, bloody diarrhea, and yin toxins in the chest. Some of these include special moxibus-

tion points not listed in the earlier sections. These passages also describe the use of various medicinals in ironing, as a steam-wash, or a powder placed inside the umbilicus.

ZJDC: 9-18 and 9-19: These sections discuss special methods for applying moxibustion:

- **9-18** is Yang's recipe for thunder-fire needle (moxa stick).
- **9-19** is another recipe for powdered medicinals to place in the umbilicus as an isolating substance for moxibustion. This method is to be practiced at specific times.

ZJDC: 9-20 through **9-35** are basically a techniques class in moxibustion. These sections discuss the timing of application, preventive moxibustion, moxa sores, the characteristics of mugwort, supplementation and draining techniques, the size and number of cones, lighting the cones, etc.

ZJDC: 9-36 contains Yang Jizhou's case studies. Four are translated here as representative.

ZJDC: 4-27 lists points contraindicated for moxibustion.

ZJDC: 4-31 discusses day selection regarding moxibustion.

> **Note:** It appears that Yang didn't often use ginger or garlic as isolating substances. Neither is prescribed in any of these passages. For the most part, he suggested direct moxibustion, although a few passages describe isolating moxibustion using other medicinals.

---

[11] 危亦林 《世醫得效方》 published in 1345.
[12] 孫思邈 (Tang, 581-682), 《千金要方》, published in 652. Hereafter known as *Prescriptions*.
[13] 羅天益 (Yuan, 1220-1290), 《衛生寶鑒》. Hereafter known as *Precious Mirror*.
[14] 王惟一 (Song, c. 987-1067), 《銅人腧穴針灸圖經》, published in 1026. Hereafter known as the *Bronze Man*.

COMMENTS ON ZHANG JIEBIN'S USE OF MOXIBUSTION

Zhang discussed moxibustion in many places throughout his books. In the *Illustrated Supplement*, he wrote about:

- General guidelines for moxibustion: **LJTY: 4-27** and **11-2**
- Treatment of various diseases: There is one large section on moxibustion treatment for twenty-four categories of disease. Sometimes the points listed for a condition are a prescription. At other times, they are a selection from which to choose. For example, under **LJTY: 11-3-7** *Accumulations, Gatherings, and Glomus Lumps*, Zhang said, "Apply moxibustion to any of the above points for accumulation lumps. You can select the function according to the pattern."
- Specific points used in moxibustion: In Volumes 6 through 8, Zhang went over the points of the main channels one by one. A sampling of the most important points used for moxibustion is included. Information on location, needling techniques, etc. is not translated here. In Volume 10, Zhang also discussed a number of non-channel points that are important for moxibustion.

In addition, scattered throughout *Jingyue's Complete Works*, he discussed the treatment of various conditions with moxibustion.

While Yang Jizhou compiled a large amount of information on the topic, the majority of it was simply passed through; Yang often copied almost verbatim from his sources. Only occasionally did he edit the passages a little or add his own thoughts. On the other hand, Zhang seemed to digest the ideas as he passed them on. His passages are harder to trace back to their source, as Zhang often rewrote the information into his own words. However, it is obvious that Zhang favored Sun's *Supplement* and certain other works because they were frequently cited.

While Zhang Jiebin is known for his development of

theory, his use of medicinals, and his annotation of the *Inner Canon*, we can see he also favored the use of moxibustion. If we can quantify his interest in acupuncture by the number of pages written, we must conclude that Zhang did not use it nearly as often.

COMMENTS ON LI SHIZHEN'S USE OF MOXIBUSTION

Li Shizhen's writings on moxibustion are scattered throughout the *Great Pharmacopeia*.

In Volume 6, Li discussed the various types of fire: from mugwort, from moxa rolls, from other sources. We find a lot of relevant information here.

Of course, Li's description of mugwort contains a lot of information about moxibustion; so does his entry on garlic. The entries on aconite, salt, and many other substances used in moxibustion contain additional information.

Finally, Volumes 3 and 4 compile many small items on the treatment of various conditions. We find many items on moxibustion and related methods here.

Most of Li's writings on moxibustion are passed down from previous sources. Fortunately, Li names the source most of the time. Only the sections on mugwort and on the moxa rolls seem to reflect Li's personal experience.

Li Shizhen is well-known as an herbalist, so his emphasis is more on the materials used in moxibustion than the clinical practice. Through Li's writings, we understand more about variety of materials and techniques. However, much of it is passed through from older books without regard to clinical efficacy or practicality.

With this background, we can now begin examining the translations to see what the practice of moxibustion looked like late in the Ming dynasty. However please note that not all treatments used at that time are considered safe, effective, or appropriate today.

CHAPTER 5
GENERAL GUIDELINES AND TECHNIQUES FOR MOXIBUSTION

The authors examined in this section assumed their reader had a certain familiarity with medical concepts and techniques. None of them defined moxibustion or wrote an introduction to to its use. However, Zhang Jiebin wrote two fairly brief summaries or general guidelines on moxibustion translated below. Both come from *Illustrated Supplement*. Even though **LJTY: 4-27** is entitled *Various Rules of Acupuncture and Moxibustion*, the focus is on the latter. Most of it is quoted or paraphrased from Volume 28 of Sun Simiao's *Supplement*.[1] The other section, **LJTY: 11-2** *Important Points Used for Applying Moxibustion to All Patterns*, comes just before Zhang's moxibustion treatment formulary. Zhang's ointment for moxa sores from his *Complete Works* is also included here.

In *Great Compendium*, Yang Jizhou wrote a longer section that could perhaps be considered a basic techniques class in moxibustion. He covered most of the material a beginner might need to know in order to practice. In **ZJDC: 9-24** through **9-35**,[2] Yang gathers writings from many previous authors. These sections describe appropriate uses of moxibustion: supplementation and draining, the size and number of cones, how to light the cones, the position of the patient in locating points, and the importance of moxa sores. In the last passage, Yang gives guidelines for post-moxibustion care of the patient; only this section seems to be written by Yang himself.

Li Shizhen wrote little on moxibustion techniques, but he did discuss the lighting of moxa cones, which is also presented here.

Through the writings of these authors, we can learn what must have been standard procedure for moxibustion treatment during the Ming dynasty. The translations are followed by a summary and discussion.

---

1 《千金翼方·卷第二十八針灸下·雜法》
2 Except **ZJDC: 9-30**, which has been moved to the chapter on treatment as it discusses moxibustion for chills and fever.

ZHANG'S GENERAL GUIDE-LINES FOR MOXIBUSTION

LJTY: 11-2 Important Points Used for Applying Moxibustion to All Patterns,[3] (Zhang 1991, 931)

《類經圖翼・十一卷・諸證灸法要穴》

LJTY: 11-2-1 Generally, the functions of moxibustion are to scatter cold evils, eliminate yin toxins, open depression, break stagnation, reinforce qi, and return yang. When the power of fire arrives, its merits are not insignificant.

凡用灸者，所以散寒邪，除陰毒，開鬱破滯，助氣回陽，火力若到，功非淺鮮

LJTY: 11-2-2 The ancients applied moxibustion in sessions,[4] from two or three up to years running without stopping. The earlier and later sessions hasten each other. Their [cumulative] effect is especially fast. Some add cones gradually, from three or five up to a hundred or a thousand cones, increasing the good effects more and more.

故古人灸法，有二報、三報，以至連年不絕者，前後相催，其效尤速，或自三壯、五壯，以至百壯、千壯者，由漸而增，多多益善也

LJTY: 11-2-3 It is suitable to apply small mugwort cones on the head and face. It is also unsuitable to use a lot. Multiply this amount a few times to apply moxibustion on the hands and feet. Multiply it again to apply moxibustion on the abdomen and back.

然灸頭面者，艾炷宜小，亦不宜多，灸手足者，稍倍之，灸腹背者，又倍之。

LJTY: 11-2-4 When using moxibustion on both the upper and the lower body, you must apply it first to the upper and then to the lower. You cannot apply it first to the lower and then to the upper.

若上下俱灸，必須先上而後下，不可先下後上也。

LJTY: 11-2-5 Overall, when using fire to supplement, do not blow on the fire. You must wait for it to naturally and thoroughly extinguish itself. When the moxibustion is finished, you can apply ointment to the site. If you intend to have more sessions while using the nourishment of fire qi, wait until all the sessions are finished before applying the ointment.

When using fire to drain, you can blow on the fire to transmit the mugwort [qi]. It is appropriate for it to burn rapidly. You must wait for the moxa sore to ulcerate and then apply ointment. This is the method of supplementing and draining.[5]

凡用火補者，勿吹其火，必待其從容徹底自滅，灸畢即可用膏貼之，以養火氣，若欲報者，直待報畢貼之可也；用火瀉者，可吹其火，傳其艾，宜于迅速，須待灸瘡潰發，然後貼膏，此補瀉之法也。

LJTY: 11-2-6 When there is a rapid pulse, agitated vexation, dry mouth, throat pain, and a red face-fire exuberance or yin vacuity internal heat patterns, etc. all this is unsuitable for moxibustion which on the contrary would reinforce the fire. You should not apply moxibustion again and again or else calamity and harm will immediately arrive. Volume 4 of the *Illustrated Supplement* has a section entitled *Various Rules of Acupuncture and Moxibustion*, which should also be examined.

---

3. This passage was originally written as one section without breaks. I have broken it down into smaller sections for convenience of discussion.

4. This passage introduces the word 報 *bao*, which Zhang uses here and there throughout his writings. I have translated it as "session." It is a moxibustion term meaning the regular re-application of a treatment. Instructions might say "up to 30 cones, one session every three days" or "if it is a light case, give three sessions; if it is serious, nine sessions." Sun Simiao also frequently used this term (Li 1995, 728).

5. This technique of using moxibustion to drain or supplement originated in *Magic Pivot*, Chapter 51. 《靈樞・背腧》

其有脈數躁煩，口} 咽痛，面赤火盛，陰虛內熱等證，俱不宜灸，反以助火，不當灸而灸之，災害立至矣。《圖翼》四卷，有針灸諸則，所當並察。

> **Note:** At the end of this passage, Zhang refers the reader to a section of Volume 4 which is translated next.

LJTY: 4-27 Various Rules of Acupuncture and Moxibustion,[6] (Zhang 1991, 800-801) 《類經圖翼・四卷・針灸諸則》

LJTY: 4-27-1 Item: Generally all disease is made from blood congestion and qi stagnation, and the inability to diffuse and flow freely. Acupuncture is used to open and guide the qi and blood. Moxibustion is used to warm it. To treat disease thoroughly, the patient must properly tend and nourish himself, avoiding things that engender cold, vinegar, things that are slippery, etc.; on the contrary, disease will be engendered if he does not understand caution.

LJTY: 4-27-2 Item:[7] In order to be able to cure disease, all moxibustion on the head and four limbs must have sufficient fire for the qi to arrive. However, the flesh is thin on the head and the four limbs; so if moxibustion is applied to them in the same amount as the rest of the body, blood and qi will expire in the lower body. At times, it is suitable to give the fire a rest. Perhaps repeat the moxibustion every other day to make the blood vessels

unobstructed. As fire qi flows and moves, accumulates and becomes plentiful, it will naturally eliminate illness.[8]

Moreover, regarding needling methods, the *Classic* often says something like "prick to enter three *fen* and use three cones of moxibustion." This is the generally cited outline, but not the complete heart method.[9]

Since the skin of the hands and feet is thin, it is suitable to use small cones, few in number. The flesh of the abdomen and back is thick, so it is suitable to use many big cones there. This is the idea you should always use to infer the size and number of cones. When applying moxibustion to the back, it is suitable to cook[10] this region well.

Whenever applying moxibustion, examine for symptoms of becoming [overly] cooked. You should take the person's condition as a criterion: exuberance or debility, old or young, fat or thin.

It is suitable to use big mugwort cones whenever applying moxibustion below the umbilicus for enduring cold, mounting [*shan*], conglomerations, strings, aggregations, qi lumps, deep-lying beams, and accumulations of qi. Moreover, *Short Sketches of All Formulas*[11] says:

> On the abdomen and back, it is suitable to apply 500 cones of moxibustion. However, when [points on] the four limbs are used to eliminate wind evils,

---

6 Most of **LJTY: 4-27** is taken from ideas expressed in Sun's *Supplement*, Volume 28.
7 The first four paragraphs in **LJTY: 4-27-2** are parallel to a section in Sun's *Supplement*, Volume 28 (Sun 1994, b262). Zhang paraphrases, but follows Sun point by point.
I have not found a source for the fifth paragraph (regarding the use of big cones below the umbilicus) but it is similar to part of **ZJDC: 9-25** where it is attributed to the *Upper Canon of the Bright Hall*.
8 In other words, take your time and let the cure come naturally. If you push it, you can cause damage.
9 A "heart method" is an oral transmission from master to disciple. Note also that "prick" (刺 *ci*) is frequently used in Ming dynasty books when we would say "needle" today. It does not mean prick to bleed unless this is specifically stated.
10 In both Zhang's and Sun's books, some editions have 熟 *shu* cook and others have 熱 *re* heat here and in the next paragraph.
11 *Short Sketches of All Formulas* by Chen Yanzhi (dates unknown, Sui dynasty) 陳延之 《小品方》. This book is lost, but much of it appears in quotes in Sun Simiao's writings or in the Japanese *Medical Heart Formulas* 《醫心方》. I have not been able to locate this passage in the books that have passed along glimpses of *Short Sketches*. This *Short Sketches* quote is quite similar to **ZJDC: 9-25**; the idea is much the same as in **LJTY: 11-2-3** above and **ZJDC: 9-27**.

they are not suitable for a lot of moxibustion: Use seven cones, up to seven times seven cones,[12] and then stop. You must not exceed this. The number of cones is based on the years of age.[13]

You should not exceed seven times seven cones when applying moxibustion to Ju Que [Ren 14] or Jiu Wei [Ren 15], even though they are points on the chest and abdomen. The mugwort cones must not be big. Use the head of bamboo chopsticks as a gauge [of size] to make cones. Apply moxibustion to these points right on the [conception] vessel. Applying a lot of moxibustion with big cones on these sites will always give the patient a feeble heart.

Using a lot of moxibustion on points on the top of the head will make the patient lose essence-spirit. Using a lot of moxibustion on the arms and legs will desiccate the patient's blood vessels and the four limbs will become thin, lean, and feeble. When a patient repeatedly loses essence-spirit and also becomes thin and lean, it means his true qi is about to desert him.

一，凡灸頭與四肢，必火足氣到，方能愈病；然頭與四肢肉薄，若併灸之，則血氣絕于下，宜時為歇火，或隔日再灸，使血脈通達，火氣流行，積數充足，自然除疾。又如本經針法多云刺入三分、灸三壯之類，乃概舉大綱，未盡心法；且手足皮薄，宜炷小數少，腹背肉厚，宜炷大壯多，皆當以意推測。若灸背者，宜熟斯佳也。凡灸察生熟之候，當以人之盛衰老少肥瘦為則。凡灸臍下久冷、疝瘕痃癖、氣塊伏梁積氣，

宜艾炷大。又《小品諸方》云：腹背宜灸五百壯。四肢則但去風邪，不宜多灸，七壯至七七壯止，不得過，隨年數。如巨闕、鳩尾、雖是胸腹之穴，灸不過七七壯。艾炷不須大，以竹筋頭作炷，正當脈上灸之。若灸此處而炷大灸多，令人永無心力。如頭頂穴若灸多，令人失精神；臂腳穴灸多，令人血脈枯竭，四肢細瘦無力，既復失精神，又加于細瘦，即脫人真氣也。

LJTY: 4-27-3 Item: Avoid moxibustion whenever the pulse is faint and rapid, or when a patient has recently sweated.[14]

一，凡人年三十以上，若灸頭不灸三里，令人氣上眼闇，以三里穴能下氣也。凡一切病，皆灸三里三壯，每日常灸，氣下乃止。

LJTY: 4-27-4 Item: Whenever someone 30 years or older applies moxibustion on the head but doesn't apply it to San Li [ST 36], it makes their qi ascend, causing dim vision. This is because San Li is able to lower qi.

In each and every disease, apply three cones of moxibustion to San Li every day. Qi will descend and the disease will stop.

一，凡人年三十以上，若灸頭不灸三里，令人氣上眼

闇，以三里穴能下氣也。凡一切病，皆灸三里三壯，每日常灸，氣下乃止。

---

[12] It is common in various ancient Chinese medical books to recommend the amount of cones in a format like "seven times seven cones," meaning 49 cones. This may just be a convention; however it is also possible that it is significant. One reason may be the numerology: odd numbers are yang and even numbers are yin. Most often, at least one of the numbers is yang (odd), which may add to the yang of moxibustion. Seven seems to be the most common multiplier.
 Another possible reason may be that moxibustion was sometimes given in sessions (報 bao), as described in **LJTY: 11-2-2** above. When two times seven cones were recommended, perhaps it meant "two sessions with seven cones each time." I have not found a clear statement to this effect, but in some cases, it seems to be implied. For example, **LJTY: 11-3-18** says, "If the condition is mild, use seven cones. If wind cold is exuberant, 14 cones is the usual dose, or divide the treatment into two or three sessions."
[13] "The number of cones is based on the years of age" is a common idea in the old books. If the patient is 37 years old, then use 37 cones. This tradition goes back at least as far as the *Elementary Questions*, Chapter 60.
[14] This is also in Sun's *Supplement*, Volume 28 (Sun 1994, b262). It is rooted in Zhang Zhongjing's *Treatise on Cold Damage*, which says, "When the pulse is faint and rapid, be careful as moxibustion cannot be applied." 《傷寒論·辨太陽病脈證并治》微數之脈，慎不可灸。

LJTY: 4-27-5 Item: Whenever applying moxibustion, you must first start in the upper body, and then go to the lower body. You must first begin in the yang, and then go to the yin.

Overall, a fundamental law of acupuncture is that it is more suitable after noon [*wu* hour, 11 AM-1 PM] and it is not desirable before noon [*wu* hour].

一，凡灸法，須先發于上，後發于下；先發于陽，後
發于陰。凡針刺大法，多宜在午時之後，不欲在午時
之前。

ZHANG'S OINTMENT FOR MOXA SORES

JYQS: 64-324 Jasper [Colored] Oil Ointment (324),[15] (Zhang 1995, 1791-2)
《景岳全書・碧油膏三二四・卷之六十四》

Stops pain, expels pus, suitable to use after moxibustion.

Tao Zhi [peach twig], Liu Zhi [willow twig], Sang Zhi [Ramulus Mori, mulberry twig], Huai Zhi [Sophora twig] (each two *liang*); Ru Xiang [Olibanum] (grind finely separately), Xue Jie [Sanguis Draconis] (each five qian); Huang Dan [Minium[16]] (four *liang*, cleaned)

Use 10 *liang* of sesame oil to decoct the above ingredients. After the ointment is made, add the Ru Xiang and Xue Jie.

止痛排膿，灸後宜用之。　桃枝，柳枝，桑枝，槐枝，
各二兩。　乳香另研，血竭，各五錢。　黃丹，四兩，

淨。　右用麻油十兩煎，膏成後下乳香，血竭。

YANG'S GENERAL GUIDELINES FOR MOXIBUSTION

ZJDC: 9-24 Supplementation and Draining with Mugwort Moxibustion (Huang 1996, 991) 《針灸大成・艾灸補瀉・卷之九》

When qi is exuberant, drain it. When it is vacuous, supplement it.[17]

Moxibustion is suitable for what the needle cannot do. When yin and yang are both vacuous, fire is naturally appropriate for it. When the channels are sunken down, fire is appropriate for it. When the channels and network vessels are hard and tight, fire is what treats it.[18]

When sunken down, apply moxibustion to it.[19]

When the network vessels are full, the channels are empty. Apply moxibustion to yin and prick yang. When the channels are full, the network vessels are vacuous. Prick yin and apply moxibustion to yang.[20]

To use fire for supplementation, do not blow on the fire. You must wait for the fire to extinguish itself. Then press the point. To use fire to drain, quickly blow on the fire and leave the point open.[21]

氣盛則瀉之，虛則補之。針所不為，灸之所宜。陰陽
皆虛，火自當之，經陷下者，火則當之。經絡堅緊，
火所治之。陷下則灸之。絡滿經虛，灸陰刺陽，經滿

---

[15] For Yang Jizhou's ointment for moxa sores, see **ZJDC: 9-33** below.

[16] Minium has lead oxide and should not be used topically or internally today.

[17] All of this section is quoted or paraphrased from *Magic Pivot* and *Elementary Questions*. Gao Wu's *Gatherings*, Part 1, Volume 2 has the same sentences but in a different order (Huang 1996, 641). This first paragraph is from *Magic Pivot*, Chapter 51.
《靈樞・背腧第五十一》

[18] This paragraph is from *Magic Pivot*, Chapter 73. 《靈樞・官能第七十三》

[19] This sentence is repeated many times in *Magic Pivot*, Chapter 10. 《靈樞・經脈第十》

[20] This paragraph is from *Elementary Questions*, Chapter 28. 《素問・通評虛實論篇第二十八》 Note that "prick" (刺 *ci*) is frequently used when we would say "needle" today. It does not mean prick to bleed unless this is specifically stated.

[21] This paragraph is adapted from *Magic Pivot*, Chapter 51. 《靈樞・背腧第五十一》

絡虛，刺陰灸陽。以火補者，毋吹其火，須待自滅，即按其穴。以火瀉者，速吹其火，開其穴也。

ZJDC: 9-25 The Size of Mugwort Cones,[22] (Huang 1996, 991)
《針灸大成・艾炷大小・卷之九》

The Yellow Emperor said:[23] If a moxibustion cone is not three *fen* wide, it is only a waste. Make sure the cones are big enough. If the patient is small or weak, then make them smaller. He also said: For children seven days and older up to their first birthday, make cones the size of sparrow feces.

The *Lower Canon of the Bright Hall*[24] says: Generally, for moxibustion, you should make the base of the cone three *fen* wide. If it is not three *fen*, the fire qi will not extend and you will not be able to cure the disease; so these moxibustion cones should be big. Only cones for the head and four limbs should be small.

The *Upper Canon of the Bright Hall* then says: Make mugwort cones the size of the end of a small chopstick when the size of the disease pulse is like a thin thread, but you should apply moxibustion right on the vessel.[25] Cones that are the size of sparrow feces are also able to cure illness. There is another route: If there is abdominal distention, mounting, conglomerations, strings, aggregations, deep-lying beam qi, etc., you must use big mugwort cones.

That is why *Short Sketches* says: The abdomen and back can be burnt a lot, but just eliminate wind evils on the four limbs and then stop; they are not suitable for big cones. When moxibustion is applied to Ju Que [Ren 14] or Jiu Wei [Ren 15], it should not exceed four or five cones the size of the head of a bamboo chopstick. However, just apply moxibustion right on the vessel. If the mugwort cones are big and you repeatedly apply more moxibustion, the person will always have a weak heart. If you apply a lot of moxibustion to the head, it makes the person lose essence-spirit. If you apply a lot of moxibustion to the back and legs, it makes the person's blood and vessels desiccated, and it makes the four limbs weak and feeble. If the patient has already lost essence-spirit and additionally has thin joints, it shortens his lifespan.

Wang Jiezhai[26] said: Moxibustion cones on the face must be small. On the arms and legs, they still can be thick.

黃帝曰：灸不三分，是謂徒冤，炷務大也。小弱乃小作之。又曰：小兒七日以上，周年以還，炷如雀糞。《明堂下經》云：凡灸欲炷下廣三分，若不三分，則火氣不達，病未能愈，則是灸炷欲其大，惟頭與四肢欲小耳。《明堂上經》乃曰：艾炷依小箸頭作，其病脈粗細狀如細線，但令當脈灸之。雀糞大炷，亦能愈疾。又有一途，如腹脹、疝瘕、痃癖、伏梁氣等，須大艾炷。故《小品》曰：腹背爛燒，四肢但去風邪而已，不宜大炷。如巨闕、鳩尾、灸之不過四五壯，炷依竹箸頭大，但令正當脈上灸之，艾炷若大，復灸多，其人永無心力。如頭上灸多，令人失精神；背腳灸多，令人血脈枯竭，四肢細而無力，既失精神，又加細節，令人短壽。王節齋云：面上灸炷須小，手足上猶可粗。

---

[22] This whole section is from Gao Wu's *Gatherings*, Part 2, Volume 3 (Huang 1996, 731). Much of it is also found in *Nourishing Life*, Volume 2 (Huang 1996, 268-9). Gao said the first paragraph comes from Sun's *Prescriptions*: both short quotes are from Volume 29 (Sun 1994, a415). The first sentence is also stated in *Short Sketches* (Chen 1993, 171). The next to the last paragraph in this section, also found in **LJTY: 4-27-2**, is attributed to *Short Sketches*.

[23] The original source is unknown. Certainly, it is not in the *Inner Canon* that came to us today. It must be from some other book written as a dialogue between the Yellow Emperor and his advisors.

[24] The *Lower Canon of the Bright Hall* refers to Volume 100 and the *Upper Canon of the Bright Hall* refers to Volume 99 of *Sage-like Prescriptions of the Taiping Era* by Wang Huaiyin 王懷隱《太平聖惠方》(Huang 1996, 235). This book was published in 1992, on the orders of the Song Emperor Taizong.

[25] Here, "vessel" means the "channel" associated with the disease pulse. In the old books, vessel was often used for what we call channel today.

[26] Wang Jiezhai, also known as Wang Lun 王綸, was active around 1500 (Ming). He wrote *Important Collection of the Materia Medica* 《本草集要》 and *Miscellaneous Writings Clarifying Medicine* 《明醫雜著》.

ZJDC: 9-26 Lighting Mugwort Fire,[27] (Huang 1996, 991) 《針灸大成・點艾火・卷之九》

The *Lower Canon of the Bright Hall* says: Since ancient times, people have avoided using the eight types of wood for making fire when using moxibustion to treat disease: pine, cedar [or cypress], bitter orange, mandarin orange, elm, Chinese date, mulberry, and bamboo. It is appropriate to avoid all of these.

The fire bead is used so that the mugwort receives sunshine. It is superior for obtaining fire. Next, there is the fire mirror which attracts and obtains the fire from sunshine into the mugwort. These fires are both good.[28]

Various minority peoples use a piece of iron to strike a stone on the steps to obtain fire, using mugwort to attract the fire. Generally, when in a hurry, it is difficult to prepare this. It is not as good as fire made without using wood.

Light a mugwort stem over a lamp that burns clear sesame oil to light the moxibustion cones. At the same time it enriches and moistens the moxa sores so that they are not painful while they heal. Using a candle is better.

《明堂下經》曰：古來灸病，忌松、柏、枳、橘、榆、棗、桑、竹八木火，切宜避之。有火珠耀日，以艾承之，得火為上。次有火鏡耀日，亦以艾引得火，此火皆良。諸番部用鑌鐵擊階石得火，以艾引之。凡倉卒難備，則不

如無木火，清麻油點燈上燒艾莖，點灸，兼滋潤灸瘡，至愈不疼，用蠟燭更佳。

ZJDC: 9-27 The Number of Cones,[29] (Huang 1996, 991) 針灸大成・壯數多少・卷之九》

Thousand Pieces of Gold says: Generally speaking about the number of cones, if the patient is an able-bodied man or if the root of the disease is serious, the number in the formula can be doubled. If old, young, emaciated, or weak, it can be halved. Bian Que's method of moxibustion uses up to 300 or 500 cones, or 1,000 cones. This is also excessive. Master Cao's method[30] of moxibustion sometimes calls for 100 cones, sometimes 50 cones. All the formulas of *Short Sketches* are also like that. Only the *Original Classic of the Bright Hall* says, "Needle to a depth of six *fen*; apply three cones of moxibustion." It does not have treatments that go beyond this.

That is why people who came after do not allow [making specific rules for the number of cones]. Only increase or decrease it based on the degree of seriousness of disease.

Whenever applying moxibustion to the head and nape, stop at seven cones or stop when up to seven times seven cones are accumulated, according to *Bronze Man*.[31]

However, when treating wind, apply up to 200 cones of moxibustion to Shang Xing [Du 23], Qian Ding

---

[27] This section is from Gao Wu's *Gatherings*, Part 2, Volume 3 (Huang 1996, 731). Gao's section is longer. Before that, this passage was found in *Nourishing Life*, Volume 2 (Huang 1996, 269).
[28] The fire bead and fire mirror are also mentioned in **ZJDC: 9-18** and **BCGM: 06-06**. A fire mirror is a concave metal reflecting device to focus the sun's rays and start a fire. The fire bead resembles a crystal; it also focuses the sun's rays to start a fire, similar to using a magnifying glass or lens. Li Shizhen also discussed the quality of fire that comes from metal, stone, lamps, and candles in **BCGM: 06-06**.
[29] This section is adapted from Gao Wu's *Gatherings*, Part 2, Volume 3 (Huang 1996, 731-2). It also occurs in Volume 6 of *Great Completion* (Huang 1996, 537) and Volume 2 of *Nourishing Life* (Huang 1996, 268). It has remained virtually unchanged since the Song dynasty when Wang Zhizhong wrote *Nourishing Life*.
   The whole first paragraph is from Volume 29 of Sun's *Prescriptions* 《千金要方・卷三十九・灸例》 (Sun 1994, a414). Therefore, the references to Bian Que, Master Cao, *Short Sketches*, and *Original Classic of the Bright Hall* were made by Sun. The rest of this section was added by a later author, probably by Wang Zhizhong.
[30] Master Cao is 曹翁 Cao Weng, who wrote 《曹氏灸經》 *Master Cao's Moxibustion Classic*, Han (lost).
[31] The *Bronze Man* suggests no more than seven cones for Shang Xing (Du 23). If more cones are used, it makes qi ascend to the head and dims the eyes. It suggests three cones, up to seven times seven cones for Qian Ding (Du 21) and Bai Hui (Du 20) (Huang 1996, 181-2).

[Du 21], and Bai Hui [Du 20]. Generally apply 500 cones of moxibustion to the abdomen and back, but, if using Jiu Wei [Ren 15] or Ju Que [Ren 14], it is still inappropriate to apply a lot of moxibustion. When a lot of moxibustion is used, the four limbs become thin and lack strength.

Regarding Zu San Li [ST 36], *Prescriptions Worth a Thousand Pieces of Gold* says to use a lot, up to 300 cones. Moxibustion is prohibited on Xin Shu [UB 15], but for wind stroke, quickly apply up to 100 cones of moxibustion.[32]

All this is applying it based on observing the degree of seriousness of the disease. You cannot be tied down by one theory, and not move with the changes.

《千金》云：凡言壯數者，若丁壯病根深篤，可倍於方數，老少羸弱可減半。扁鵲灸法，有至三五百壯、千壯，此亦太過。曹氏灸法，有百壯、有五十壯。《小品》諸方亦然。惟《明堂本經》云：針入六分、灸三壯，更無餘治。故後人不准，惟以病之輕重而增損之。凡灸頭項，止於七壯，積至七七壯止《銅人》。治風，灸上星、前頂、百會、至二百壯，腹背灸五百壯。若鳩尾、巨闕、亦不宜多灸。灸多則四肢細而無力。《千金方》於足三里穴，乃云多至三百壯。心擴禁灸：若中風，則急灸至百壯，皆視其病之輕重而用之，不可泥一說，而不通其變也。

> **Note:** This paragraph states that books such as the *Bronze Man* recommend a certain number of cones, but, depending on the disease, you can go beyond the recommended number. It also explains that while generally you may be able to use a lot of moxibustion on the abdomen or back, specific points may need a more cautious approach.

The overall message is that different authors suggest different quantities of moxa cones or even prohibit moxibustion on certain points, but a good doctor must use these guidelines flexibly, not as rigid rules. To get the best results, you must treat each patient and condition individually.

ZJDC: 9-28 Moxibustion,[33] (Huang 1996, 991)
《針灸大成・灸法・卷之九》

Prescriptions Worth a Thousand Pieces of Gold says:[34] Overall for moxibustion, when a point is found while the patient is sitting, apply moxibustion sitting. When a point is found while lying down, apply moxibustion lying down. When a point is found standing, apply moxibustion standing. The four limbs must be level and straight. Do not let the patient lean to the side. If he leans to the side, the point location is not correct. You will break good flesh in vain.

The *Bright Hall* says: You must get the body level and straight. Do not let it curl up or contract. When a point is found while sitting, do not let the patient bend forward or look up. When found while standing, do not let him lean to the side.

《千金方》云：凡灸法，坐點穴，則坐灸；臥點穴，則臥灸；立點穴，則立灸；須四體平直，毋令傾側。若傾側穴不正，徒破好肉耳。《明堂》云：須得身體平直，毋令捲縮，坐點毋令俯仰，立點毋令傾側。

---

[32] Sun's *Prescriptions* says to use up to 500 cones on Zu San Li (ST 36) in Volume 30 (Sun 1994, a433). Sun recommends 100 cones of moxibustion on Xin Shu (UB 15) for wind stroke in Volume 8 of Prescriptions (Sun 1994, a122). I cannot find a place where Sun prohibits moxibustion on Xin Shu. It is not among the points he lists as contraindicated for moxibustion (Sun 1994, a411). However, the *Bronze Man* prohibits moxibustion on Xin Shu (Huang 1996, 188). It is also prohibited by both Yang and Zhang in their memorization poems of contraindicated points. Please refer to the chapter on *Points Contraindicated for Moxibustion*.

[33] This section is from Gao Wu's *Gatherings*, Part 2, Volume 3 (Huang 1996, 3). It is also in Volume 2 of *Nourishing Life* (Huang 1996, 268).

[34] Volume 29 《千金要方・卷三十九・灸例》, although, as transmitted here, it has been edited a little by later authors (Sun 1994, a414).

ZJDC: 9-29 The Order of Burning Cones,[35] (Huang 1996, 991)

《針灸大成・炷火先後・卷之九》

Nourishing Life says:[36] "Whenever applying moxibustion, you should first treat yang and afterwards treat yin." It continues, "Proceed from the head towards the left and gradually down. Next, proceed from the head towards the right and gradually down. Treat the upper first and then treat the lower."

The *Bright Hall* says: "First apply moxibustion to the upper and then apply moxibustion to the lower. First apply less moxibustion and then apply more moxibustion. It is appropriate to be careful in all of this."

Wang Jiezhai said: "Moxibustion fire must be applied from the upper to the lower. Moxibustion cannot be applied to the lower first and applied to the upper afterwards."

《資生》云：凡灸當先陽後陰，言從頭向左而漸下，次從頭向右而漸下，先上後下。《明堂》云：先灸上，後灸下，先灸少，後灸多，皆宜審之。王節齋曰：灸火須自上而下，不可先灸下，後灸上。

ZJDC: 9-31 Important Method for Moxibustion Sores,[37] (Huang 1996, 992)

《針灸大成・灸瘡要法・卷之九》

Nourishing Life says:[38] Generally, when you are touched by mugwort, sores erupt. Whatever the mugwort affects is promptly healed. If sores do not erupt, the disease will not recover. The *Systematic Classic* says:[39] If moxibustion sores do not erupt, heat the sole of an old shoe and iron it [at the site

where the sores should erupt]. Within three days, moxa sores will erupt.

Modern people use red-skinned scallions: three times five stalks, removing the green. Roast them in warm ashes, beat them to break them open, and use them to hot iron the sores ten or more times. The sores will then erupt within three days.

Another method: use fresh sesame oil to soak the site of the moxibustion and the sores will erupt.

Also, some use a decoction of gleditsia [zaojiao]. Wait until it is cold, and drip it on the sores frequently.

There is also the possibility that blood and qi are debilitated so the sores do not erupt. Take Si Wu Tang [Four Agents Decoction] to enrich and nourish blood and qi.

It is impossible to discuss all the possibilities without exception.

Some repeat one or two cones of moxibustion until the sores erupt. Some eat hot fried things such as fried fish, deep-fried tofu, or lamb to make the sores erupt. Use different ideas to seek assistance, depending on the person. You cannot go along with their nature, or in the end the sores will not erupt.

《資生》云：凡著艾得瘡發，所患即瘥，若不發，其病不愈。《甲乙經》曰：灸瘡不發者，故履底灸令熱，熨之，三日即發。今人用赤皮蔥三五莖，去青，於｝灰中煨熱，拍破，熱熨瘡上十餘遍，其瘡三日遂發。又以生麻油漬之而發，亦有用皂角煎湯，候冷頻點之，而亦有恐血氣衰不發，服四物湯，滋養血氣，不可一概論也。

---

[35] This section is from Gao Wu's *Gatherings*, Part 2, Volume 3 (Huang 1996, 733).

[36] Volume 2 (Huang 1996, 268). Wang Zhizhong attributes it to Sun's *Prescriptions*. It is found there in Volume 29 (Sun 1994, a414).

[37] This section is from Gao Wu's *Gatherings*, Part 2, Volume 3 (Huang 1996, 732) but Yang edited it a little. He took out a few sentences and added his own ideas on dietary therapy.

[38] In Volume 2 (Huang 1996, 269). It attributes the first line to the *Lower Canon of the Bright Hall*. *Nourishing Life* also has the whole passage, except Yang's dietary advice. The discussion of "modern people" using red-skinned scallions was first mentioned in *Nourishing Life*.

[39] At the end of Volume 3 (Huangfu 1997, 34). It is paraphrased here.

有復灸一二壯遂發，有食熱炙之物，如燒魚，煎豆腐，
羊肉之類而發，在人以意取助，不可順其自然，終不發
矣！

ZJDC: 9-32 Applying Medicinal Paste to Moxibustion Sores,[40] (Huang 1996, 992)
《針灸大成・貼灸瘡・卷之九》

The ancients did not apply medicinal pastes to moxibustion sores. They thought it was important to let a lot of pus out in order to eliminate the disease. *Nourishing Life* says: In the spring, use willow cotton. In the summer, use bamboo membrane.[41] In the autumn, use new cotton. In the winter, use the fine white hair from the underbelly of a rabbit or hair from a cat's belly.[42]

Modern people often apply medicinal paste to moxa sores, changing it two or three times a day. They want quick recovery. This is not the idea of treating the root of the disease. However, in the present era, they apply medicinal pastes. They still seek convenience. But the paste cannot be changed quickly. If medicinal paste is applied, there is no decay. It can only be applied a long time after [the moxibustion treatment]. If the paste is quickly changed, there will be quick recovery of the moxa sores, and it is possible that the disease root is not entirely eliminated.

古人貼灸瘡，不用膏藥，要得膿出多而疾除。《資生》云
：春用柳絮，夏用竹膜，秋用新綿，冬用兔腹下白細毛，
或用貓腹毛。今人多以膏藥貼之，日兩三易，而欲其速愈
也。此非治疾之本意也。但今世貼膏藥，亦取其便，不可

易速，若膏藥不壞，惟久久貼之可也。若速易，即速愈，
恐病根未盡除也。

ZJDC: 9-33 Moxibustion Sores Ointment Method,[43] (Huang 1996, 992)
《針灸大成・灸瘡膏法・卷之九》

Use Bai Zhi [Radix Angelicae Dahuricae], Jin Xing Cao [Herba Lepidogrammitis], Dan Zhu Ye [Herba Lophatheri], [Fu] Ling [Poria], [Huang] Lian [Rhizoma Coptidis], Ru Xiang [Olibanum], Dang Gui [Radix Angelicae Sinensis], Chuan Xiong [Rhizoma Chuanxiong], Bo He [Herba Menthae Haplocalycis], Cong Bai [Bulbus Allii Fistulosi], stir-fried processed Qian Fen [Galenite],[44] and Xiang You [fragrant, *i.e.*, roasted, sesame oil]. Boil into an ointment.

If you use other ointments, they will not counteract the pathocondition. If perchance the moxa sore opening closes easily, the disease qi is unable to exit. If you use other things to treat moxa sores, dryness will cause pain. This is also inappropriate.

用白芷, 金星草，淡竹葉，苓，連，乳香，當歸，川芎，
薄荷，蔥白等，炒鉛粉，香油煎膏貼。如用此膏不對症
。倘瘡口易收，而病氣不得出也。如用別物，乾燥作疼
，亦且不便。

ZJDC: 9-34 Washing Moxibustion Sores,[45] (Huang 1996, 992)
《針灸大成・洗灸瘡・卷之九》

The ancients applied large mugwort cones for moxi-

---

[40] This whole section was basically taken from Gao Wu's *Gatherings*, Part 2, Volume 3 (Huang 1996, 732). Gao revised it from *Nourishing Life*, where it is found in Volume 2 (Huang 1996, 269). The discussion of the impatience of "modern people" was first mentioned in *Nourishing Life*. The first two sentences and some of the commentary in the last paragraph appear to be Yang's. Yang felt strongly that moxa sores must suppurate because the root of the disease will not be eliminated if shortcuts are taken.

[41] This is a membrane from inside the bamboo.

[42] These are applied to the moxibustion sore to make more pus.

[43] In Gao Wu's *Gatherings*, a note follows the previous entry giving a recipe for an ointment for moxa sores (Huang 1996, 732). Yang took all the medicinals that Gao suggested and added a few more to make his own formula. Yang's distain for other ointments is parallel to Gao's. However, the statement that the disease evils exit through the moxa sore is given only by Yang.

[44] This contains lead. So it is not appropriate for topical or internal use today.

[45] This whole section is from Gao Wu's *Gatherings*, Part 2, Volume 3 (Huang 1996, 732). It originated in *Nourishing Life*, Volume 2 (Huang 1996, 269).

bustion. Therefore, it was fitting to use a washing method. This method uses a warm decoction of red-skinned scallions and Bo He [Herba Menthae Haplocalycis] to wash around the sores for about a double-hour. It allows the wind evils to be expelled, exiting from the opening of the sore. In addition, it allows smooth going and coming inside the channels and vessels, and, hence, recovery is naturally quick.

If you use a decoction of the fresh green tender skin from a branch on the southeast side of a peach tree as a warm wash after the moxa sores abate and scab over, the sores will be protected from any strikes by wind.

If the sores are black and putrid, add Hu Sui [Fructus Coriandri] to the decocted wash.

If there is insufferable pain, add Huang Lian [Rhizoma Coptidis] to the decoction. It is miraculously effective.

古人灸艾炷大，便用洗法。其法以赤皮蔥，薄荷煎湯，溫洗瘡周圍，約一時久，令驅逐風邪於瘡口出，更令經脈往來不澀，自然疾愈。若灸火退痂後，用東南桃枝青嫩皮煎湯溫洗，能護瘡中諸風；若瘡黑爛，加胡荽煎洗；若疼不可忍，加黃連煎神效。

ZJDC: 9-35 Nursing Health after Moxibustion,[46] (Huang 1996, 992)
《針灸大成・灸後調攝法・卷之九》

After moxibustion, you cannot drink tea right away, as it is possible that it will undo the fire qi. In addition, you cannot eat, as it is possible that it will make the channel qi stagnate. You must pause for a little while: one or two double-hours. It is appropriate to enter a room and quietly lie down. Stay distant from human affairs. Stay distant from sexual desire. Level your heart and settle your qi. Overall, you must release all emotional pressure. Especially

avoid great anger, great taxation, great hunger, great satiety, and contracting heat or catching cold.

It is also appropriate to avoid fresh cold melons and fruits. Eat only bland things that nourish the stomach and make qi and blood flow freely. Mugwort fire expels disease qi. If you consume excessively thick toxic flavors or drink to intoxication, it results in the generation of phlegm-drool, obstruction and disease qi. Because fresh fish, chicken, and lamb are able to effuse fire, they can only be used during the initial 10-plus days after moxibustion. You cannot add them in after a half month.

Many modern people do not know how to tranquilly nourish themselves. Even if they use moxibustion, how can they boost themselves? So they carry on using moxibustion, but, on the contrary, it results in harm. How can they pointlessly reproach mugwort moxibustion as ineffective!

灸後不可就飲茶，恐解火氣；及食，恐滯經氣，須少停一二時，即宜入室靜臥，遠人事，遠色慾，平心定氣，凡百俱要寬解。尤忌大怒、大勞、大饑、大飽、受熱、冒寒。至於生冷瓜果，亦宜忌之。惟食茹淡養胃之物，使氣血通流，艾火發出病氣。若過厚毒味，酗醉，致生痰涎，阻滯病氣矣。鮮魚雞羊，雖能發火，止可施於初灸十數日之內，不可加於半月之後。今人多不知恬養，雖灸何益？故因灸而反致害者，此也。徒責灸艾不效，何耶！

LI'S GENERAL GUIDELINES FOR MOXIBUSTION

BCGM: 06-06 Fire from Mugwort (Li 1996, 203) 《本草綱目・第六卷・火部・艾火》

Indications: Moxibustion for hundreds of diseases. If you use moxibustion on the various wind and cold diseases, add a little Liu Huang [Sulfur] powder. This is especially good. *Li Shizhen*

---

[46] *Nourishing Life*, Volume 2 (Huang 1996, 269) has a smaller section of things to avoid after moxibustion which Gao Wu expands (Huang 1996, 733). However, Yang's discussion does not seem like it is based on any earlier writing. It was probably written with Yang's own brush.

【主治】灸百病。若灸諸風冷疾，入硫黄末少許，尤良
。時珍

Explanation: Li Shizhen says: Whenever the mugwort fire is used for moxibustion, you should use a yang speculum or fire bead[47] to carry the sun to obtain greater yang[48] true fire. Second best is boring Huai [Sophora] wood to obtain fire [by friction]. This is good. If it is an emergency and it is difficult to prepare this type of fire, you can promptly use a sesame oil lamp or a candle flame. Use a mugwort stem to light the cone of mugwort. This will nourish and moisten the moxa sores so that there will be no pain while the patient is recovering.

The fire of tapping metal, striking stone, or boring into wood: none of them can be used. Shaozi[49] said: "Fire lacks its own body. It relies on other things to use as its body." The fire of metal or stone is fiercer than the fire of grasses and wood.

The eight types of wood are:[50]

- Fire from pine makes it difficult to recover.
- Fire from cedar [or cypress] damages the spirit and causes a lot of sweating.
- Fire from mulberry damages the flesh.
- Fire from silkworm oak damages qi and the vessels [or pulse].
- Fire from Chinese date damages the interior and causes vomiting of blood.
- Fire from mandarin orange damages construction and defense, and the channels and vessels.
- Fire from elm damages the bones and makes the recipient lose his will [or mind].

- Fire from bamboo damages the sinews and harms the eyes.

The Southern Qi Book records that in the time of Emperor Wu [of Liang], there was a Buddhist monk from Northern Qi who came to make an offering of red fire. The fire was redder and smaller than normal fire. He said it could be used to cure illness. Both the eminent and the humble people contended to get it. When seven cones of moxibustion were applied, it was quite effective. Yang Daoqing of Wuxing had vacuity disease for 20 years. He received this moxibustion and immediately recovered. All called it "fire of the sages." Even a royal decree forbidding it did not stop it. It is not known what kind of fire this was.

【發明】時珍曰：凡灸艾火者，宜用陽燧、火珠承日，取太陽真火。其次則鑽槐取火，為良。若急卒難備，即用真麻油燈，或蠟燭火，以艾莖燒點于炷，滋潤灸瘡，至愈不痛也。其夏金、擊石、鑽燧入木之火，皆不可用。邵子云：火無體，因物以為體，金石之火，烈于草木之火，是矣。八木者，松火，難瘥；柏火，傷神多汗；桑火，傷肌肉；柘火，傷氣脈；棗火，傷內吐血；橘火，傷營衛經絡；榆火，傷骨失志；竹火，傷筋損目也。《南齊書》載武帝時，有沙門從北齊赤火來，其火赤于常火而小，云以療疾，貴賤爭取之，灸至七炷，多得其驗。吳興楊道慶虛疾二十年，灸之即瘥。咸稱為聖火，詔禁之不止。不知此火，何物之火也。

Appended records:

Yang speculum: This is a fire mirror, cast from iron. The face is concave. Rub it until hot and then face it towards the sun. When mugwort receives its heat, it catches fire...

---

[47] For yang speculum, see the appended record below, under this heading. According to Volume 8 of **BCGM**, a fire bead is something resembling a crystal that can focus the rays of the sun to light a fire, similar to a magnifying glass or a lens.

[48] Tai yang, greater yang, refers to the sun, among other things.

[49] Shao Kangjie, the Song dynasty philosopher 邵康節《皇極經世 • 觀物外篇衍義 • 卷六》.

[50] Warnings about these eight kinds of wood are common in the old books. It also occurs in *Short Sketches* (Chen 1993, 171). Li Shizhen discussed it in more detail than Yang did in **ZJDC: 9-26**, above. Li reported the type of trouble that could be expected if the wrong wood was used. In addition, the two authors did not have identical lists: Li mentioned silkworm oak (柘 zhe4) while Yang prohibited bitter orange (枳 zhi3) instead.

【附錄】陽燧：時珍曰：火鏡也。以銅鑄成，其面凹，摩熱向日，以艾承之，則得火。……

A SUMMARY OF GUIDELINES AND TECHNIQUES

Generally, the origin of disease is the lack of free flow of qi and blood. Acupuncture opens up this flow and moxibustion warms it. Warmth causes qi and blood to move faster, so it helps promote uninhibited flow. **LJTY: 4-27-1**

The functions of moxibustion are to scatter cold evils, eliminate yin toxins, open depression, break stagnation, reinforce qi, and return yang. It is effective for this. **LJTY: 11-2-1**

However, there are cases where moxibustion is contraindicated. Zhang said to avoid its use for internal heat patterns—fire exuberance or yin vacuity—rapid pulse, agitated vexation, dry mouth, throat pain, sweating, red face, etc. **LJTY: 11-2-6** and **LJTY: 4-27-3**

Zhang was one of the founders of the school of warm supplementation. Because of this view, he felt moxibustion was quite useful. However, unlike Zhu Danxi, Zhang did not find the use of moxibustion in heat conditions generally appropriate.

The materials and method of lighting a fire modify the effects of medicinals, food, or moxibustion. Fire from the sun, greater yang (tai yang) fire, is more powerfully yang. This reinforces the yang of moxibustion. However, fire from a sesame oil lamp or a candle has a moistening effect, which helps moxa sores to heal more comfortably.

Certain materials should not be used to light moxa cones. If metal or stone is used (as in flint), the fire is too "fierce." There are eight kinds of wood to avoid, commonly mentioned in the old books, although the details may vary. **ZJDC: 9-26, BCGM: 06-06**

THE EIGHT TYPES OF WOOD		
TYPE OF WOOD	DAMAGE	DOCTOR
Pine	difficult to recover	both
Cedar (or Cypress)	damages the spirit and causes a lot of sweating	both
Mulberry	damages the flesh	both
Silkworm Oak	damages qi and the vessels (or pulse)	Li
Bitter Orange	not given	Yang
Chinese Date	damages the interior and causes vomiting of blood	both
Mandarin Orange	damages construction and defense, the channels and vessels	both
Elm	damages the bones and makes the recipient lose his will (or mind)	both
Bamboo	damages the sinews and harms the eyes	both

When you locate points for moxibustion, the patient's body must be level and straight. You should apply moxibustion to the patient in the same position as when you located the points. **ZJDC: 9-28**

Zhang said it is better to apply moxibustion after-noon. **LJTY: 4-27-5.** Yang disagrees in **ZJDC: 9-20.** Their discussion of this topic is in the chapter on timing.

Moxibustion must be applied on the upper body first and the lower body last. Because so many doctors recorded these guidelines, it must have been standard practice. If too much moxibustion is applied to the head or upper body, heat will accumulate above since heat rises. Using points on the lower body afterwards helps the hot qi to circulate. This will be discussed in detail later. **ZJDC: 9-29, LJTY: 11-2-4** and **LJTY: 4-27-5**

Moxibustion on Zu San Li (ST 36) descends qi. It is especially useful after applying moxibustion to the head or upper body. In a related statement, Zhang said, "Avoid applying moxibustion to [Zu] San Li in children. Those beyond 30 years can apply moxibustion to it. Otherwise, on the contrary, it will produce illness."[51] However, in adults, moxibustion on Zu San Li can be used preventively. **LJTY: 11-27-4**

Moxibustion must be strong enough to have effect. It must be noted that generally moxibustion as it is used today is much weaker than during the Ming dynasty.

However, too much moxibustion can have side effects. More can be used on the limbs than on the head and face. Even more moxibustion can be used on the back and abdomen (but use fewer cones on Ju Que, Ren 14, or Jiu Wei, Ren 15). This is an old idea. It was discussed back as far as in *Short Sketches* (*Xiao Pin Fang*), more than a thousand years earlier. **LJTY: 11-2-3, LJTY: 4-27-2, ZJDC: 9-25,** and **ZJDC: 9-27**

The above restrictions are to prevent an accumulation of yang or heat from damaging the patient. Caution is needed when applying moxibustion to the more yang areas or at the more yang times of the day.

LJTY: 4-27-2 lists some of the possible side effects of excessive moxibustion.

SIDE EFFECTS OF EXCESSIVE MOXIBUSTION		
REGION	STANDARD NUMBER OF CONES	SIDE EFFECT
Ju Que (Ren 14) Jiu Wei (Ren 15)	no more than 14 small cones	weak heart
top of head	small cones, few cones	lose essence-spirit
arms and legs	7-14 small cones	dessicate the blood & vessels, thin weak limbs
head & four limbs	see above	qi and blood expire in lower body

Different authors disagree on the appropriate number of cones to use on a particular point. Stay within reason, but use your own judgment based on the individual patient: age, body type, strength, gravity of the illness, etc. **LJTY: 11-27-2** and **ZJDC: 9-27**

The effects of moxibustion treatment are cumulative, and treatments can be spread out into sessions. **LJTY: 11-2-2**

To supplement with moxibustion, let the cones burn themselves out and close the point. Apply ointment only after all the sessions are finished. **LJTY: 11-2-5, ZJDC: 9-24**

To drain with moxibustion, blow on the cones so they burn rapidly, and leave the point open. Do not apply ointment until the sores appear. Zhang recommends the use of ointments on the moxa sores here, but Yang is generally opposed to the use of ointments. **LJTY: 11-2-5, ZJDC: 9-24**

Pastes or ointments that help moxa sores heal too quickly may reduce the efficacy of treatment. **ZJDC: 9-32.** Yang felt strongly that moxa sores must suppu-

---

[51] **LJTY: 6-3-36** 小兒忌灸三里，三十外方可灸，不爾反生疾。《類經圖翼・卷六・經絡四》

rate and that the root of the disease will not be eliminated if shortcuts are taken. Zhang is more favorable to ointments. **LJTY: 11-2-5**

Yang gave a formula for an ointment for moxa sores that won't reduce the efficacy of the treatment. There is also an effective herbal wash for moxa sores. If the sores have trouble healing, there are some modifications for this wash. **ZJDC: 9-33** and **9-34**

Zhang Jiebin also gave recipe for an ointment to treat moxa sores. **JYQS: 64-324**

> **Note:** Some ingredients of these ointments may be considered inappropriate for use today. The formulas need modification for modern use.

Since moxibustion treatments were generally stronger in the past due to the emphasis on making moxa sores, it was considered important for the patient to take good care of himself afterwards. It was also important that he not do things that would counteract the effects of treatment. Therefore, the patient should rest quietly for a few hours after treatment, without drinking tea or eating. Sex, stress, and emotional upset should be avoided. The diet should be bland for some days afterwards. A patient who does not care for himself in this way should blame himself if the treatment is not effective. **ZJDC: 9-35**

MOXA SORES

According to our Ming dynasty masters, moxa sores are necessary for moxibustion to be effective in treating disease. There are a number of methods to help them erupt if they are reluctant. **ZJDC: 9-31** and **9-32**

The mention of moxa sores occurs throughout the writings of these three authors. This is a subject we will revisit often. **ZJDC: 9-31** through **9-34**, above, all discuss moxa sores so this is a good time for a preliminary investigation.

Yang declares in **ZJDC: 9-31**, "If sores do not erupt, the disease does not recover," and then proceeds to list seven different ways to help the sores to develop. It is not enough for the sores to erupt; in **ZJDC: 9-32**, we learn that if you apply a paste or ointment to the sores, making them heal too quickly, the root of the disease may not be completely eliminated.

Yang prescribes the application of medicinals to moxa sores that will not impede the treatment. In these passages, Yang hints at the mechanism for the healing actions of moxa sores. In **9-33**, he said, "If perchance the moxa sore opening closes easily, the disease qi is unable to exit." In **9-34**, he adds that the medicinal wash "allows the expulsion of wind evils, exiting from the opening of the sore." From this we can see that, at least for repletion evils, moxa sores create an opening for the evil qi to exit from the body. This idea is analogous to the concept of opening the interstices [or pores] to expel wind evils from the exterior of the body. In the case of moxa sores, the opening is into the channel system, as moxibustion is frequently applied to points on the channels, while sweating affects the most superficial layers of the body. Moxibustion is also frequently used on an affected site, for example on an abscess. In that case, it can directly allow the evil qi to exit.

The ingredients for the ointment and medicinal wash that Yang recommended include medicinals to release the exterior and expel wind, such as Bo He (Herba Menthae Haplocalycis), Bai Zhi (Radix Angelicae Dahuricae), and Cong Bai (Bulbus Allii Fistulosi). These help expel the evil from the body through the opening of the sore.

The idea of the sore being an opening where evils can exit is also confirmed in **ZJDC: 9-24**, where Yang instructs the practitioner in draining and supplementing with moxibustion. To drain, blow on the fire and leave the point open. Fire has a quality of radiating outward. Blowing on the fire makes it strong, bright, and quick; it is better able to force the evil to scatter. This is why Yang wrote in **ZJDC: 9-35**, "Mugwort fire expels disease qi."

According to **ZJDC: 9-24**, letting the fire extinguish itself and closing the hole is a supplementation technique. If the patient is vacuous, you do not want their right qi to escape through the hole. So it must be closed. Yet it seems moxa sores are still necessary, perhaps for the qi of the mugwort to enter the patient deeply.

Note that *Elementary Questions*, Chapter 5 says, "Vigorous fire scatters qi; lesser fire generates qi." This helps explain why we let the fire burn slowly to supplement and blow on it it drain.

Our three doctors discuss moxa sores further in the sections on treatment.

CHAPTER 6
POINTS USED FOR MOXIBUSTION

Chapter Contents

While moxibustion may be applied on most points, some points are frequently treated with moxibustion. In fact, certain points are virtually never needled; moxibustion is the only treatment applied to them. The majority of points in this category are non-channel points, but a few, like Shen Que (Ren 8) and Gao Huang Shu (UB 43), are points of the 14 channels.

Below, we will explore some of the points commonly used for moxibustion as described by Yang Jizhou and Zhang Jiebin. Li Shizhen is not represented in this chapter since he never discussed moxibustion by points; he only described the materials used or the condition that was to be treated.

After the translations there is a discussion of some of the more important points that are especially reserved for moxibustion and how this type of point developed.

YANG JIZHOU ON SPECIAL MOXIBUSTION POINTS

Introduction

Section 9-6 of the *Great Compendium* describes the use of a number of special points for moxibustion, most of them non-channel points. This whole section was copied almost word for word from Li Chan's *Entering the Gate of Medicine*, Volume 1 where they were also condensed into one section, although in a different order (Li 1999, 278-81). Earlier mention of many of these points can be found in Wei Yilin's *Effective Formulas Obtained from Generations of Doctors* (published in 1345); there, they were spread out in various chapters.

Unfortunately, the location of some of these points is in question. They were probably popular during the late Ming dynasty, since authors like Li Chan and Yang Jizhou included them in their books. If the written location was not perfectly clear, a teacher could demonstrate the exact location to his student. Afterwards, the text would be adequate for the student to remember how to find the point. Another possibility is that even though the author was not sure of the exact location, he was reluctant to remove information that had been passed down. Perhaps other sources can be found with a better description of the location of these points.

ZJDC: 9-6 Quick Essentials of Moxibustion (*Entering the Gate of Medicine*) (Huang 1996, 987)

《針灸大成・捷要灸法《醫學入門》・卷之九》

ZJDC: 9-6-1 Ghost Crying point:
Treats ghosts, evil spirits, hu huo [see glossary], abstrac- tion [see glossary] and shivering. Take the patient's two thumbs side by side and bind them securely. Use mugwort cones on the corners of the two nails as well as on the flesh proximal to the nails, riding the seam. There are a total of four places. When the fire for applying the moxi-bustion is lit, the sufferer will mournfully declare [as if the ghost were speaking]: "I myself will go." It is effective.1

鬼哭穴：治鬼魅狐惑，恍惚振噤。以患人兩手大指，相並縛定，用艾炷於兩甲角，及甲後肉四處騎縫，著火灸之，則患者哀告：我自去。為效。

ZJDC: 9-6-2 Moxibustion for sudden death:
For all acute oppressive ghost dreams and fulmin-ant expiry, apply moxibustion to the inside of both big toes, the distance of a Chinese leek leaf from the nail.2

灸卒死：一切急魘暴絕，灸足兩大指內，去甲一韭葉。

ZJDC: 9-6-3 Moxibustion on Jing Gong [UB 52]:3
This is special for treating dream emissions. It is below the 14th vertebra [L2], three *cun* lateral. Apply seven cones of moxibustion. It is effective.

灸精宮：專主夢遺，十四椎下各開三寸，灸七壯效。

ZJDC: 9-6-4 Ghost Eye point:4
Especially dispels consumption worms. Make the patient raise up his arms. When they are rotated a little towards the back, two visible depressions appear in the lumbar region. These are the Yao Yan [Lumbar Eyes, non-channel]. Mark them with ink. Apply moxibustion during the 6th lunar month on a gui hai evening during the hai hour.5 Do not let people know. The Four Flowers, Gao Huang [UB 43]6 and Fei Shu [UB 13], can also dispel worms.

鬼眼穴：專祛癆蟲。令病人舉手向上，略轉後些，則腰上有兩陷可見，即腰眼也，以墨點記。於六月癸亥夜亥時灸，勿令人知。四花，膏肓，肺俞，亦能祛蟲。

ZJDC: 9-6-5 Pi Gen [Glomus Root, non-channel]:7
This is special for treating glomus lumps. It is below the 13th vertebra [L1], 3.5 *cun* lateral on both sides. Frequently apply moxibus-tion to the left side. If there is a glomus lump on both the left

---

1 This point should be Shao Shang (LU 11), also known as the ghost eye point of the hand. It is the second of Sun Simiao's ghost points. See also **LJTY: 10-1-4-32** where this point is explained in more detail.

2 Expiry is critical exhaustion. This point should be in the vicinity of Yin Bai (SP 1), also known as foot ghost eye. It is the third of Sun Simiao's ghost points. See also **LJTY: 10-1-4-32** where this point is explained in more detail.

3 UB 52 is more commonly known as *Zhi Shi* [Will Chamber].

4 This method is also in *Generations of Doctors* (Wei 1964, 152). See also **LJTY: 10-1-2-20** below and the chapter on timing of treat-ment for more discussion.

5 The sixth lunar month is usually around July in the Western calendar, shortly after the summer solstice. *Gui hai* is the last day in the cycle of sixty. *Gui* and *hai* both correspond to yin water. A *gui hai* day will not occur every year in the sixth month, as it occurs only once every sixty days. The *hai* hour is 9-11 pm.

6 See below, **LJTY: 9-7** for the Four Flowers and **LJTY: 9-8** for Gao Huang (UB 43).

7 This passage has three different points used to treat glomus lumps. A glomus lump is a palpable abdominal mass. The character for glomus consists of the disease radical with *pi* 否, which means blockage, among other things (Wiseman 1998, 242). *Pi* 否 is also the name of the twelfth double-*gua* in the *Yi Jing (Classic of Changes)* which represents a time when everything is obstructed and out of place. In Western medicine, a glomus lump may be a tumor or enlarged organ (Wiseman 1998, 242). There are many subtypes of glomus lumps. This passage does not specify a particular type. For Pi Gen (Glomus Root, non-channel M-BW-16), see also **LJTY: 11-3-7** where it is discussed in more detail.

and right, apply moxibustion to both the left and right.

Another treatment: Use a straw that is cleaned of debris. Measure the distance from the end of the patient's big toe to the center of the back of the heel and cut it. Then take this straw and measure from the tip of the coccyx to the site at the far end of the straw. The point is on both sides, about the distance of a Chinese leek leaf from the midline. If the lump is on the left, apply moxibus-tion to the right. If the lump is on the right, apply moxibus-tion to the left. Needle it to a depth of three *fen*. Apply seven cones of moxibustion. It is miracu-lously effective.[8]

Another treatment: Apply five times seven cones of moxibustion to the site at the fork of the se-cond toe. If the left is affected, apply moxibustion to the right. If the right is affected, apply moxi-bustion to the left. One evening after applying moxibustion, the sound of something stirring will be perceived in the abdomen. This is proven.[9]

痞根穴：專治痞塊。十三椎下各開三寸半，多灸左邊，如左右俱有，左右俱灸。又法：用程心量患人足大指齊，量至足後跟中截斷，將此程從尾骨尖量至程盡處，兩旁各開一韭葉許，在左灸右，在右灸左，針三分，灸七壯，神效。又法：於足第二指歧叉處灸五七壯，左患灸右，右患灸左，灸後一晚夕，覺腹中響動，是驗。

ZJDC: 9-6-6 Zhou Jian [Elbow Tip, non-channel]: Treats scrofula. If the left is affected, apply moxibustion to the right. If the right is affected, apply moxibustion to the left. During the initial onset of scrofula, apply moxibustion to Feng Chi [GB 20] on the left for males and on the right for females.[10]

Another treatment: Use a straw that is cleaned of debris and compare it to the two corners of the patient's mouth as a template. Break the straw and make two segments. Use it to measure from the wrist crease. The points are the four places at the far ends: up, down, left, and right. Apply moxibus-tion to these four points. They also are effective.[11]

肘尖穴：治瘰癧。左患灸右，右患灸左，如初生時，男左女右，灸風池。又法：用程心比患人口兩角為則，折作兩段，於手腕窩中量之，上下左右四處盡頭是穴，灸之亦效。

ZJDC: 9-6-7 Moxibustion for infixation and hostility [see glossary]: For patterns such as cadaverous infixation, visiting hostility, and malignity stroke. Apply moxibustion three *cun* behind the breast, on the left for males, and on the right for females. Or, [apply moxibustion] at the ends of the two thumbs.[12]

灸痓忤：尸痓客忤，中惡等症。乳後三寸，男左女右灸之。或兩大拇指頭。

ZJDC: 9-6-8 Moxibustion for mounting pain: For unilateral sag [sagging of one testicle],

[8] On me, this point came out approximately level with the lower border of the spinous process of L3. There is no governing vessel point at this level. It is in between Yao Yang Guan (DU 3) and Ming Men (DU 4). This point is located slightly lateral to the gov-erning vessel.
[9] The location of this point is not clear. Perhaps it is Nei Ting (ST 44). Since there is a lump or accumulation, perceiving something stirring in the abdomen is a sign of the lump dispersing.
[10] For Zhou Jian (M-UE-46) see also **LJTY: 10-1-4-13**. Males are associated with the left (yang) and females with the right (yin) in clas-sical medicine.
[11] These points also treat scrofula. These four points are apparently in the shape of a cross with one end at Da Ling (PC 7) and the other end more proximal on the pericardium channel, the length of the width of the mouth. The other piece is turned 90 degrees, with its midpoint at the center of the first piece. Perhaps these two points end up on the heart channel and the lung channel. It is also possible that these four points are on the yang side of the arm. The number of cones is not specified, but it would probably be a small quantity as some of the points would be over the region of the radial artery.
[12] The location of these points is not precisely given. This could possibly mean the ends of the two big toes instead of the thumbs.

use a straw that is cleaned of debris to measure the two corners of the patient's mouth as a template. Bend it to make three segments in the shape of a △. Place one corner in the center of the umbilicus. The two corners are placed below the umbilicus to the two sides. The points are the sites at the end of the angles. If the left is affected, apply moxibustion to the right. If the right is affected, apply moxibustion to the left. If both the left and the right are affected, apply moxibustion to both the left and right. Apply 40 mugwort cones the size of a grain of millet. It is miraculously effective.[13]

Another treatment: Apply moxibustion below the second toe, right in the center of the horizontal crease of the middle joint, on the left for males and on the right for females. It simultaneously treats all qi [patterns of *shan*], pain of the heart region and abdomen, swollen pendulous external kidneys [male genitals], and acute pain of the smaller abdomen.[14]

灸疝痛：偏墜用稈心一條，量患人口兩角為則，折為三段如△字樣，以一角安臍中心，兩角安臍下兩旁，尖盡處是穴。左患灸右，右患灸左，左右俱患，左右俱灸。炷艾如粟米大，灸四十壯，神效。又法：取足大指次指下，中節橫紋當中，男左女右灸之。兼治諸氣，心腹痛，外腎吊腫，小腹急痛。

ZJDC: 9-6-9 Moxibustion for stomach reflux: One *cun* below the two breasts, or three fingers below the medial malleolus, somewhat obliquely towards the front.[15]

灸翻胃：兩乳下一寸，或內踝下三指，稍斜向前。

ZJDC: 9-6-10 Moxibustion for intestinal wind and all hemorrhoids: Below the 14th vertebra [L2], one *cun* to each side. It is most effective for disease that has lasted for years.[16]

灸腸風諸痔：十四椎下各開一寸，年深者最效。

ZJDC: 9-6-11 Moxibustion for swelling and fullness: On the seams of the two thumbs, or 1.5 *cun* above the second toe.[17]

灸腫滿：兩大手指縫，或足二指上一寸半。

ZJDC: 9-6-12 Moxibustion for patch wind [see glossary]: In the depression on the joint of the middle finger of the left and right hands. Whenever there are blemishes and various moles, apply moxibustion to it. No one does not receive immediate effects.[18]

灸癜風：左右手中指節宛宛中，凡贅疣諸痣，灸之無不立效。

---

[13] See also **LJTY: 11-3-19-8**. Today, this point is called San Jiao Jiu 三角灸 Triangle Moxibustion (M-CA-23). Deadmen et al. (1998, 575) says the *Great Compendium* gave the first description of the Triangle Moxibustion point, but this passage is also found in the earlier book, *Entering the Gate*. An even older source is *Generations of Doctors* (Wei 1964, 46). The directions in this passage are a little ambiguous. It could be read that the width of the mouth is broken into three sections to make a very small triangle. However, *Generations of Doctors* clearly states that these are three sections, each the width of a mouth.

[14] This point also treats mounting or *shan* pain. It is from *Generations of Doctors* (Wei 1964, 46).

[15] The location of the first point should be between Ru Gen (ST 18) and Qi Men (LV 14). The location of the second should be around the spleen channel, fairly close to Gong Sun (SP 4). While the channel points listed here are not necessarily identical to the moxibustion points that Yang described, all three treat stomach reflux. If the moxibustion points are not identical to Ru Gen, Qi Men, or Gong Sun, being nearby may lend them similar functions.

[16] *Acupuncture: A Comprehensive Text* (O'Connor and Bensky 1981, 378) calls this point Intestinal Wind (Chang Feng 腸風, M-BW-18). It is slightly medial to the kidneys' transport point, Shen Shu (UB 23).

[17] Both these points are given in *Generations of Doctors* (Wei 1964, 160). There, Wei said they treat "water qi and swelling and fullness of the whole body." Wei said the first point is at the *end* of the thumb seam and that seven cones should be used. Unfortunately, the exact location is still not clear. The first point may be slightly distal to Yu Ji (LU 10). The second point is related to the stomach channel, perhaps near Xian Gu (ST 43). Xian Gu also treats edema, abdominal pain, distention, and fullness (Deadman 1998, 170). Wei said to use the age as a guide to the number of cones on the second point.

[18] This comes from *Generations of Doctors* (Wei 1964, 231). It may be a depression in the center of the middle phalange of the finger, or it may be two points in the center of both interphalangeal joints.

ZJDC: 9-7 Master Cui's Method of Applying Treatment to the Four Flowers (Huang 1996, 988) 《針灸大成・崔氏取四花穴法・卷之九》

Treats the five taxations and seven damages in males or females, qi vacuity and blood weakness, steaming bones, tidal fever, cough, phlegm panting, emaciation, and intractable disease.

Use a waxed string to measure the length of the patient's mouth. Cut out a paper square in accordance with the string[19] and cut a small hole in the center. Use another long waxed string. Place it below the foot and step on it. Make it even with the big toe in front. In back, cut it at the knee crease. If a woman has bound feet, this comparative measurement is not appropriate. In that case, apply the waxed string to the flesh of the right arm and measure from Jian Yu [LI 15] to the end of the middle finger. Cut it.

Next, wind the string around the neck below the laryngeal prominence, both ends hanging down towards the back. Use a brush to mark the place at the far ends of the string. Then take the paper square made earlier and place the small hole on the mark. Mark the four sides and apply moxibustion to the site of the corners of the paper, seven cones on each corner.

Notes on the Four Flowers' points: The ancients feared people did not know how to locate points so they established this quick method. The points are probably equivalent to the transport points of the five viscera. Today, we depend on this method to find these points. If they are equivalent to the second line on the back,[20] they are the four points of Ge Shu (UB 17) and Dan Shu (UB 19) on the foot greater yang urinary bladder channel.

The *Classic of Difficulties*[21] says, "The meeting point of the blood is Ge Shu." Shu[22] said, "This point treats blood disease." Steaming bones and tidal fever are usually due to blood vacuity with effulgent fire; thus, we select this point [Ge Shu, UB 17] in order to supplement the blood. The gallbladder is the bowel of the liver and the liver is able to store blood. That is why we also select this point [Dan Shu, UB 19].

Master Cui just called them the Four Flowers. He did not call them the four points of Ge Shu and Dan Shu. He described the location in this way for the vulgar healer. However, people's mouths have differences in width. Because of this, comparative measurement of the Four Flowers is not standardized; no one is correct who tries to figure it out by feeling the vertebrae for Ge Shu and Dan Shu.

In addition, there is no one who does not respond to the application of moxibustion to the two Gao Huang [UB 43] points.

Ge Shu is located below the 7th vertebra [T7], 1.5 *cun* bilateral.

Dan Shu is located below the 10th vertebra [T10], 1.5 *cun* bilateral.

Gao Huang Shu is located one *fen* below the 4th vertebra [T4], two *fen* above the 5th vertebra [T5], three *cun* bilateral, in the 4th intercostal space.[23]

治男婦，五勞七傷，氣虛血弱，骨蒸潮熱，咳嗽痰喘，尪羸癲疾。用蠟繩量患人口長，照繩裁紙四方，中剪小孔，別用長蠟繩踏腳下，前齊大趾，後大曲[月+秋]橫紋截斷。如婦人纏足，比量不便，取右膊肩髃穴貼肉，量至中指頭截斷，卻絡在結喉下，雙垂向背後，繩頭盡處，用筆點記，即以前紙小孔安點中，分

---

[19] Each side of the square is the length of the string.

[20] The governing vessel is counted as the first line; the inner urinary bladder line is the second.

[21] In the 45th Difficulty.

[22] A commentator on the *Classic of Difficulties*.

[23] This section is basically from Gao Wu's *Gatherings*, Part 2, Volume 2 (Huang 1996, 708). Before that, a similar passage appeared in *Nourishing Life*, Volume 3 (Huang 1996, 272). Yang rewrote it a little and updated the technique, for example suggesting a waxed string rather than a straw. Otherwise, the location technique is the same. See **LJTY: 10-1-6** and the discussion below for a comparison of the variations on Master Cui's Four Flowers.

四方，灸紙角上，各七壯。按：四花穴，古人恐人不
知點穴，故立此捷法，當必有合於五臟俞也。今依此
法點穴，果合足太陽膀胱經行背二行：膈俞膽俞四穴
。《難經》曰：血會膈俞。疏曰：血病治此。蓋骨蒸
勞熱，血虛火旺，故取此以補之。膽者，肝之腑，肝
能藏血，故亦取是俞也。崔氏止言四花而不言膈俞，
膽俞四穴者，為粗工告也。但人口有大小，闊狹不同
，故比量四花亦不準，莫若揣摸脊骨膈俞，膽俞為正
。再取膏肓二穴灸之，無不應矣。膈俞：在七椎下兩
旁，去脊各一寸五分。膽俞：在十椎下兩旁，去脊各
一寸五分。膏肓俞：在四椎下一分，五椎上二分兩旁
，去脊各三寸，四肋一間。

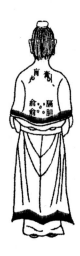

This diagram of Gao Huang (UB 43), Ge Shu (UB 17), and Dan Shu (UB 19) is included in the *Great Compendium* (Huang 1996, 988).

ZJDC: 9-8 Method for Applying Treatment to Gao Huang [UB 43] (*Entering the Gate of Medicine*) (Huang 1996, 988)
《針灸大成・取膏肓穴法《醫學入門》・卷之九》

Indicated for hundreds of patterns of depleted and weak yang qi, all wind and intractable cold, dream emissions, ascending qi, hiccough, dysphagia-occlusion [see glossary], and mania bewilderment with raving.

To find the point, you must make the patient sit evenly on the bed bending his knees so they are even with the chest. Wrap his two arms around his legs and knees. Make his shoulder blades open up and separate. Do not let the patient move or shake. Use your finger to press slightly below (one *fen*) the 4th vertebra, slightly above (two *fen*) the 5th vertebra. Mark it with ink. Then draw a line level with the ink mark, about six *cun* bilateral.[24] It is located in the 4th intercostal space, about a finger-breadth medial to the shoulder blades. Rub outside the paravertebral muscles and press the empty places in the sinews and bones. If the patient feels a pulling pain in the chest and ribs upon palpation, it is the true point.

Apply up to 100 or 1,000 cones of moxibustion to it. If the patient feels congestion and fullness after applying moxibustion, you can apply moxibustion to Qi Hai [Ren 6] and Zu San Li [ST 36] to drain down fire repletion. After applying moxibustion, it makes the person's yang exuberant. The patient should consider whether to safeguard and nourish himself. He cannot indulge in sensual pleasures.[25]

主治陽氣虛弱，諸風瘤冷，夢遺上氣，呃逆膈噎，狂
惑妄誤百症。取穴須令患人就床平坐，曲膝齊胸，以
兩手圍其足膝，使胛骨開離，勿令動搖，以指按四椎
微下一分，五椎微上二分，點墨記之，即以墨平畫相
去六寸許，四肋三間，胛骨之裏，肋間空處，容側指
許，摩脊肉之表，筋骨空處，按之患者覺牽引胸肋中
手指痛，即真穴也。灸至百壯，千壯，灸後覺氣壅盛
，可灸氣海及足三里，瀉火實下，灸後令人陽盛，當
消息以自保養，不可縱慾。

ZJDC: 9-9 Ride the Bamboo Horse Moxibustion Point Method (Master Yang) (Huang 1996, 988)
《針灸大成・騎竹馬灸穴法（楊氏）・卷之九》

These two points especially treat all disease patterns such as abscesses, malign sores, back eruptions, toxic boils, scrofula, and all wind.

---

[24] Meaning three *cun* on each side of the spine.
[25] This is almost word for word from *Entering the Gate*, Volume 1 (Li 1999, 278). See also **LJTY: 7-1** and the discussion, below.

First, begin from the center of the elbow crease, using the left on males, and the right on females. Measure with a thin bamboo strip up to the end of the flesh of the middle finger; do not measure the fingernail. Cut it. Next, use a bamboo strip to find one *cun* from the same body. Then make the patient remove his clothing and securely straddle a big bamboo pole. Have two people slowly raise it until the patient's feet leave the ground by three *cun*. For stability, have two people support the patient on the sides. Raise the previously measured length of bamboo strip vertically from the bamboo pole along the sacrum, sticking it securely to the spine and measure up to the site at the end of the strip. Mark it with a brush. Then take the bamboo strip that is the length of a body *cun*. The point is one *cun* bilateral. Apply seven cones of moxibustion. This is the Yang family's method of moxibustion.

Note that in the *Divinely Responding Classic*,[26] two people raise the patient up to carry him on their shoulders. This is not stable. You should put the bamboo carrying pole on two wooden stools. Let the patient's feet lightly touch the ground. Use two people on the sides to support him. This is especially wonderful.

Also, note that *Gatherings from Eminent Acupuncturists* says it is one *cun* bilateral. I suspect it is 1.5 *cun*. It should be on the same course as Ge Shu [UB 17] and Gan Shu [UB 18].[27]

此二穴，專治癰疽惡瘡，發背，瘤毒，瘰癧諸風，一切病症。先從男左女右臂腕中橫紋起，用薄篾一條，量至中指齊肉盡處，不量爪甲，截斷。次用篾取前同身寸一寸；卻令病人脫去衣服，以大竹扛一條跨定，兩人隨徐扛起，足離地三寸，兩旁兩人扶定，將前量長篾，貼定竹杠豎起，從尾骶骨貼脊量至篾盡處，以筆點記，後取身寸篾，各開一寸是穴。灸七壯。此楊氏灸法。按《神應經》：兩人抬扛不穩，當用兩木凳

，擱竹扛頭，令患人足微點地，用兩人兩旁扶之，尤妙。又按《聚英》言：各開一寸，疑為一寸五分。當合膈俞，肝俞穴道。

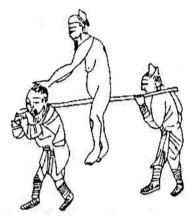

This drawing of the bamboo horse method is included in the *Great Compendium* (Huang 1996, 988). Although Yang criticized the directions in the *Divinely Responding Classic*, his illustration depicts the same method: raising the pole up on the shoulders of the carriers. Perhaps it was added in a later printing.

ZJDC: 9-10 Applying Moxibustion to the Taxation Point (*Gatherings from Eminent Acupuncturists*) (Huang 1996, 989)
《針灸大成・灸勞穴法《聚英》・卷之九》

The *Classic of Nourishing Life* says: The condition of enduring taxation manifests as heat of the hands, feet, and heart; night sweating, exhausted essence-spirit, and pain and coldness of the bones and sinews. It initially emerges as cough, gradually developing into spitting blood and pus, thinning of the flesh, yellow face, reduced food intake, and reduced strength.

Make the patient stand erect. Using the left side on males and the right side on females, measure with a

---

[26] Written by Chen Hui 陳會 and revised by 劉瑾 Liu Jin, published in 1425 (Ming).

[27] Up until Yang's note, this section is basically from Gao Wu's *Gatherings*, Part 2, Volume 2 (Huang 1996, 708). Yang changes or adds a few details. For example, Yang includes toxic boils, scrofula, and all wind in the list of indications. Gao said to lift the patient about 5 *cun* from the ground, while Yang reduces it to three *cun* and then in his note said to let the patient's feet touch the ground lightly. Gao said to use three cones, while Yang said to use seven. Even though Yang claims this as his family tradition, his treatment is quite similar to the doctors that came before him. See also **LJTY: 10-1-7** and the discussion, below.

straw from the tip of the middle toe, passing through the heart of the lower leg, upwards to the knee crease. Cut the straw there. Then, take this straw and measure from the tip of the nose vertically over the head, parting the hair at the exact center, and measure to the spine. Mark the place at the far end of the straw with ink. Take another straw. Make the person close his mouth naturally. Measure its width and cut the straw. Then place this straw [horizontally] on the ink mark, evenly dividing the two ends. The point is the place measured at the ends.

When applying moxibustion, base the number of cones on the age plus one. If the person is 30 years old, apply 31 cones of moxibustion. It is repeatedly effective.

> **Note:** This point is equal to the two points of Xin Shu [UB 15], each 1.5 cun lateral to the 5th vertebra. The heart governs blood. That is why moxibustion is applied to this point.[28]

《資生經》云：久勞其狀手腳心熱，盜汗，精神困頓，骨節疼寒，初發咳嗽，漸吐膿血，肌瘦面黃，減食少力。令身正直，用草於男左女右自腳中指尖，量過腳心下，向上至曲[月+秋]大紋處，截斷；卻將此草，白鼻尖量，從頭正中，分開髮，量至脊，以草盡處，用墨點記。別用草一條，令病人自然合口，量闊狹，截斷。卻將此草於墨點上，平折兩頭，盡處量穴。灸時隨年紀，多灸一壯。如人三十歲，灸三十一壯，累效。按此穴，合五椎兩旁，各一寸五分，心俞二穴也。 心主血，故灸之。

ZJDC: 9-11 Method to Apply Treatment to Shen Shu [UB 23] (Huang 1996, 989)
《針灸大成・取腎俞穴法・卷之九》

Stand on a level place. Use a stick to measure roughly up to the umbilicus. Use this stick again to measure up the spine. Know that this site is level with the umbilicus. Then, find the point 1.5 *cun* bilateral to it. This is Shen Shu [UB 23].[29]

在平處立，以杖子約量至臍，又以此杖，當背脊骨上量之，知是與臍平處也。然後左右各寸半，取其穴，則腎俞也。

ZHANG JIEBIN ON POINTS USED FOR MOXIBUSTION
Introduction

In the *Illustrated Supplement to the Categorized Classic*, Volumes 6-8, Zhang goes over the points of the 14 channels one by one. A sampling is included of his relevant comments about four of the most important points used for moxibustion: Shen Que (Ren 8), Qi Hai (Ren 6), Gao Huang Shu (UB 43), and Zu San Li (ST 36). These are exerpts; information on location, needling techniques, etc. is not translated here. In addition, brief references to moxibustion on a variety of other channel points follows.

In Volume 10 of the same book, Zhang discussed a number of non-channel points that are important for moxibustion. Some of these will also be presented below.

LJTY: 6-3-36 San Li [ST 36] (Zhang 1991, 832):[30] Someone said, "Avoid applying moxibustion to San Li [ST 36] in children. Those beyond 30 years can receive moxibustion. Otherwise, on the contrary, it will produce illness."… *Secret Necessities of a Frontier Official* [*Waitai Miyao*] says, "If a person over 30 years of age does not apply moxibustion to San Li, it allows qi to ascend and surge into the eyes, making the eyes lack brilliance." San Li seems to be able to descend qi.

---

[28] This passage is virtually identical to Gao Wu's *Gatherings*, Part 2, Volume 2 (Huang 1996, 708). Gao quoted it from the *Classic of Nourishing Life*, Volume 3 (Huang 1996, 273). The speculation that it is the same as Xin Shu UB 15 seems to have originated with Gao Wu. This point is equivalent to Zhang's Suffering Gate (*Huan Men*) point. See **LJTY: 10-1-6** and the discussion, below.

[29] This passage is virtually identical to Gao Wu's *Gatherings*, Part 2, Volume 2 (Huang 1996, 709). Earlier, it came from Sun's *Prescriptions* as a method to apply moxibustion on Shen Shu UB 23 to treat lumbar pain (Sun 1994, a275). It is also given in *Generations of Doctors* (Wei 1964, 47, 119). See also **LJTY: 11-3-17.**

[30] See also **LJTY: 4-27-4.**

三里：一云：小兒忌灸三里，三十外方可灸，不爾反生疾……《外臺・明堂》云：人年三十已外若不灸三里令氣上衝目使眼無光，蓋以三里能下氣也。

LJTY: 7-1-35 Gao Huang Shu [UB 43] (Zhang 1991, 857-8): Apply up to 100 cones each on the left and right Gao Huang [UB 43]. Some apply three or five hundred [or] even more, up to 1,000 cones. It makes qi move down, gurgling like the descent of flowing water… After applying moxibustion to this point, it makes yang qi flourish more each day. The patient should consider whether to supplement and nourish himself. It allows the patient to obtain a cure. So there is no disease it does not treat… Someone said after applying moxibustion to Gao Huang, moxibustion should be applied to Zu San Li [ST 36] in order to guide fire repletion downward.[31]

膏肓俞：左右各灸至百壯，或三五百，多至千壯。當氣下嘽嘽然如流水之降……此穴灸後，令陽氣日盛，當消息自為補養，令得平復，則諸病無所不治……一云：灸後常灸足三里，以引火實下……

LJTY: 8-3-6 Qi Hai [Ren 6] (Zhang 1991, 898): In ancient times, Liu Gongdu[32] said, "I nourish life with no other method besides not allowing original qi to aid joy and anger, and I constantly warm Qi Hai [Ren 6]. That's all. Today people are already incapable of avoiding the use of original qi to aid joy and anger. If they have time, they apply moxibustion to Qi Hai to make it warm, also using this as a secondary measure. In the past, I had a lot of illness. The doctor often instructed me to apply moxibustion to Qi Hai when I had shortness of breath. Consequently, my breath is not short. From this idea, I applied moxibustion to it [Qi Hai, Ren 6] once or twice each year because of my weak qi."

昔柳公度曰：吾養生無他術但不使元氣佐喜怒，使氣海常溫爾。今人既不能不以元氣佐喜怒，若能時灸氣海使溫，亦其次也。予舊多病，常若氣短，醫者，教灸氣海，氣遂不促，自是每歲一二次灸之，則以氣怯故也。

LJTY: 8-3-8 Shen Que [Ren 8] (Zhang 1991, 899):[33] (Also named Qi She [Qi Abode]), [this point is] located right in the navel.

Apply three cones of moxibustion. Piercing is contraindicated. Piercing it makes the person have malign open ulcerating sores. They will die if it is not treated.

Someone said to fill the umbilicus with dry, clean, stir-fried salt. On top, cover it with a thick slice of ginger. Apply 100 cones of moxibustion. Some use Chuan Jiao [Pericarpium Zanthoxyli] in place of the salt. This is also wonderful.

This point is indicated for yin patterns, cold damage, wind stroke, loss of consciousness, vacuity cold in the abdomen, damage from exhaustion, borborygmus, unceasing diarrhea, water swelling, drum distention, unceasing milk dysentery in children with enlarged abdomens, wind epilepsy, arched-back rigidity, and prolapse of the anus. There will never be a miscarriage if moxibustion is applied to this point in females with infertility due to cold in the blood.

Not all doctors discuss application of moxibustion to this point. Some only say it is contraindicated for acupuncture. The *Bronze Man* says,[34] "It is appropriate to apply 100 cones of moxibustion."

---

[31] See also **ZJDC: 9-8** and the discussion below.

[32] Liu Gongdu (778-865) was a statesman and calligrapher (Liu 1999, 166). He said that the way to nourish life is not to let emotions consume original qi and to frequently apply moxibustion to Qi Hai (Ren 6). The idea that emotions consume original qi is common. For example, Li Dongyuan said, "Overall, anger, resentment, sadness, thought, fear, and dread all harm original qi" (Li 1993, 98). 凡怒、忿、悲、思、恐、懼、皆損元氣。李東垣《脾胃論・卷中・安養心神調治脾胃論》

[33] In this passage, Zhang put forth the idea that large amounts of moxibustion on Shen Que (Ren 8) not only treats disease, but also promotes long life. In treating disease, he felt it was important to apply a large quantity of moxibustion. Otherwise, the patient may have a relapse.

[34] The *Bronze Man* is by Wang Weiyi. This citation is from Volume 2 (Huang 1996, 193).

There was someone named Xu Ping who suffered sudden stroke with loss of consciousness. Tao Yuanbu applied 100 cones of moxibustion on his umbilicus, and he began to revive. After another few months, Xu Ping had not relapsed. Zheng Jiu said [regarding this], "I had a relative who suffered sudden windstroke. When the doctor applied 500 cones of moxibustion, he revived. This occurred after he was over 80 years old. If Xu Ping really received up to 300 or 500 cones of moxibustion, how do we know he didn't achieve longevity?"

Thus, to apply moxibustion to Shen Que, you must fill up the umbilicus with fine salt and then apply moxibustion to it. Using a lot of moxibustion is good. If you apply 300 or 500 cones of moxibustion to it, you will not only cure disease, but you will also promote longevity. Sometimes when you apply less moxibustion, someone will recover for the short-term, but later the disease may re-emerge and it will be difficult to rescue the patient.

However, the human spirit[35] is in the umbilicus in the summer months. Therefore, it is not appropriate to apply moxibustion at that time.

A Thousand Pieces of Gold says, "Put salt in the umbilicus and apply 3 cones of moxibustion. This treats strangury." It also says, "Whenever someone has sudden turmoil [cholera], put salt in the umbilicus and apply two times seven cones of moxibustion. It also treats distention and fullness."

神闕一名氣舍：當臍中。〇灸三壯，禁刺，刺之令人惡瘍潰矢，死不治。一曰納炒乾淨鹽滿臍，上加厚薑一片蓋定，灸百壯，或以川椒代鹽亦妙。主治陰證傷寒中風，不省人事，腹中虛冷傷憊，腸鳴泄瀉不止，水腫臌脹，小兒乳痢不止，腹大風癇，角弓反張，脫肛。婦人血冷不受胎者，灸此永不脫胎。〇此穴在諸家俱不言灸，只云禁鍼。《銅人》云：宜灸百壯。有徐平者，卒中不省，得桃源簿為灸臍中百壯始甦，更數月復不起。鄭紏云：有一親卒中風，醫者為灸五百壯而甦，後年逾八十。向使徐平灸至三五百壯，安知

其不永年耶？故神闕之灸，須填細鹽，然後灸之，以多為良。若灸之三五百壯，不惟愈疾，亦且延年；若灸少，則時或暫愈，後恐復發，必難救矣。但夏月人神在臍，乃不宜灸。《千金》云：納鹽臍中灸三壯治淋病。〇又云：凡霍亂，納鹽臍中，灸二七壯，並治脹滿。

ADDITIONAL BRIEF REFERENCES TO MOXIBUSTION ON VARIOUS POINTS

LJTY: 6-1-6 Kong Zui [LU 6] (Zhang 1991, 818): Kong Zui [LU6] is indicated for febrile disease without sweating. Apply three cones of moxibustion and the patient will promptly sweat.

LJTY: 6-1-7 Lie Que [LU 7] (Zhang 1991, 818): If someone suffers hemilateral wind, apply up to 100 cones of moxibustion. If someone suffers taxation of the wrist, applying seven times seven cones of moxibustion is very wonderful.

LJTY: 6-1-10 Yu Ji [LU 10] (Zhang 1991, 819): A treatment handed down for toothache, unable to eat or drink: If the left is affected apply moxibustion to the right. If the right is affected, apply moxibustion to the left. Three cones for males; four cones for females.

LJTY: 6-2-4 He Gu [LI 4] (Zhang 1991, 821): The *Shennong Classic* [*Shen Nong Jing*] says, "To treat nosebleeds, painful eyes that are not bright, toothache, throat impediment, scabs and sores, you can apply three cones or up to seven cones of moxibustion."

LJTY: 6-2-15 Jian Yu [LI 15] (Zhang 1991, 824): If moxibustion is applied to this point for hemilateral wind paralysis, use from seven up to seven times seven cones and then stop. You cannot use too much moxibustion or it may make the arms thin. If the sinews and bones are feeble in wind dis-

---

[35] The human spirit is a prohibition for acupuncture and moxibustion based on the time or season.

ease and it is not cured for a long time, you should apply a lot of moxibustion. Do not fear thinning of the arms.

LJTY: 7-1-12 Feng Men [UB 12] (Zhang 1991, 851): This point is able to drain hot qi from the whole body. When moxibustion is frequently applied, you never suffer the likes of abscesses, sores, and scabs.

LJTY: 7-1-16 Ge Shu [UB 17] (Zhang 1991, 853): This is the meeting point of blood. It is appropriate to apply moxibustion to this point in all blood diseases, such as unceasing vomiting of blood, nosebleeds, vacuity detriment, clouding dizziness, frenetic movement of hot blood, retching of blood due to both the heart and lung channels, and visceral toxins causing bloody stool that does not stop.

LJTY: 6-3-4 Di Cang [ST 4] (Zhang 1991, 826): If someone suffers wind [in the channels of the face] for a long time… apply seven or two times seven cones of moxibustion. If it is severe, apply seven times seven cones. If the disease is on the left, treat the right. If the disease is on the right, treat the left. Small mugwort cones are suitable, the size of the leg of a coarse hairpin. If they are too big, the mouth will become deviated, but if moxibustion is applied to Cheng Jiang [Ren 24], it will promptly recover.

LJTY: 6-3-28 Shui Dao [ST 28] (Zhang 1991, 830): *A Thousand Pieces of Gold* says, "It governs hot qi in the the triple burner, urinary bladder, and kidneys. Apply the number of moxibustion cones according to the years of age."

LJTY: 6-6-3 Hou Xi [SI 3] (Zhang 1991, 845): A treatment handed down for vomiting at noon after eating early, or vomiting in the afternoon after eating at noon is to apply nine cones of moxibustion to this point bilaterally. There will be immediate recovery.

LJTY: 7-3-8 Lao Gong [PC 8] (Zhang 1991, 874): A treatment handed down for mania and withdrawal: the application of moxibustion to this point is effective.

LJTY: 8-1-21 Jian Jing [GB 21] (Zhang 1991, 885): If a woman has a difficult childbirth and, after expelling the fetus, there is reversal counterflow of the hands, needle it. She will immediately recover. If moxibustion is applied, it is superior.

LJTY: 8-2-10 Yin Lian [LV 11] (Zhang 1991, 893): Yin Lian [LV 11] is indicated for female infertility. If her periods are irregular and she has never been pregnant, apply three cones of moxibustion and she will promptly have a child.

LJTY: 8-4-14 Da Zhui [Du 14] (Zhang 1991, 907): Da Zhui [Du 14] is the meeting [point] of bones.[36] Moxibustion can be applied to it for bone disease… The method for fever and chills is to first apply moxibustion to Da Zhui and then Chang Qiang [Du 1]. The number of cones is based on the years of age. Someone said it treats generalized pain, fever and chills, and wind qi pain. Someone said it treats unceasing nosebleeds. Apply 20 or 30 cones of moxibustion. It severs the root so the disease will not re-emerge.

LJTY: 8-4-26 Shui Gou [Du 26] (Zhang 1991, 911): *A Thousand [Pieces] of Gold* says, "…For ghost strike and sudden death, you must promptly apply moxibustion to it."

Illustrated Supplement to the Categorized Classic, Volume 10: Non-channel points

Zhang discussed a number of non-channel points that were important for moxibustion. A sampling of them follows:

---

[36] Most sources list Da Zhu (UB 11) as the meeting point for bones.

LJTY: 10-1-1-4 Yin Tang [Hall of Impression] (Zhang 1991, 917): Located between the two eyebrows. The *Shen Nong Acupuncture Classic* [*Shen Nong Zhen Jing*] says, "Treats acute or chronic pediatric fright wind. You can apply three cones of moxibustion. Use mugwort cones the size of a grain of wheat." The *Ode to the Jade Dragon* [*Yu Long Fu*] says, "It is good to treat fright convulsions."

LJTY: 10-1-2-13 Bao Men [Uterine Gate], Zi Hu [Child Door] & Qi Men [Qi Gate] (Zhang 1991, 919): The *Supplement to a Thousand Pieces of Gold* says: When the infant's viscus [uterus] gate is blocked and does not receive essence, pregnancy is not achieved, or for miscarriage with abdominal pain and the appearance of red spotting, apply 50 cones of moxibustion to Bao Men [Uterine Gate] which is located two *cun* lateral to Guan Yuan [Ren 4] on the left. The right side is called Zi Hu [Child Door].

Needle Bao Men one *cun* deep for all of these: retention of placenta and death *in utero*, or accumulations and gatherings in the abdomen.

The *Supplement* also says: For infertility, apply 50 cones of moxibustion to each side of Qi Men [Qi Gate], which is located three *cun* lateral to Guan Yuan (Ren 4). Also, for threatened miscarriage with inability to hold in the blood, apply 100 cones of moxibustion.

胞門、子戶、氣門：《千金翼》云：子藏門塞不受精，妊娠不成，若墮胎腹痛，漏胞見赤，灸胞門五十壯，關元左邊二寸是也，右邊名子戶。若胞衣不出，及子死腹中，或腹中積聚，皆鍼入胞門一寸。又云：胎孕不成，灸氣門穴，在關元旁三寸，各五十壯。○又漏胎下血不禁，灸百壯。

LJTY: 10-1-2-20 Yao Yan [Lumbar Eyes] (Zhang 1991, 902): The method is to let the patient sleep peacefully and use a brush to mark the two points in the depressions of the two lumbar eyes. Apply seven cones of moxibustion to each. No book has these points. Someone residing at home must be used to carry it out. It is said to be effective every time it is tried.

It is indicated for all taxation consumption that is already serious and difficult to treat. On a *gui hai* day, at the end of the second watch, entering the third watch,[37] let the patient sleep peacefully. Apply three cones of moxibustion to the points.

Someone passed down a treatment for corpse transmission consumption that results in the whole family dying one by one, leaving it without posterity. Because the patient is tormented by cold and heat in this pattern, blood congeals and qi stagnates; it transforms and worms eat the internal organs. It always results in transmission to other people. Even with hundreds of formulas, it is difficult to treat. Only moxibustion can attack it.

The method: The time when the six spirits all gather is on a *gui hai* day, after the second watch as it is about to reach midnight. Do not let people know what you are doing. Make the patient take off his lower clothing. When he raises his arms and rotates them a little towards the back, tiny depressions on the two sides of the lumbar region will spontaneously appear. This is called the Ghost Eye point. It is what the laypeople call *Yao Yan* [Lumbar Eyes]. Mark it with ink while the patient stands erect. Then the patient should get in bed, close his eyes, and go to sleep. Apply moxibustion with seven or nine small mugwort cones. Eleven cones are especially good. The worms will come out in the vomit and diarrhea that follows. Destroy these excretions by burning them and discard them far away so you can avoid further transmission. This method is especially easy and effective compared to points like the Four Flowers.[38]

---

[37] *Gui hai* is the last day in the cycle of sixty. *Gui* and *hai* both correspond to yin water. The five watches are the five two-hour periods of the night, starting from 8 PM (Wiseman, 1995). The time between the second and third watch would be around midnight.

[38] For the Ghost Eye point, see also **ZJDC: 9-6-4**. This method is also in Wei Yilin's *Effective Formulas Obtained from Generations of Doctors* (Wei 1964, 152). For the Four Flowers, see below.

The *Supplement to a Thousand Pieces of Gold* says, "To treat lumbar pain, apply moxibustion to the pits at the Lumbar Eyes. They are located above the buttocks around the left and right sides." It also says, "A point is located three *cun* below Shen Shu [UB 23], 1.5 *cun* to each side of the spine. Use the fingers to press in the depression. It is indicated for wasting-thirst." These two passages both seem to indicate this point.

腰眼：其法令病人平眠，以筆於兩腰眼宛宛中點二穴，各灸七壯。此穴諸書所無，而居家必用載之，云其累試累驗。主治諸勞瘵已深之難治者，於癸亥日二更盡，入三更時，令病人平眠取穴，灸三壯。一傳治傳屍癆瘵，以致滅門絕戶者有之。此證因寒熱煎作，血凝氣滯，有化而為蟲者，內食臟腑，每致傳人，百方難治，惟灸可攻。其法：於癸亥日二更後，將交夜半，乃六神皆聚之時，勿使人知，令病者解去下衣，舉手向上，略轉後些，則腰間兩旁自有微陷可見，是名鬼眼穴，即俗人所謂腰眼也。正身直立，用墨點記，然後上床合面而臥，用小艾炷灸七壯，或九壯、十一壯尤好。其蟲必於吐瀉中而出，燒燬遠棄之，可免傳染。比四花等穴，尤易且效。《千金翼》云：治腰痛灸腰目〔穴+卯〕，在尻上約左右○又云：在腎俞下三寸，夾脊兩旁各一寸半，以指按陷中，主治消渴。此二說者，似皆指此穴。

LJTY: 10-1-4-13 Zhou Jian [Elbow Tip] (Zhang 1991, 922):[39] The *Supplement to a Thousand Pieces of Gold* says, "It treats intestinal abscess. When 100 cones of moxibustion are applied to each tip of the two elbows while the elbow is bent, it precipitates pus and blood, and the patient will recover." It also says, "Apply moxibustion directly to the end of the pointed bone on the elbow."

肘尖：《千金翼》云：治腸癰，屈兩肘尖頭骨，各灸百壯，則下膿血者愈○又云：正灸肘頭銳骨。

LJTY: 10-1-4-22 Wai Huai Jian [Tip of the Lateral Malleolus] (Zhang 1991, 923): Located three *cun* above the tip of the lateral malleolus. It is indicated for external cramping.[40] Three cones of moxibustion can be applied or prick it to bleed.

外踝尖：在外踝尖上三寸。主治外轉筋，可灸七壯，或刺出血。

LJTY: 10-1-4-32 Thumbnail & Big Toenail points (Zhang 1991, 924-5):[41] The *Supplement to a Thousand Pieces of Gold* says: To treat sudden strike by an evil spirit, apply treatment to Ren Zhong [Du 26] below the nose and to the thumbnail and big toenail. Place mugwort cones half on the nail, half on the flesh. Apply seven cones of moxibustion. If it does not stop, use 14 cones the size of sparrow feces.

Also, from the 13 Ghost Points:[42] Insert the needle into the second Ghost Point, pricking below the thumbnail, entering three *fen* into the flesh. This point is named Gui Xin {Ghost Faith].

Also, insert the needle into the third Ghost Point, pricking below the nail of the big toe, entering two *fen* into the flesh. This point is named Gui Lei [Ghost Heap].

Also, to treat frequent urination that is scant and difficult, and frequent seminal loss in males, this formula is very effective: Make the person put their palms together, bringing the two thumbs side by side. Apply moxibustion to the border of the flesh at the corner of the nails. Use one cone on the two thumbs together. Also, apply moxibustion to the big toe the same way as for the hand. Apply three cones on each. In three days, give another session.

---

[39] For Zhou Jian see also **ZJDC: 9-6-6**.

[40] External cramping means cramping in the muscles of the limbs as opposed to abdominal cramping, uterine cramping, etc.

[41] This section is related to **ZJDC: 9-6-1** and **9-6-2**. There is a similar discussion for the Ghost Crying points in Wei Yilin's *Effective Formulas Obtained from Generations of Doctors* (Wei 1996, 141).

[42] The 13 Ghost Points were first described by Sun Simiao. The second and third ghost points (Shao Shang, LU 11, and Yin Bai, SP 1) are the same as these, according to Zhang. This paragraph is paraphrased from Volume 27 of *Supplement* (Sun 1997, 272).

Also, to treat bulging disease and genital swelling, place the feet side by side. Use one mugwort cone on the joined nails of the two big toes. Apply seven cones of moxibustion to the ends of the two nails, right on the corner.

In addition, Qin Chengzu's ghost moxibustion is called the Ghost Crying Point.[43] Take the two thumbs side by side and bind them securely. Use mugwort cones to ride the seam and apply moxibustion to it. Make the fire touch the four places proximal to the two nails including the flesh. If one of the four places does not receive the fire, it is ineffective. Apply seven cones or two times seven cones of moxibustion.

Someone said: Earlier, Qin Chengzu used what was called Hand Ghost Eye.[44] You can also apply treatment to the points between the two big toes along with the hand points, using the same method. These are called Foot Ghost Eye and are used to treat withdrawal, epilepsy, oppressive ghost dreams, and ghost strike. The application of moxibustion to it is greatly effective. It also treats the five epilepsies and feeble-mindedness as well as patterns such as cold damage and mania.

手足大趾爪甲穴：《千金翼》云：治卒中邪魅，鼻下人中，及手足大指爪甲，令艾炷半在爪上，半在肉上，灸七壯，不止，十四壯，炷如雀矢〇有十三鬼穴，於第二次下鍼，刺手大指爪甲下，入肉三分，穴名鬼信〇又第三次下鍼，刺其足大指爪甲下，入肉二分，穴名鬼壘〇又治小便數而少且難，男輒失精，此方甚驗，令其人合掌，並兩大指，灸甲角肉際，兩指共此一壯，亦灸足大指與手同，各三壯，三日一報之〇又治〔疒＋頹〕病陰腫，令並足，合兩拇指爪甲，以一艾炷，灸兩爪端方角上，七壯〇又秦承祖灸鬼法，名鬼哭穴，以兩手大指相並縛定，用艾炷騎縫灸之，令兩甲後連肉四處著火，一處無火則不效，灸七壯，或二七壯〇一曰：前秦承祖所用者，是名手鬼眼。又二穴在兩足大指間，亦與取手穴同法，是名足鬼眼，用

治癲癇夢魘鬼擊，灸之大效，亦治五癇呆癡，及傷寒發狂等證。

LJTY: 10-1-6 The Four Flowers & Six Points of Master Cui (Zhang 1991, 926-7): Whenever males or females have the five taxations and seven damages, qi and blood vacuity detriment, steaming bones, tidal fever, cough, phlegm panting, vexing heat in the five hearts, fatigued and cumbersome limbs, emaciation and weakness, these points treat all such patterns equally.

First, find the first two points: Make the patient stand erect. Take a waxed string approximately three or four *chi* [Chinese feet] long. Do not let it stretch out or contract. Then, make one end of the string even with the tip of the big toe, using the left foot on men and the right on women. Make the string follow the arch until it is behind heel. The patient should step on it firmly. Then, guide the string posteriorly straight up the heel and calf, sticking it to the flesh, until it reaches the bend of the knee. Cut it off at the great horizontal crease at the center of the back of the knee.

Next, make the patient sit up straight. Part his hair, dividing it at the vertex to expose a 'seam' in the center of the head. Place one end of the previously measured waxed string even with the tip of the nose and press it securely. Guide the string up through the part in the hair, nape, and back. Stick it to the flesh, running it down to reach the site at the far end of the string. Mark it with ink. (This is not the moxibustion point.)

Again, take another small string. Make the patient close his mouth. Fold the string in half. Press it securely to the root of the nasal septum. Separate and open the left and right ends. Cut off the string where it reaches the two corners of the mouth. It will be in the shape of the 人 [ren, human] character.

---

[43] Qin Chengzu was a doctor from the Southern and Northern period (Li 1995, 1201). For the Ghost Crying Point, see also **ZJDC: 9-6-1**.
[44] For Hand and Foot Ghost Eye, see also **ZJDC: 9-6-2; LJTY: 11-3-15**.

Then, open out the string horizontally. Place its midpoint on the ink mark that was previously made on the spine. Mark the site at both of the far ends of the string with ink. This corresponds to the first two moxibustion points. It is named Huan Men [Suffering Gate].

In the above method, if a woman's feet are bound, it is difficult to use them as a standard. In that case you should select her right arm, beginning from Jian Yu [LI 15]. Mark it with ink. Extend her arm and lead the string down until it reaches the end of her middle finger. Cut off the string at that point. This can take the place of the method to measure the foot. It is probably suitable.

Second, find two more points: Make the patient sit up straight with the arms a little bent. Wind a length of waxed string behind the nape, doubled forward and hanging down. Cut off the two ends when they are even with the tip of the xiphoid process. Then, turn the string ends around to the back. Take the location of the center bend of the string and press it directly on the Adam's apple. Mark with ink the location on the spine between the lower ends of the string which are hanging down. (This is not the moxibustion point).

Take another small string. Make the patient close his mouth. Measure horizontally and cut it off even with the two corners of the mouth. Go back and add [this string] to the site of the ink mark on the spine. Measure horizontally, as in the earlier method. Mark the location of the two ends. This corresponds to the second two moxibustion points. They are the left and right two points of the Four Flowers.

Apply moxibustion to all of the previous four points at the same time. Initially, apply seven cones, or two times seven, or three times seven cones of moxibustion. Up to 100 cones is wonderful.

Wait until the moxa sores are about to recover or when the fire sores erupt. Then apply moxibustion to two additional points according to the next method.

Next, find two more points: Use the second measurement, [i.e., the corners of the mouth] with the short string. Center the short string vertically from the location of the ink mark on the spine (from the second method). You must make the upper and lower ends stop each other [i.e., make the string tight]. Mark the locations where the string ends with ink. These are the moxibustion points. They are the upper and lower two points of the Four Flowers.

On all the above six points, it is appropriate to select a *li gua* day, a fire [*bing* or *ding*] day, to apply moxibustion to them.

For 100 days after applying moxibustion, it is appropriate for the patient to be careful of sexual taxation, excessive thought and preoccupation, to take seasonable drink and food, keep a balance of cold and heat, and to support, nourish, regulate, and protect himself. If after the sores have healed, you feel that he has still not recovered, apply the previous method of moxibustion again. There is no one who does not recover. That is why it says to use moxibustion continuously until 100 cones are reached.

However, it is not appropriate to use a lot of moxibustion on the two points on the vertebrae. Generally, you can only use three times five cones on these points at one time. When a lot is used, the person may become fatigued.

When you use moxibustion on these six points, it is also appropriate to apply moxibustion to Zu San Li [ST 36] to drain fire. This method is wonderful.

I humbly note that, in the earlier method of applying moxibustion to the four points beside the spine, the upper two points are near the 5th vertebra, Xin Shu [UB 15], and the lower two points are near the 9th vertebra, Gan Shu [UB 18], Cui Zhiti did not indicate point names but instead established this method to find them. He must have wanted it to be easy to explain to people. Thus he verified this method of point location for the spine and back. The greater yang second line [on the back] should be located two *cun* bilateral to the center of the spine in order to obtain exactly the correct vessel.[45] Then, you can reap its effects. It is still appropriate for the one who uses it to examine it.[46]

崔氏四花六穴：凡男婦五勞七傷，氣血虛損，骨蒸潮熱，咳嗽痰喘，五心煩熱，四肢困倦，羸弱等證，並皆治之。第一次先取二穴：令患人平身正立，取一細繩約長三四尺者，蠟之勿令伸縮，乃以繩頭與男左女右足大拇指端比齊，令其順腳心，至後跟踏定，卻引繩向後，從足跟足肚貼肉直上，比至膝灣曲䐐中大橫紋截斷，次令病者平身正坐，解髮分頂，中露頭縫，取所比蠟繩，一頭齊鼻端按定，引繩向上，循頭縫項背，貼肉垂下至繩頭盡處，以墨記之此非灸處。別又取一小繩，令患者合口，將繩雙摺，自鼻柱根按定，左右分開，比至兩口角如人字樣截斷，卻將次繩展直取中，橫加於前記脊背中墨點之上，其兩邊繩頭盡處，以墨記之，此第一次應灸二穴，名曰患門。右法若婦人足小者，難以為則，當取右臂自肩髃穴起，以墨點記，伸手引繩向下，比至中指端截斷，以代量足之法，庶乎得宜。第二次取二穴：令患人平身正坐，稍縮臂膊，取一蠟繩繞項後向前雙垂頭與鳩尾尖齊，雙頭一齊截斷，卻䭰繩頭向後，將此繩中摺處正按結喉上，其繩頭下垂脊間處，以墨記之此非灸穴。又取一小繩，令患人合口，橫量齊兩吻截斷，還加於脊上墨點處，橫量如前法，於兩頭盡處點記之，此是第二次應灸兩穴，即四花之左右二穴也。前共四穴，同時灸之，初灸七壯，或二七、三七壯，以至百壯為妙。俟灸瘡將瘥，或火瘡發時，又依後法灸二穴。後次取二穴：以第二次量口吻短繩，於第二次脊間墨點處，對中直放，務令上下相停，於繩頭盡處以默記之，此是灸穴，即四花之上下二穴也。右共六穴，宜擇離日火日灸之，灸後百日內，宜慎房勞思慮，飲食應時，寒暑得中，將養調護。若瘡愈後，仍覺未瘥，依前再灸，無不愈者，故云累灸至百壯。但脊骨上兩穴不宜多灸，凡一次只可三五壯，多則恐人倦怠。若灸此六穴，亦宜灸足三里瀉火方妙。愚按前法，灸脊旁四穴，

上二穴近五椎，心俞也；下二穴近九椎，肝俞也。崔知悌不指穴名，而但立去法，蓋欲人之易曉耳，然稽之脊背穴法，則太陽二行者，當去脊中各開二寸，方得正脈，乃可獲效，用者仍宜審之。

LJTY: 10-1-7 Ride the Bamboo Horse Moxibustion (Zhang 1991, 927): Indicated for all abscesses, malign sores, eruptions on the back, and female breast abscess. It can treat all this.[47]

The measuring method [is to] use a thin strip of bamboo to measure on the left on males and the right on females. Measure from the horizontal crease at Chi Ze (LU 5), on the center of the elbow, to the tip of the middle finger.[48] Cut or break the bamboo strip even with the place at the extreme end of the flesh as the standard of measurement.

Then use a bamoo carrying pole. Make the patient take off his upper garments and ride the pole with his body erect, remaining stable. Make two people raise up the carrying pole, one in front and one behind. Do not let the patient's legs touch the ground while the two people support him. Do not let him bend over or sway.

Then touch the bamboo strip that was measured earlier to the place on the bamboo carrying pole where the patient sits, below his coccyx, and apply it straight up his spine. Mark the site reached by the other end of the bamboo strip. This is to find the center; it is not the moxibustion point.

Use another thin bamboo strip to measure his middle finger. Use the same body-*cun* method, seeking to determine two *cun*.[49] Each point is one *cun* lateral

---

[45] Zhang is referring to the inner line of the greater yang urinary bladder channel. The governing vessel is the first line. Zhang places the inner bladder line two *cun* lateral to the posterior midline.

[46] Zhang used the method of location given in Li Chan's *Entering the Gate of Medicine*, which followed Wang Tao's *Secret Necessities of a Frontier Official*. Yang used a different method of location. See also **ZJDC: 9-7, 9-10**, the discussion below, and the chapter on timing of treatment.

[47] **JYQS**, Volume 64, adds, "Treats all sores. There is no one who does not recover." 治一切瘡瘍，無有不愈。

[48] **JYQS**, Volume 64, tells us not to include the fingernail in the measurement.

[49] **JYQS**, Volume 64, also says, "Use a thin bamboo strip to measure the place on the middle finger joint between the two horizontal creases. Use the left on males and the right on females. Cut it off as the samebody-*cun* method." ’用薄篾量男左女右手中指節兩橫紋處，截為同身寸法。 He is saying to use the proportional body *cun*, not a standard unit of measurement.

(one edition writes that each point is two *cun* lateral), level with the ink spot on the center of the spine. Apply five times seven cones of moxibustion.

Someone said that when an abscess erupts on the left, apply moxibustion to the right; when an abscess erupts on the right, apply moxibustion to the left. When it is severe, apply moxibustion to both the left and right.

It must be that the heart vessel passes through the site of these two points. Abscesses are always toxins from retained and stagnant heart fire. When moxibustion is applied to this point, heart fire flows freely and the toxins scatter. This method has the ability to raise the dead and return them to life. It is effective every time it is tried.[50]

騎竹馬灸法：主治一切癰疽惡瘡發背，婦人乳癰，皆可治之〇量法：用薄篾一條，以男左女右手臂腕中，白尺澤穴橫紋起，比至中指端，齊肉盡處，截斷為則。卻用竹杠一條，令病者脫去上衣，正身騎定，使兩人前後杠起，令病人腳不著地，仍令二人扶之，勿使偏僂搖動。卻將前所量篾，從竹杠坐處尾骶骨下，著杠比起，貼脊直上，至篾盡處點記之，此取中，非灸穴也。更用薄篾量手中指，用同身寸法，取定二寸，平放於脊中墨點上，各開一寸是穴一本作各開二寸，灸五七壯。一曰：疽發於左則灸右，疽發於右則灸左，甚則左右皆灸。蓋此二穴，乃心脈所過之處。凡癰疽皆心火留滯之毒，灸此則心火流通而毒散矣。起死回生之功，屢試屢驗。

DISCUSSION OF SPECIAL POINTS FOR MOXIBUSTION

Traditionally, certain points were reserved for moxibustion. Other modalities, such as needling, were not discussed in the context of these points. Points of this type include the Si Hua (Four Flowers), Yao Yan (Lumbar Eyes), Zhou Jian (Elbow Tip), Qi Zhu Ma Xue (Ride the Bamboo Horse) points, and San Jiao Jiu (Moxibustion Triangle). Most are non-channel points, but a few points of the 14 channels are recommended for moxibustion only, such as Gao Huang Shu (UB 43) and Shen Que (Ren 8). Additionally, some channel points that are used for acupuncture have special functions when moxibustion is applied, for example, Zu San Li (ST 36) for nourishing life, Bai Hui (Du 20) for raising qi, and Yong Quan (KI 1) for drawing down fire from above.

Many of the traditional non-channel moxibustion points are not located by anatomical landmark. Instead, a string or a straw is used to measure one part of the body and then this measurement is used on another body part. This includes the Four Flowers, Moxibustion Triangle, and Ride the Bamboo Horse points.

Why was this method used to locate points? During the Southern and Northern dynasties (420–581 CE), Chen Yanzhi[51] wrote that moxibustion could be used as a home remedy. It was not necessary to be treated by a doctor. He said, "You must have a teacher before practicing the technique of acupuncture, but even the ordinary person can apply moxibustion. If a teacher has explained the *Classic*,[52] you can readily practice acupuncture-moxibustion. However, if a teacher has not explained the texts, you can apply

---

[50] Li Chan said that "moxibustion on this point courses and drains heart fire" (Li, Y. 1999, 279). In the section on the nineteen disease mechanisms, *Elementary Questions*, Chapter 74 says, "All painful and itching sores are ascribed to the heart." See also **ZJDC: 9-9** and the discussion below.
[51] Chen wrote 陳延之《小品方》 *Short Sketches of Formulas*. This book was lost. However, large portions of it were quoted in later works, especially in the Japanese medical classic *Medical Heart Formulas* 《醫心方》, so we still have access to much of Chen's writings (Li 1995, 129).
[52] *Yellow Emperor's Inner Canon*

moxibustion according to diagrams and explanatory texts."[53] In other words, a person does not need to know detailed theories and surface anatomy or develop skilled hand techniques to practice moxibustion as long as the directions are written so that a layman could understand.

Moxibustion is something the common people could easily use. Mugwort is readily available for free and family traditions can easily be developed and passed down.

In discussing the Four Flower points, Zhang Jiebin noted (**LJTY: 10-1-6**), "Cui Zhiti did not indicate point names but instead established this method to find them. He must have wanted it to be easy to explain to people. Therefore, he verified this method of point location for the spine and back."

Yang Jizhou noted in regard to the same point (**ZJDC: 9-7**), "The ancients feared people did not know how to locate points. So they established this quick method." He speculated that these were probably the same as some of the channel points but warned that people's bodies vary in proportion. Thus we cannot be sure that a nearby channel point is identical. Indeed, we should consider that these may be unique points found from a different perspective of the body. They may not be directly related to the channel system. Maybe the width of the mouth or the distance from the tip of the middle finger to the elbow crease has a relationship to other areas of the body.

We can only speculate on how these points were discovered. Perhaps a trained doctor tried to find a way he could teach his patients to locate a moxibustion point at home. Perhaps a patient tried to find a simple way to locate a point he had observed a doctor

using. Perhaps illiterate folk healers discovered these points on their own. While it is likely that this type of technique was passed down among the common people, some of these points were able to penetrate into the armamentarium of the scholar physicians.

Few eminent doctors spent time researching folk medicine. One notable exception was Zhao Xuemin, who wrote *Stringing Together the Refined*[54] (Unschuld 2000, 36). He wrote sections on moxibustion and the related modalities of steaming, fuming, and ironing. In his chapter on moxibustion, only one channel point was named – San Yin Jiao (SP 6). The other treatments were given directly on the affected site or by a simple anatomical description, such as "in the center of the umbilicus" or the "two depressions below the knee cap." He also included a few methods using a string or straw to aid in location, including Moxibustion Triangle and Ride the Bamboo Horse method. While this book was written approximately 200 years after Yang and Zhang, there is no reason to believe that folk methods were significantly different at an earlier time.

Below, I discuss a few of the special moxibustion points in detail.

The Four Flowers (ZJDC: 9-7 and LJTY: 10-1-6)

The first extant mention of the Four Flowers was in Volume 13 of *Secret Necessities of a Frontier Official*,[55] published in 752. The author, Wang Tao, listed their location, indications, and treatment method. Wang simply called these points the "Four Flowers." He did not equate them with regular channel points. Wang attributed them to Master Cui Zhiti,[56] an earlier Tang dynasty doctor. Unfortunately, Master Cui's writings have since been lost.

The Four Flowers were described in a number of

---

[53] 夫針術，須師乃行，其灸則凡人便施。為師解經者，針灸隨手而行，非師所解文者，但依圖，詳文則可灸。《醫心方・卷二・灸例法》 (Tamba 1993, 69)

[54] Zhao Xuemin (Qing, c. 1720-1805) 趙學敏《串雅・外篇・卷二・灸法門》 (Zhao 1998, 189-93).

[55] 王燾《外台秘要》

[56] Cui wrote *Moxibustion Formulas for Steaming Bones Disease* 崔知悌《骨蒸病灸方》.

books over the centuries, and a simplified location method appeared after a while. The *Classic of Nourishing Life* became an influential text. It contained the simplified method. In 1537, Gao Wu quoted from *Nourishing Life* when he described the Four Flowers. Gao may have been the first to name these points as Ge Shu (UB 17) and Dan Shu (UB 19). Yang Jizhou used the writings of Gao as his template for the Four Flowers passage in the *Great Compendium* about 65 years later. The wording is almost identical. Modern books generally follow Yang and Gao in saying that the Four Flowers are Ge Shu and Dan Shu.

Other authors, for example Li Chan,[57] stayed faithful to the location method described by Wang Tao. Zhang Jiebin followed this line of transmission in his *Illustrated Supplement*. Yang Jizhou also must have read Li Chan's description of the Four Flowers since he quoted Li for other point locations. However, he chose to follow Gao Wu's lineage.

Not only did Yang Jizhou and Zhang Jiebin locate the Four Flowers in different manners, but Zhang said that the Four Flowers actually consisted of six points; whereas Yang said four points belong to this cluster.

Zhang called his method "The Four Flowers and Six Points of Master Cui." He included Huan Men (Suffering Gate).[58] Zhang's Four Flowers consist of two points on the spine and two points lateral to the spine.

Yang's simplified method ends up with only four points, all lateral to the spine, in the vicinity of Ge Shu and Dan Shu. He also discussed the point Zhang called Suffering Gate, but named it Lao Xue (Taxation Point). Yang included this Taxation Point in the

same part of his book as the Four Flowers (**ZJDC: 9-10**), but it was not included as part of the grouping. Yang and Zhang both identified this point as Xin Shu (UB 15).

Both doctors described the folk method of moxibustion point location using a waxed string to measure the patient's body. The string is waxed so it can stick to the flesh; this makes the measurement more accurate as the string is less likely to slip out of place.

Based on the language used and the similarity of the method, Zhang must have taken Li Chan's *Entering the Gate* as his source (Li, Y. 1999, 279). Li discussed the theory behind these points, "Altogether there are six points. They have the image of *kan* and *li* in *Already Completed* (*Ji Ji*)." This refers to Hexagram 63 of the *Book of Changes* (*Yi Jing*). *Already Completed* is considered an auspicious hexagram. Every line is in order. Fire (*li*) and water (*kan*) communicate with each other. Water is located above and descends; fire is below and ascends. In this way, they move toward each other.[59]

TRIGRAMS	HEXAGRAM 63 ALREADY COMPLETED
kan (water)	
li (fire)	

Suffering Gate point

the Four Flowers

---

[57] Li Chan (16th c., Ming) wrote *Entering the Gate of Medicine*, published in 1575.

[58] The name, Suffering Gate (悲門 Huan Men) seems to come from Li Chan's *Entering the Gate*. Wang Tao did not give this point a name. However, he discussed it in the same section as the rest of the Four Flowers.

[59] Think of this like a pot of water on a stove. The water will boil. If the fire were on top and the water below, they would move away from each other. There would be no interaction, no circulation.

While a hexagram has six lines and the six points of the Four Flowers only have four lines, the image is there. In Hexagram 63, *Already Completed*, the top line is yin. From there down, yin and yang lines alternate.[60] Suffering Gate and the horizontal two points of the Four Flowers resemble yin lines since they are bilateral. The two points on the spine in the Four Flowers resemble yang lines as they have only one component. In addition, they are located on the governing vessel, the most yang part of the channel system.

Hexagram 63 has every line in its proper position.[61] In addition, the image of fire and water communicating signifies the proper interaction of heart and kidneys or the balance of yin and yang. This image is a confirmation that the six points of the Four Flowers have the ability to put all aspects of the body in proper order.

Li Chan also discussed the simplified method of finding the Four Flowers, the same method Yang used. He called this configuration the "channel gate four flowers"[62] and said that in this case, "the meaning is that the *li gua* [or trigram] has mutated into the *kun gua* [or trigram], downbearing heart fire to engender spleen earth. Like this, it is appropriate for all yang vacuity."[63]

So, according to Li Chan, the original method is better used to harmonize fire and water, yin and yang, heart and kidneys. The simplified (Channel Gate) method is more for supplementation of the spleen, especially spleen yang, but is unlikely to have the side effect of fire flaring upward. This because it simultaneously downbears heart fire.

Zhang suggested applying moxibustion to these six

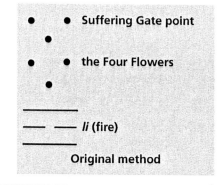

Original method

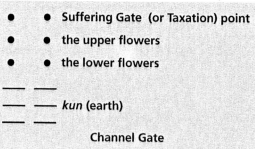

Channel Gate

points on fire days based on the heavenly stems. This would increase the amount of yang or fire that the moxibustion engenders in the treatment. Even though this point is often used in yin vacuity, we can apply Zhu Danxi's theory of moxibustion: "This is to supplement yang, because when yang is generated, yin is [also] generated."[64] Or as Dou Cai stated during the Song dynasty, "Qi is yang, which is life. This is why you must die when yang qi is exhausted."[65]

Zhang was aware that this treatment could have side effects due to heat. He noted that after applying moxibustion to these six points, moxibustion should also be applied to Zu San Li (ST 36) to drain any resulting fire that might flare up.

---

[60] A yin line is broken, and has two components. A yang line is unbroken, and has one component.

[61] In other words, yin lines are in yin positions and yang lines are in yang positions. The 1st (bottom), 3rd, and 5th positions are yang. The 2nd, 4th, and 6th (top) positions are yin.

[62] 經門四花

[63] 以離卦變作坤卦，降心火生脾上之意也，　然此皆陽虛所宜。(Li, Y. 1999, 279)

[64] 大病虛脫，本是陰虛，用艾丹田者，所以補陽，陽生則陰生故也。《金匱鉤玄・腳氣》 *Probing into the Subtleties of the Golden Cabinet* (Zhu 2000, 114). The idea that "when yang is generated, yin is [also] generated" comes from *Elementary Questions*, Chapter 5 (Wu and Wu 1997, 31).

[65] 氣者陽所生也。故陽氣盡必死。《扁鵲心書・卷上・須識扶陽》(Dou 2000, 8)

Ride the Bamboo Horse Moxibustion

"Riding the Bamboo Horse" is the name of a non-channel point on the back. To find the point, measure the patient from the tip of the middle finger (not counting the nail) to the elbow crease. Use this length to measure from the tip of the coccyx straight up, while the patient straddles a bamboo pole. The point is one *cun* bilateral, although Yang and Zhang note that it might be 1.5 or two *cun* lateral. A modern doctor, Li Zhiming, speculates that this point is equivalent to Ge Shu (UB 17) (Chen and Deng, 1989, 217).

Bamboo Horse moxibustion is a type of direct suppurating moxibustion. Its earliest mention was during the Song dynasty, in Dongxuan Jushi's *Precious Book of Protecting and Aiding* (He 2003, 36-7).[66] This one-volume book discusses treatment of external diseases such as abscesses (Li, 1995, 398).

When Wenren Qi'nian wrote *Moxibustion for Emergencies*,[67] he also included the Bamboo Horse method for treating acute patterns with abscesses (Li, 1995, 1151). The Bamboo Horse method caught on and later doctors, such as Xu Feng (Huang 1996, 540-1), Li Chan (Li, C. 1999, 279-80), Yang (**ZJDC: 9-9**), and Zhang (**LJTY: 10-1-7, LJTY: 11-3-23**) included it in their books.

Dongxuan Jushi explained how these points could treat abscesses (Dongxuan Jushi 1989, 29-30):

> It must be that these two points are where the heart vessel arises. Generally all abscesses are engendered from heart fire that is retained and stagnant. When moxibustion is applied to these two points, heart fire immediately flows freely. Recovery will come before three days pass. It can raise the dead and rescue someone from danger. It has uncommon merits. If tried repeatedly, it will have repeated results. *Elementary Questions* says, 'All painful and itching sores are ascribed to the heart.'[68] It also says that when construction qi is not harmonious, it counterflows into the flesh and consequently engenders abscesses and swellings.[69] Construction qi is blood. The heart is able to move blood. When blood is already stagnant, the vessels do not move, so it counterflows into the flesh and consequently engenders abscesses and swellings. Applying moxibustion to these two points regulates and extends heart fire, the blood vessels spontaneously flow freely, and recovery is better than with medicinals.

Wenren Qi'nian agreed that stagnant heart fire is the cause of abscesses and that applying moxibustion on these points assists heart fire to become unblocked. He added (Zhang 1994, 66):

> There must be something wonderful in suspending the whole body by riding on the bamboo pole so that the twin passes of the coccyx do not allow flowing and pouring. As soon as the moxibustion is finished on the two points and the patient gets off the bamboo pole, the moxibustion fire promptly accompanies the flowing and pouring, first reaching the coccyx with heat like steam, also passing through the two external kidneys [male genitalia], which completely feel the steaming heat. In a little while it resumes its flow into the foot and the Yong Quan [KI 1] point, and then ascends from below, little by little circulating through the entire body. It has remarkable merits and uncommon efficacy. The source [of its efficacy] must be in this.

The coccyx is one of the three passes where qi circulation in the governing vessel is easily obstructed (Deadman *et al.* 1998, 535). The deer is a symbol of immortality or longevity. Certain types are said to live for one or two thousand years (Li 1989, 15). In Volume 51 of the *Great Pharmacopeia*, Li Shizhen tells us, "When a deer sleeps, its mouth faces its coccyx in order to allow free passage through the

---

[66] 東軒居士, literally, "Scholar who Resides on the Eastern Veranda" (12th c.), 《衛濟寶書》.
[67] 聞人耆年, literally, "Knowledgeable Aged Person" (Song, dates unknown), 《備急灸法》, one volume, published in 1226.
[68] Chapter 74 (Wu and Wu 1997, 457)
[69] Paraphrased from Chapter 3 (Wu and Wu 1997, 20).

governing vessel" (Li 1996, 1191). The anterior branch of the governing vessel also passes through the heart (Deadman *et al.* 1998, 530).

Wenren Qi'nian seems to theorize that stagnant heart fire engenders abscesses. By placing the patient on the pole, the lower pass of the coccyx is blocked by the pressure of the pole. However, sitting on a pole like this would open up the governing vessel by curving the spine like a sleeping deer. When the patient gets off the pole, the combination of the opening of the spine, the qi of the moxibustion, and the sudden release of the pass at the coccyx enables the stagnant heart fire to break through and circulate through the entire body. This also has the image of the communication of fire and water, heart and kidneys, as it involves the governing vessel, the genitals and Yong Quan (KI 1). When fire and water circulate, yin and yang are harmonious, and there is health.

Since the time when the Bamboo Horse method was devised, doctors who use it have tried to design an easier way to achive the correct posture in the patient. Yang discussed this problem, feeling it was better to rest the pole on two stools, rather than on the shoulders of two men. He Puren (2003, 36) includes a drawing for a modern "horse." It looks like a padded sawhorse with handlebars for the patient to lean on:

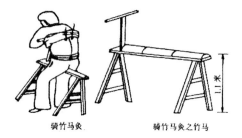

骑竹马灸   骑竹马灸之竹马

Gao Huang Shu (UB 43)

The above points are non-channel points that are reserved for moxibustion only. Some channel points also have a special relationship with moxibustion. Two examples are discussed here: Gao Huang Shu (UB 43), a point that is rarely used with acupuncture, and Zu San Li (ST 36), a point that is commonly treated with acupuncture as well as moxibustion.

Moxibustion has been applied to Gao Huang Shu for centuries to treat vacuity taxation and emaciation. It is located three *cun* lateral to the lower border of the spinous process of the 4th thoracic vertebra, on the medial border of the scapula.

What does the name mean? It comes from the old histories. *Zuo's Commentary on the Spring and Autumn Annals* recounts that in 518 BCE, Doctor Huan said of Prince Jing of Jin, "His illness cannot be handled. The disease is located above the *huang* and below the *gao*.[70] It cannot be attacked. Penetrating cannot reach it. Medicinals cannot treat it." It is generally agreed that "penetrating" indicates the needle stone and "attacking" refers to moxibustion (He 2003, 2; Duan 1984, 4; Wang 1984, 2).

Sun Simiao was the first to mention the point called Gao Huang Shu (Li 1995, 1667). He said that the Prince of Jin could not be saved because Doctor Huan did not know this point. Sun recommended moxibustion, not acupuncture, as the treatment of choice for Gao Huang Shu. He stated, "There is nothing that Gao Huang Shu does not treat... When this moxibustion is completed, it allows a person's yang qi to become healthy and prosperous."[71] Sun recommended 600 or 1,000 cones on each side.

Since Sun Simiao described Gao Huang Shu, it has been included in almost every book about acupuncture and moxibustion. A book called *Moxibustion on Gao Huang Shu [UB 43]* was written by Zhuang Chuo[72] during the Southern Song dynasty. It is a treatise on the treatment of consumption with moxibustion. He included textual research, diagrams,

---

[70] The *gao* is the region below the heart; the *huang* is the region above the diaphragm, so the *gao huang* is "the region below the heart and above the diaphragm. When a disease is said to have entered the *gao huang*, it is difficult to cure" (Wiseman 1998, 239).
[71] 《千金要方・卷四十・雜病》 *Prescriptions*, Volume 30 (Sun 1997b, 1088).
[72] 莊綽 《灸膏肓俞穴法》 published in 1127.

and his own comments on the location and treatment methods for Gao Huang Shu (He 2003, 6). This book was included as one of the *Four Books on Acupuncture-moxibustion* during the Yuan dynasty[73] (Huang 2003, 633).

Wei Yilin wrote *Effective Formulas Obtained from Generations of Doctors*, an encyclopedic treatment manual. He collected numerous moxibustion formulas, for example: "To treat extreme vacuity, apply moxibustion to Gao Huang Shu and Qi Hai [Ren 6]; the more cones, the more wonderful."

During the Ming dynasty, Li Chan shortened the name of this point to Gao Huang. Afterwards, many used this as the point's name (Li 1999, 278). Yang Jizhou directly quoted Li Chan when he wrote about Gao Huang Shu (**ZJDC: 9-8**) and declared, "No one does not respond to the application of moxibustion to the two points of Gao Huang." However, Yang also worried about a side effect of moxibustion on this point, "After applying moxibustion, if the patient feels congestion and fullness of qi, you can apply moxibustion to Qi Hai [Ren 6] and Zu San Li [ST 36] to drain down fire repletion."

Many Ming dynasty doctors recommended the application of moxibustion to points on the lower body for this reason. For example, Gao Wu suggested using Qi Hai (Ren 6), Dan Tian (Ren 5), Guan Yuan (Ren 4), Zhong Ji (Ren 3), or Zu San Li (ST 36) in *Gatherings from Eminent Acupuncturists*.

Yang explained in Volume 6 of his *Great Compendium,* "Just after 20 years of age a person can apply moxibustion to these two points (Gao Huang). They should still apply moxibustion to San Li [ST 36] bilaterally. This draws fire qi to move downward in order to secure the root. If one has not yet left childhood and applies moxibustion to Gao Huang, fire qi may become exuberant and the upper burner will become hot."

Zhang Jiebin also wrote with enthusiasm about Gao Huang (**LJTY: 7-1**). The most striking thing in the writings of all these doctors is the amount of confidence they had in the ability of moxibustion on Gao Huang Shu to cure intractable and serious disease. As Yang Jizhou said, "Generations all take this point as having the marvel of raising the dead and returning life." It is certainly a point we should keep in our armamentarium.

The Four Flowers, the Bamboo Horse points, and Gao Huang serve as representatives of special moxibustion points in general. It can be seen that they have their own history and development, methods for location, and functions. They also were very effective in treatment, prevention, and nourishing life in the eyes of many respected doctors of the past.

---

[73] 《針灸四書》 published in 1312.

CHAPTER 7
POINTS CONTRAINDICATED FOR MOXIBUSTION

Both Yang and Zhang presented memorization poems regarding points contraindicated for moxibustion. Li Shizhen did not discuss point contraindications. In these poems, none of the words are important except the point names. The other words are only there to help with the rhythm and rhyme. The poems from Zhang Jiebin and Yang Zizhou list the points in a different order. A discussion and comparison will follow.

FORBIDDEN POINTS ACCORDING TO YANG JIZHOU

ZJDC: 4-27 Contraindicated Moxibustion Points Song (45 Points) (Huang 1996, 871)
《針灸大成・禁灸穴歌・卷之四》

Introduction

This is a poem of seven characters per line. It has two parts. The first part, on acupuncture contraindications, is not translated here. What follows is the second part

which lists points contraindicated for moxibustion. Yang attributes it to *Great Completion of Unified Ancient and Modern Medicine* by Xu Chunfu. (Li 1995, 373)[139] This poem is also identical to the corresponding section of Li Chan's *Entering the Gate of Medicine*.

Ya Men [Du 15], Feng Fu [Du 16], and Tian Zhu [UB 10] are elevated;
Cheng Guang [UB 6], Lin Qi [GB 15], and Tou Wei [ST 8] are at the same level.
Si Zhu [SJ 23], Zan Zhu [UB 2], and Jing Ming [UB 1] points,
Su Liao [Du 25], He Liao [LI 19], and Ying Xiang [LI 20] are a sequence.
Quan Liao [SI 18], Xia Guan [ST 7], and Ren Ying [ST 9] go.
Tian You [SJ 16], Tian Fu [LU 3], up to Zhou Rong [SP 20],
Yuan Ye [GB 22], Ru Zhong [ST 17], and Jiu Wei [Ren 15] below.

---

¹ 徐春甫《古今醫統大全》, published in 1556 (Ming).

Fu Ai [SP 16], seek for Jian Zhen [SI 9] behind the arm.

Yang Chi [SJ 4], Zhong Chong [PC 9], and Shao Shang [LU 11] points,

Yu Ji [LU 10] and Jing Qu [LU 8] move forward as one.

Di Wu [GB 42], Yang Guan [GB 33], and Ji Zhong [Du 6] govern.

Yin Bai [SP 1], Lou Gu [SP 7], passing through Yin Ling [SP 9].

Tiao Kou [ST 38], Du Bi [ST 35], and Yin Shi [ST 33] above,

Fu Tu [ST 32], Bi Guan [ST 31], and Shen Mai [UB 62] welcome.

Wei Zhong [UB 40], Yin Men [UB 37], and Cheng Fu [UB 36] above,

Bai Huan [UB 30] and Xin Shu [UB 15] are on the same channel.

Apply moxibustion and do not needle, needle and do not apply moxibustion.

Because of this, when needling the channels, always repeat the instructions.

The vulgar healer uses acupuncture and moxibustion at the same time,

Making the patient endure fire torture punishment[2] in vain.

啞門風府天柱擎，承光臨泣頭維平，
絲竹攢竹晴明穴，素髎禾髎迎香程，
顴髎下關人迎去，天牖天府到周榮，
淵液乳中鳩尾下，腹哀臂後尋肩貞，
陽池中沖少商穴，魚際經渠一順行，
地五陽關脊中主，隱白漏谷通陰陵，
條口犢鼻上陰市，伏兔髀關申脈迎，
委中殷門承扶上，白環心俞同一經。
灸而勿針針勿灸，針經爲此嘗叮嚀，
庸醫針灸一齊用，徒施患者炮烙刑。

FORBIDDEN POINTS ACCORDING TO ZHANG JIEBIN

LJTY: 4-26 Song of Contraindicated Moxibustion Points (47 Points) (Zhang 1991, 800)
《類經圖翼・四卷・禁灸穴歌》〔四十七穴〕

Introduction

In Volume 4 of the *Illustrated Supplement*, Zhang discusses points and times that are contraindicated for acupuncture and moxibustion, and some guidelines for using acupuncture and moxibustion. This poem, like Yang's has seven characters per line.

There are 47 points that are contraindicated for moxibustion.

Cheng Guang [UB 6], Ya Men [Du 15], and Feng Fu [Du 16] are contrary,

Jing Ming [UB 1], Zan Zhu [UB 2], below them Ying Xiang [LI 20],

Tian Zhu [UB 10], Su Liao [Du 25], above them Lin Qi [GB 15],

Nao Hu [Du 17], Er Men [SJ 21], and Chi Mai [SJ 18] flow freely,

He Liao [LI 19], Quan Liao [SI 18], and Si Zhu Kong [SJ 23],

Tou Wei [ST 8], Xia Guan [ST 7], and Ren Ying [ST 9],

Jian Zhen [SI 9], Tian You [SJ 16], and Xin Shu [UB 15] together,

Ru Zhong [ST 17], Ji Zhong [Du 6], and Bai Huan Shu [UB 30],

Jiu Wei [Ren 15], Yuan Ye [GB 22], like Zhou Rong [SP 20],

Fu Ai [SP 16], Shao Shang [LU 11], and Yu Ji [LU 10],

Jing Qu [LU 8], Tian Fu [LU 3], and Zhong Chong [PC 9],

Yang Chi [SJ 4], Yang Guan [GB 33], and Di Wu Hui [GB 42],

Lou Gu [SP 7], Yin Ling [SP 9], and Tiao Kou [ST 38] meet,

---

[2] 炮烙刑 *pao lao xing*: "An ancient torture or punishment by ordering a prisoner to walk on a slippery metal beam kept hot by coal underneath" (Zhang 1992, 824). The metal beam must represent acupuncture and the hot coals represent moxibustion when used improperly.

Avoid Yin Men [UB 37], Shen Mai [UB 62], and
Cheng Fu [UB 36],
Fu Tu [ST 32], Bi Guan [ST 31], including Wei
Zhong [UB 40],
Yin Shi [ST 33] flowing down to seek Du Bi [ST 35],
Cease attacking all these points by means of mug-
wort fire.

禁灸之穴四十七，承光啞門風府逆。
睛明攢竹下迎香，天柱素髎上臨泣。
腦戶耳門瘈脈通，禾髎顴髎絲竹空。
頭維下關人迎等，肩貞天牖心俞同。
乳中脊中白環腧，鳩尾淵液如周榮。
腹哀少商并魚際，經渠天府及中衝。
陽池陽關地五會，漏谷陰陵條口逄。
殷市申脈承扶忌，伏兔髀關連委中。
陰市下行尋犢鼻，諸穴休將艾火攻。

DISCUSSION

Yang and Zhang agreed on 44 of the points that are
forbidden for moxibustion. There were four points
that were listed by only one of these two authors.

Many of these points are on the head or face near
the sense orifices. Others are over major arteries or
sensitive structures such as the nipples. Reasons for
prohibiting moxibustion at some of these points are
not so obvious.

In the *Illustrated Supplement to the Categorized Classic*,
Volumes 6-8, Zhang goes over the channel points
one by one. In some of these he gives the reason
that a point is contraindicated for moxibustion or
discusses the original source forbidding that point.
Zhang describes the adverse affect if moxibustion is
applied to the following points:

- **Tian Fu (LU 3):** Applying moxibustion to it
makes a person's qi counterflow. **LJTY: 6-1-3**

- **Jing Qu (LU 8):** When moxibustion is applied,
it damages a person's spirit brightness. **LJTY: 6-1-8**

- **Ru Zhong (ST 17):** Zhang said that "the notes
[of Wang Bing] for *Elementary Questions*, Chapter 59 say, 'Pricking and moxibustion on it engender consuming sores.'" **LJTY: 6-3-17**

POINTS CONTRAINDICATED IN THE *GREAT COMPENDIUM* AND THE *ILLUSTRATED SUPPLEMENT TO THE CATEGORIZED CLASSIC*		
CONTRAINDICATED BY BOTH	YANG ADDS	ZHANG ADDS
LU 3, LU 8, LU 10, LU 11		
LI 19, LI 20		
ST 7, ST 8, ST 9, ST 17, ST 31, ST 32, ST 33, ST 35, ST 38		
SP 7, SP 9, SP 16, SP 20	SP 1	
SI 9, SI 18		
UB 1, UB 2, UB 6, UB 10, UB 15, UB 30, UB 36, UB 37, UB 40, UB 62		
PC 9		
SJ 4, SJ 16, SJ 23		SJ 18, SJ 21
GB 15, GB 22, GB 33, GB 42		
Ren 15		
Du 6, Du 15, Du 16, Du 25		Du 17
Total	45	47

- **Tian You (SJ 16):** Not suitable for moxibustion. Moxibustion makes people's face swell up. The *Classic of Nourishing Life* says, "Apply one cone of moxibustion." The *Systematic Classic* says, "Apply three cones of moxibustion." **LJTY: 7-4-16**

- **Si Zhu Kong (SJ 23):** Moxibustion is contraindicated. Applying moxibustion to it is not fortunate. It makes people's eyes small and blind. **LJTY: 7-4-23**

- **Yuan Ye (GB 22):** Moxibustion is contraindicated. Applying moxibustion to it is not fortunate. It engenders swollen consuming saber lumps and open sores. When they ulcerate internally, the patient will die. **LJTY: 8-1**

- **Di Wu Hui (GB 42):** Moxibustion is contraindicated. The *Systematic Classic* says, "Applying moxibustion to it makes a person thin. They will die before three years have passed." **LJTY: 8-1-41**

- **Ji Zhong (Du 6):** Moxibustion is contraindicated. When moxibustion is applied, it makes a person hunchbacked. **LJTY: 8-4-6**

- **Ya Men (Du 15):** Moxibustion is contraindicated. Applying moxibustion to it makes a person mute. **LJTY: 8-4-15**

- **Feng Fu (Du 16):** Moxibustion is contraindicated. When moxibustion is applied, it makes a person lose his voice. **LJTY: 8-4-16**

- **Nao Hu (Du 17):** Zhang said acupuncture and moxibustion are both contraindicated, and moxibustion makes a person lose their voice. **LJTY: 8-4-17**

- Without giving any details, Zhang simply said moxibustion is contraindicated on Ying Xiang (LI 20), Tou Wei (ST 8), Ren Ying (ST 9), Quan Liao (SI 18), Cheng Guang (UB 6), Xi Yang Guan (GB 33), and Su Liao (Du 25), all listed in the poem above.

There are also a number of points not mentioned by the poem that are said by Zhang or another source to be forbidden for moxibustion. Zhang described the side effects of moxibustion or contraindications for some of these points. Most of these are based on the patient's condition, and are not universal contraindications.

- **Qi Chong (ST 30):** The *Systematic Classic* says, "Moxibustion is not fortunate. It makes a person unable to get his breath." **LJTY: 6-3-30**

- **Da Du (SP 2):** Overall, in the case of pregnant women, regardless of which month they are in, and women less than 100 days after childbirth, moxibustion is not appropriate. **LJTY: 6-4-2**

- **Da Dun (LV 1):** Pregnant women before and after childbirth are unsuitable for moxibustion. **LJTY: 8-2-1**

- **Ming Men (Du 4):** Someone said, "… Apply 27 cones of moxibustion. If 20 years old or above, applying moxibustion may terminate childbearing." **LJTY: 8-4-4**

- **Xia Guan (ST 7):** Zhang said three cones are allowed. He adds, "If there is dried wax in the ear, moxibustion is contraindicated." **LJTY: 6-3-7**

- **Xi Yan (Eyes of the Knee) (Zhang 1991, 922-3):** In the past, there were people with knee pain who applied moxibustion to this point resulting in failure to rise [impotence]. Because of this, moxibustion is contraindicated. **LJTY: 10-1-4-14**

For the following points, Zhang mentioned that some sources say the point is contraindicated and others do not.

- **Shao Shang (LU 11):** Moxibustion is unsuitable. The *Systematic Classic* says, "Apply one cone of moxibustion." Another [unnamed book] says three cones. **LJTY: 6-1-11**

- **Bi Guan (ST 31):** Zhang said three cones are allowed but adds, "Someone said, 'Prick three fen. Moxibustion is contraindicated.'" **LJTY: 6-3-31**

- **Fu Tu (ST 32):** Zhang said moxibustion is contraindicated but adds that "*Thousand Pieces of Gold* says, 'For mania evil with ghost talk, apply 100 cones of moxibustion. You can also apply 50 cones.'" **LJTY: 6-3-32**

- **Yin Shi (ST 33):** Zhang said moxibustion is contraindicated, but added that "the notes [of Wang Bing] on *Elementary Questions*, Chapter 41 say, 'In the depression below Fu Tu [ST 32], apply three cones of moxibustion,' meaning this point." **LJTY: 6-3-33**

- **Zan Zhu (UB 2):** Zhang wrote, "Moxibustion is not appropriate" but added that the *Systematic Classic* recommends three cones. LJTY: 7-1-2

- **Da Zhu (UB 11):** Apply five or seven cones of moxibustion. Someone said that moxibustion is contraindicated. If there is no great urgency, you cannot apply moxibustion to it. **LJTY: 7-1-11**

- **Xin Shu (UB 15):** "Note that the *Systematic Classic* says moxibustion is contraindicated. Thus, generations of doctors all say that that Xin Shu can be needled but moxibustion cannot be applied to it. It is remarkable they do not know that when pricking hits the heart, the patient will die in one day. This is a warning from *Elementary Questions* [Chapter 52], so how can it be easy to needle? *Prescriptions Worth a Thousand Pieces of Gold* says for wind striking the heart, quickly apply 100 cones of moxibustion to Xin Shu and take Xu Ming Tang [Life-prolonging Decoction]. This book also said to apply 100 cones of moxibustion for counterflow vomiting with inability to eat. You also must determine whether it is urgent or not." Zhang also quoted the *Shennong Classic* as recommending five grains of wheat-size cones for certain conditions. **LJTY: 7-1-15**

- **Bai Huan Shu (UB 30):** Zhang said you can apply three cones of moxibustion but added that the *Systematic Classic* says that moxibustion cannot be used. **LJTY: 7-1-27**

- **Yang Chi (SJ 4):** Zhang said you can apply three cones of moxibustion but that the *Bronze Man Classic* says moxibustion is contraindicated. However, *Thousand Pieces of Gold* allows 50 cones for dry mouth from wasting-thirst. **LJTY: 7-4-4**

- **Jiu Wei (Ren 15):** Zhang said acupuncture and moxibustion are both contraindicated but an unnamed book allows three cones. **LJTY: 8-3-15**

- Zhang noted that a small amount (three or seven cones) are allowed on the following points but that some other unnamed source said moxibustion is contraindicated: Jing Ming (UB 1), Tian Zhu (UB 10), Wei Zhong (UB 40), Chi Mai (SJ 18), Er Men (SJ 21) (three cones for each of the above). Lin Qi (GB 15) (seven cones).

Zhang's *Song of Contraindicated Moxibustion Points* does not seem to be rigorously applied. Zhang discussed the application of moxibustion for the following points without even noting that it was listed as contraindicated in the poem:

- **Yin Ling (SP 9):** Zhang said three cones are allowed. He also quoted Sun Simiao and the *Shennong Classic* as recommending different amounts of cones for different ailments. **LJTY: 6-4-9**

• **Shen Mai (UB 62):** Zhang said you can apply three cones of moxibustion and that the *Shen Nong Classic* recommends five cones for lumbar pain. **LJTY: 7-1-59**

• **Zhong Chong (PC 9):** Zhang said one cone of moxibustion can be applied and that the *Shen Nong Classic* recommends one grain of wheat-size cone for certain pediatric conditions. **LJTY: 7-3-9**

• Without discussing the fact that elsewhere the point is listed as contraindicated, Zhang noted that a small amount of moxibustion is allowed on the following points: Yu Ji (LU 10), He Liao (LI 19), Du Bi (ST 35), Tiao Kou (ST 38), Lou Gu (SP 7), Jian Zhen (SI 9), Cheng Fu (UB 36), and Yin Men (UB 37) (all the above, three cones each). Fu Ai (SP 16) and Zhou Rong (SP 20) (these last two, five cones each).

From this, it seems clear that there is no consensus on points forbidden to moxibustion. The best method is probably to avoid most points that are contraindicated when possible. If moxibustion is to be applied, common sense says that only a small number of cones should be used in more urgent situations.

CHAPTER 8

THE MATERIALS OF MOXIBUSTION

This section contains passages regarding the materials used in moxibustion. Obviously, mugwort is discussed. However, sometimes other materials are applied as moxibustion. In addition, certain medicinals are used as isolating substances for indirect moxa or powdered and mixed with the mugwort.

The majority of the passages in this chapter were authored by Li Shizhen. However, Yang Jizhou and Zhang Jiebin also discussed the properties of mugwort in regard to moxibustion, and Zhang examined a few other medicinals in this context.

In the *Great Pharmacopoeia*, Li Shizhen not only described the method of gathering, the properties, preparation, and functions of each substance, he also gave sample formulas. These are included below if they involve moxibustion, fuming, ironing, or related external heat treatments.

MUGWORT

Mugwort is the main substance burned in moxibustion. All three authors wrote sections on mugwort and its use in moxibustion.

Chapter Contents

Li Shizhen on Mugwort

BCGM: 15-05 Mugwort (*Records of Famous Doctors:*[1] Medium Grade) (Li 1996, 435)

《本草綱目・草部第十五卷・草之四・艾》
（《別錄》中品）

Explanation of the name

- Ice Platform [Bing Tai], *Er Ya;*[2]

---

[1] 《名醫別錄》 [*Ming Yi Bie Lu*] *Records of Famous Doctors* is frequently mentioned in Li Shizhen's writings. The name of the compiler has been lost, although some say it is a Dr. Tao, perhaps Tao Hongjing. It was probably written at the end of the Han dynasty (Li 1995, 601). From now on, I will not include the Chinese and pinyin for this source.

[2] *Er Ya* is an ancient book containing commentaries on the classics.

- Medicinal Herb [Yi Cao], *Records of Famous Doctors*;
- Yellow Herb [Huang Cao], *Pi Ya*;
- Mugwort Wormwood [Ai Hao].

Li Shizhen says: Wang Anshi's *Character Explanation* [*Zi Shuo*] said: Mugwort can *cut out* illness [like cutting weeds].[3] If it is aged for a long time, it is better quality. That is why the character for mugwort is from *cutting out*.

Lu Dian, the author of *Pi Ya* said: *Records of Nature Studies* [*Bo Wu Zhi*] says that in ancient times, ice was cut to make a sphere. It was raised towards the sun, and mugwort was held under it to receive the "shadow." This was how they obtained fire. Therefore, mugwort was named "ice platform." This might be possible.

Medical doctors use it to apply moxibustion to hundreds of diseases. Thus it is called "moxibustion herb." One burning of it is called one "invigoration" [*zhuang*], taking the invigoration of a person as the standard.[4]

【釋名】冰臺《爾雅》、醫草《別錄》、黃草《埤雅》、艾蒿。時珍曰：王安石《字說》云：艾可疾，久而彌善，故字從 。陸佃《埤雅》云：《博物志》言削冰令圓，舉而向日，以艾承其影則得火。則艾名冰臺，其以此乎？醫家用灸百病，故曰灸草。一灼謂之一壯，以壯人為法也。

Gathering explanation

Records of Famous Doctors says: Mugwort leaf grows in the wild. Pick it on the third day of the third lunar month and dry it in the sun.

Su Song[5] said: Every place has it. The mugwort from Fudao and Siming is best. It is said that when this type is used in moxibustion of the hundred diseases, it is especially superb. At the beginning of spring, its sprouts spread across the earth. The stalks resemble Hao [Herba Artemisiae Scopariae]. The back of the leaf is white. It is better to use the short sprouts. Pick the leaf on the third day of the third lunar month or the fifth day of the fifth lunar month and dry it in the sun. It can only be used when it has been aged.

Li Shizhen says: The ancient pharmacopeias did not write about the location where mugwort leaf originated. They only said it grows in the wild. During the Song times, they took mugwort from Fudao of Tangyin as the best. The mugwort from Siming was illustrated in an old book. In modern times, the mugwort from Tangyin is called "mugwort of the north." The mugwort from Siming is called "mugwort of the sea."

Since the reign of Chenghua (1465 CE), the mugwort from Qizhou has been regarded as superior. It serves as the standard ingredient for formulas. All under heaven value it and call it Qizhou mugwort [Qi Ai]. Tradition has it that mugwort from other places is unable to penetrate a wine jug when used for moxibustion, but one application of moxibustion using Qizhou mugwort will penetrate directly into it. This is extraordinary.[6]

This herb often grows in a mountainous wilderness. In the second month, the perennial roots grow sprouts, forming groves. The white-colored stalks grow straight, four or five *chi* high. The leaves spread in groups of four and look like sweet wormwood [Hao]. Each leaf is separated into five points, and forks into smaller points. The face of the leaf is green [*qing*] and the back is white. It has soft, thick fuzz. In the seventh or eighth lunar month, it sends out

---

3   The character for mugwort is 艾. It consists of 乂 (*yi4* cutting out) with the signific for herbs and grasses on top.

4   This term 壯 *zhuang* is translated into English as cone, but its real meaning is something like "invigoration" or "strengthening." If a book says, "three cones" in English, it would literally be "three invigorations" in Chinese.

5   Su Song 蘇頌 (1019-1101, Northern Song) was the author of *Illustrated Classic Materia Medica* 《圖經本草》. This book has been lost (Li 1995, 708).

6   This passage seems to be saying that if a closed jug is nearby when moxibustion is performed using Qizhou mugwort, the odor of the moxibustion will be able to penetrate into the jug. Since the qi from moxibustion needs to penetrate into the channels, this means that Qizhou mugwort is very potent.

spikes of tiny flowers between the leaves, like the spikes of Che Qian [Plantago]. It forms branches with clusters full of fruit. There are tiny seeds inside. After a frost it begins to wither.

On the fifth day of the fifth lunar month everyone cuts the stalks with the leaves and dries this harvest in the sun.

My late father, named Li Yuechi, also called Li Chanwen, wrote one volume called *Transmission on Qizhou Mugwort* [*Qi Ai Chuan*]. In it, there is song of praise that says:

> It is produced on the sunny side of the mountain,
> And picked at the Dragon Boat Festival.[7]
> It treats diseases and is applied to illness as
>   moxibustion.
> It results in benefits that are not small.

Also, Zong Lin said in *Jingchu Suishi Ji*: On the fifth day of the fifth lunar month, before the rooster crows, pick mugwort that appears in the shape of the human form,[8] grasp, and take it. Harvest it for the application of moxibustion to treat disease. It is extremely effective.

On this day, pick mugwort that is in the shape of a man, and hang it over the doorway. It can exorcise toxin qi.

Dry the stalks and soak them in sesame oil to kindle fire for lighting moxa cones. This enriches and moistens moxa sores so they will not hurt while recovering. It can also can substitute for yarrow strips [for *Yi Jing* divination] and make candle wicks.

【集解】《別錄》曰：艾葉生田野，三月三日采，曝乾。頌曰：處處有之，以複道及四明者為佳，云此種灸百病尤勝。初春布地生苗，莖類蒿，葉背白，以苗短者為良。三月三日，五月五日，采葉曝乾。陳久方

可用。時珍曰：艾葉本草不著土產，但云生田野。宋時以湯陰複道者為佳，四明者圖形。近代惟湯陰者謂之北艾；四明者謂之海艾。自成化以來，則以蘄州者為勝，用充方物，天下重之，謂之蘄艾。相傳他處艾灸酒罈不能透，蘄艾一灸則直透徹，為異也。此草多生山原。二月宿根生苗成叢，其莖直生，白色，高四五尺。其葉四布，狀如蒿，分為五尖，丫上復有小尖，面青背白，有茸而柔濃。七、八月，葉間出穗如車前穗，細花，結實纍纍盈枝，中有細子，霜後始枯。皆以五月五日連莖刈取，曝乾收葉。先君月池子諱言聞，嘗著《蘄艾傳》一卷。有贊云：產于山陽，采以端午。治病灸疾，功非小補。又宗懍《荊楚歲時記》云：五月五日雞未鳴時，采艾似人形者攬而取之，收以灸病，甚驗。是日采艾為人，懸于戶上，可禳毒瓦斯。其莖乾之，染麻油引火點灸炷，滋潤灸瘡，至愈不疼。亦可代蓍策，及作燭心。

BCGM: 15-05-1 The leaf

Preparation

Kou Zongshi said: Pound dry mugwort leaves with a pestle. Remove the green residue and take the white. Add a little Liu Huang [Sulfur] powder into it. This is called sulfured mugwort. Moxibustion specialists use it. You can also grind a little rice flour into a powder with the mugwort and put it into food and medicinals for use.

Li Shizhen says: Generally, you must use aged mugwort leaves. When treated to make them fine and soft, it is called mugwort floss. Moxibustion fire from fresh mugwort damages a person's flesh and vessels. Thus, Mencius said, "For diseases of seven years, seek three year-old mugwort."

Pick the clean leaves, winnow them to remove the dust and scraps, put them inside a stone mortar, and pound them into floss with a wooden pestle. Remove the residue with a sieve, take the white, and pound it again. It meets the standard when it is soft and mashed like silk floss. At the time of use, stone-

---

[7] The Dragon Boat Festival is held on the fifth day of the fifth lunar month.

[8] If you can find a stalk of mugwort that resembles the shape of a man, it would have a greater affinity for treating conditions of man. The resemblance of an image shows a natural connection or reflection according to Chinese medical thought. This same principle is used in selecting ginseng roots.

bake it until it is dry so that the fire of moxibustion will be potent.

When put in a woman's pills and powders, you must use mugwort floss. Boil it with vinegar until dry and pound it into cakes. Bake it dry and pound it again to make a powder to use. Some mix in glutinous rice paste to make the cakes or stir-fry with wine. Neither of these is good.

Master Hong Mai said in *Rong Zhai Sui Bi*: It is difficult to apply enough force to process mugwort, but if three or five slices of white Fu Ling [Poria] are added into it and ground together, you can immediately make a fine powder. This is also something strange.

葉：
【修治】宗曰：艾葉乾搗，去青滓，取白，入石硫黃末少許，謂之硫黃艾，灸家用之。得米粉少許，可搗為末，入服食藥用。
時珍曰：凡用艾葉，須用陳久者，治令細軟，謂之熟艾。若生艾灸火，則傷人肌脈。故《孟子》云：七年之病，求三年之艾。揀取淨葉，揚去塵屑，入石臼內木杵搗熟，羅去渣滓，取白者再搗，至柔爛如綿為度。用時焙燥，則灸火得力。入婦人丸散，須以熟艾，用醋煮乾，搗成餅子，烘乾再搗為末用。或以糯糊和作餅，及酒炒者，皆不佳。洪氏《容齋隨筆》云：艾難著力，若入白茯苓三、五片同碾，即時可作細末，亦一異也。

Qi & flavor: Bitter, slightly warm, nontoxic

Su Gong said: The fresh is cold; the floss is hot.

Zhang Yuansu said: Bitter and warm, yang within yin.

Li Shizhen says: Bitter and acrid. The fresh is warm and the floss is hot. It can upbear or downbear. It is yang. It enters the foot greater yin, reverting yin, and lesser yin channels. Vinegar and Xiang Fu [Rhizoma Cyperi] are its couriers.

【氣味】苦，微溫，無毒。恭曰：生寒；熟熱。元素曰：苦溫，陰中之陽。時珍曰：苦而辛，生溫熟熱，可升可降，陽也。入足太陰、厥陰、少陰之經。苦酒、香附為之使。

Indications

Applying moxibustion to hundreds of diseases. You can make a decoction to check vomiting of blood, dysentery, invisible-worm sores in the lower regions, and females spotting blood. It disinhibits yin qi, engenders flesh, repels wind cold, and allows people to have children. Do not allow exposure to wind while taking mugwort. *Records of Famous Doctors*

Pounded into a juice and taken internally, it stops damage to the blood and kills roundworms. *Tao Hongjing*

It governs nosebleed, bloody stool, and dysentery with pus and blood. Boil it in water or make pills and powders. *Su Gong*

It stops flooding of blood, bleeding intestinal hemorrhoids, and open incised wounds. It stops abdominal pain and quiets the fetus. It is extremely good when decocted in vinegar to treat lichens. Pound it into juice to drink for treating cold qi and ghost qi of the entire heart region and abdomen. *Zhen Quan*

It treats vaginal discharge, stops sudden turmoil [*i.e.*, cholera] with cramping, and fever and chills after dysentery. *Da Ming*[9]

It treats diseases of the girdling vessel, abdominal distention and fullness, and the lumbar region when it is unable to contain itself so the patient feels like he is sitting in water.[10] *Wang Haogu*

---

[9]   Da Ming's *Ri Hua Ben Cao* 大明《日華本草》 [*Da Ming Ri Hua Ben Cao*]
[10]   This last refers to a symptom of the girdling vessel in the *Classic of Difficulties*, Chapter 29.

It warms the center, expels cold, and eliminates dampness. *Li Shizhen*

【主治】灸百病。可作煎，止吐血下痢，下部〔匿+虫〕瘡，婦人漏血，利陰氣，生肌肉，辟風寒，使人有子。作煎勿令見風。《別錄》搗汁服，止傷血，殺蛔蟲。弘景
主衄血、下血 ，膿血痢，水煮及丸散任用。蘇恭
止崩血、腸痔血，拓金瘡，止腹痛，安胎。苦酒作煎，治癬甚良。搗汁飲，治心腹一切冷氣、鬼氣。甄權
治帶下，止霍亂轉筋，痢後寒熱。大明
治帶脈為病，腹脹滿，腰溶溶如坐水中。好古
溫中、逐冷、除濕。時珍

Explanation

Meng Xian said: In the spring months, pick young mugwort to eat as a vegetable or mix it with flour to make dumplings shaped like pellets. Swallow three or five of them and follow it down with cooked rice. It treats all ghosts and malign qi. Taking it regularly stops cold dysentery. You can also use young mugwort to make dry cakes. Boil them with fresh ginger and take them. This stops diarrhea and postpartum bloody diarrhea. It is quite wonderful.

Su Song's *Illustrated Classic* says: Recent generations take mugwort alone, or mix it with steamed *Mu Gua* [Fructus Chaenomelis] to make pills, or make a decoction to drink on an empty stomach. It strongly supplements vacuity with emaciation. Since this is so, [if it is misused] it can cause toxins to erupt, hot qi to surge upward, and uncontrollable manic agitation. It will eventually attack the eyes and there will be bleeding sores. You really cannot take it recklessly.

Zhu Zhenheng[11] said: Often female infertility is due to reduced blood. Therefore, the woman is unable to contain essence [semen]. Vulgar healers call it "vacu-

ity cold of the uterus." They throw acrid, hot medicinals at it or give mugwort leaf. They do not know that the nature of mugwort is extremely hot. When it enters the patient through the fire of moxibustion, its qi moves downward. When it enters the patient through medicinals, its qi moves upward. The *Materia Medica* only says it is warm. It does not say it is hot. The common people like warm medicinals, hastily taking a lot of them. After a long time, toxins erupt. How could they ever blame mugwort?! I have researched Su Song's *Illustrated Classic* and have been influenced by it.[12]

Li Shizhen said: When mugwort leaf is fresh, it is slightly bitter and very acrid. When processed into floss, it is pure yang. It can be used to take greater yang [the sun's] true fire. It can be used to return falling or expiring original yang. When taken internally, it runs through the three yin channels and expels all cold damp evils, shifting the awful qi so it becomes balanced. When applying moxibustion with mugwort, it penetrates through all the channels and treats hundreds of types of disease evils, raising up people who have chronic disease so they can become healthy and free of trouble. Its merits are also great.

Su Gong said the fresh is cold. Su Song said it is toxic. On the one hand, they view it as able to check all bleeding, but, on the other hand, they view it as causing hot qi to surge upward and then calling its nature cold or toxic. This is erroneous. They must not have known that blood follows the movement of qi. When qi moves, blood scatters. The reason there is heat is because taking it internally for a long time sends fire surging upward. Since medicinals are used to treat disease, you should stop taking them once they hit the disease.

---

11 Also known as Zhu Danxi, one of the four great masters of the Jin-Yuan period.
12 For discussion of Zhu's analysis of the differences between the qi of mugwort when used internally or as moxibustion, see also **ZJDC: 9-23** p. 105 and the discussion below.

If you simply have intractable cold due to vacuity or if a female has damp depression with vaginal discharge or spotting, why not use mugwort mixed with medicinals like Dang Gui [Radix Angelicae Sinensis] and Fu Zi [Radix Lateralis Praeparata Aconiti] to treat their disease? But it is a reckless idea to seek descendents by taking mugwort assisted by acrid, hot medicinals for an indefinite period of time. When taken for a long time, the nature of these medicinals becomes unbalanced, resulting in fire and agitation. Who is to blame for this? How is mugwort at fault?

Ai Fu Wan [Mugwort & Aconite Pills] treat all pain of the heart region, abdomen, and lesser abdomen and regulate all diseases of females. They have quite profound merits.

Jiao Ai Tang [Ass Hide Glue & Mugwort Decoction] treats vacuity dysentery as well as pregnancy and postpartum bleeding. It is especially apparent that it is extraordinarily effective.

When qi is weak in the *dan tian* [cinnabar field] of the elderly and the umbilical region is averse to cold, place a cloth sack of mugwort floss on the umbilical region. It is not possible to say just how wonderful this is! It is also appropriate to use mugwort floss inside the socks for leg qi caused by cold food.

【發明】詵曰：春月采嫩艾作菜食，或和麵作餛飩如彈子，吞三、五枚，以飯壓之，治一切鬼惡氣，長服止冷痢。又以嫩艾作乾餅子，用生姜煎服，止瀉痢及產後瀉血，甚妙。
頌曰：近世有單服艾者，或用蒸木瓜和丸，或作湯空腹飲，甚補虛羸。然亦有毒發則熱氣沖上，狂躁不能禁，至攻眼有瘡出血者，誠不可妄服也。
震亨曰：婦人無子，多由血少不能攝精，俗醫謂子宮虛冷，投以辛熱，或服艾葉。不知艾性至熱，入火灸則氣下行；入藥服，則氣上行。本草止言其溫，不言其熱。世人喜溫，率多服之，久久毒發，何嘗歸咎於艾哉！予考蘇頌《圖經》而因默有感焉。
時珍曰：艾葉生則微苦太辛，熟則微辛太苦，生溫熟熱，純陽也。可以取太陽真火，可以回垂絕元陽。服

之則走三陰，而逐一切寒濕，轉肅殺之氣為融和。灸之則透諸經，而治百種病邪，起沉疴之人為康泰，其功亦大矣。蘇恭言其生寒，蘇頌言其有毒。一則見其能止諸血，一則見其熱氣上沖，遂謂其性寒有毒，誤矣。蓋不知血隨氣而行，氣行則血散，熱因久服致火上沖之故爾。夫藥以治病，中病則止。若素有虛寒痼冷，婦人濕鬱帶漏之人，以艾和歸、附諸藥治其病，夫何不可？而乃妄意求嗣，服艾不輟，助以辛熱，藥性久偏，致使火躁，是誰之咎歟，于艾何尤？艾附丸治心腹、少腹諸痛，調女人諸病，頗有深功。膠艾湯治虛痢，及妊娠產後下血，尤著奇效。老人丹田氣弱，臍腹畏冷者，以熟艾入布袋兜其臍腹，妙不可言。寒食腳氣，亦宜以此夾入襪內。

Appended formulas [abridged] 【附方】

BCGM: 15-05-3 Wind cold during pregnancy: Sudden stroke, loss of consciousness, it appears like wind stroke. Use three *liang* of mugwort floss. Stir-fry it with rice vinegar until extremely hot. Wrap it with thin silk and iron it below the umbilicus. After a very long time, the patient will revive. *Good Gynecology Formulas*

妊娠風寒卒中，不省人事，狀如中風：用熟艾三兩，米醋炒極熱，以絹包熨臍下，良久即蘇。《婦人良方》

BCGM: 15-05-4 Wind stroke with deviated mouth: Use a reed tube that is five *cun* long. One end is inserted into the ear. Seal it with flour dough on all sides so wind cannot penetrate. Use seven cones of mugwort moxibustion on the other end. If the right ear is affected, apply moxibustion to the left. If the left is affected, apply moxibustion to the right. *Formulas Superior to Gold*

中風口歪：以葦筒長五寸，一頭刺入耳內，四面以麵密封，不透風，一頭以艾灸之七壯。患右灸左，患左灸右。《勝金方》

BCGM: 15-05-5 Wind stroke with clenched jaw: Apply five cones each of mugwort wool moxibustion to Cheng Jiang [Ren 24] (one point) and Jia Che [ST 6] (bilateral). *Prescriptions Worth a Thousand Pieces of Gold*

中風口噤：熟艾灸承漿一穴，頰車二穴，各五壯。
《千金方》

BCGM: 15-05-6 Wind stroke with pulling pain:
Numbness and paralysis. Knead about a *hu* of dried
mugwort into a ball and put it into an earthenware
steamer that has all the holes stopped up except
one. Place the painful site above the opening in the
steamer and burn the mugwort to fume it. In a little
while, the patient will perceive sensation. *Emergency
Prescriptions to Keep Up Your Sleeve*

中風掣痛，不仁不隨：並以乾艾斛許，揉團
納瓦甑中，並下塞諸孔，獨留一目，以痛處著甑目，
而燒艾熏之，一時即知矣。《肘後方》

BCGM: 15-05-10 All kinds of wind epilepsy: Use
mugwort wool right in between the scrotum and the
main gate of the grain path [*i.e.,* the anus]. Apply
moxibustion to it based on the years of age. *Constellation Gate Formulas*

癲癇諸風：熟艾于陰囊下穀道正門當中間，隨年歲灸
之。《斗門方》

BCGM: 15-05-12 Pediatric umbilical wind: Pursed
mouth. Fill up the umbilicus with the burnt ash of
mugwort leaf. Bind it securely with silk. This is effective. Or apply garlic-isolated moxibustion to it. Wait
until there is mugwort qi [the smell of mugwort] in
the mouth. There will be immediate recovery. Yang
Qi's *Simple and Convenient Formulas*

小兒臍風撮口：艾葉燒灰填臍中，以帛縛定效。或隔
蒜灸之，候口中有艾氣立愈。《簡便方》

BCGM: 15-05-13 Hu huo & invisible-worm disease:[13]
The patient's teeth are colorless and the top of the
tongue is white. Some like to sleep and do not perceive pain or itching at the sites. Some have dysen-

tery. It is appropriate to quickly treat the lower region of his body. If you do not know about it, this
just seems to attack the upper. However, if the lower
region is growing worms that eat the anus, with erosion appearing on the five viscera, then the patient
will die. Burn mugwort in a tube, and fume the
lower region, making the smoke penetrate. Adding a
little Xiong Huang [Realgar] is even more wonderful.
You can also burn the smoke in a vase. *Prescriptions
to Keep Up One's Sleeve*

狐惑蟲〔匿+虫〕，病人齗無色，
舌上白，或喜睡不知痛癢處，或下痢，宜急治下部。
不曉此者，但攻其上，而下部生蟲，食其肛，爛見五
臟，便死也。燒艾于管中，熏下部令煙入，或少加雄
黃更妙。罌中燒煙亦可。《肘後方》

BCGM: 15-05-25 Pheasant hemorrhoidal disease:[14]
First use Huai Yang Tang [Sophora & Willow Decoc-
tion] to wash the site. Then apply seven cones of
moxibustion to it. It is effective. Official Wang Ji
rode a donkey to western Sichuan. After some days,
hemorrhoids erupted. It felt to him like a cucumber
[*hu gua*] was piercing the end of his intestines. It was
as hot as fire. He suddenly collapsed. He was at his
wit's end. There was a postal official who said, "You
must apply moxibustion for a prompt cure." He
then used the above method to apply three or five
cones of moxibustion. The patient suddenly perceived a path of hot qi entering into the intestines
causing great cramping and diarrhea. Blood and filth
came out together. After the diarrhea, he lost the
feeling of a cucumber at the site. *Good Formulas from
Experience*

野雞痔病：先以槐柳湯洗過，以艾灸上七壯，取效。
郎中王及乘騾入西川，數日病痔大作，如胡瓜貫于腸
頭，其熱如火，忽至僵仆，無計。有主郵者云：須灸
即瘥。乃用上法灸三五壯，忽覺一道熱氣入腸中，因
大轉瀉，血穢並出，瀉後遂失胡瓜所在矣。《經驗良
方》

---

13 See the glossary for discussion of *hu huo* and invisible-worm disease. These terms come from Zhang Zhongjing's *Golden Cabinet*.
14 There are related entries in **BCGM: 35-16** and **35-29** and *Generations of Doctors* (Wei 1964, 122). Pheasant hemorrhoidal disease
probably refers to hemorrhoids that appear multicolored.

BCGM: 15-05-31 Postpartum abdominal pain: The patient feels like she is about to die. It arises because of contracting cold. Bake two *jin* of aged Qizhou mugwort until it is dry. Pound it and spread it on the umbilicus. Use silk to cover it and iron it. Wait for mugwort qi [or smell] to come out of her mouth. Then the pain will spontaneously stop. *Yang's True Experience Formulas*

產後腹痛欲死，因感寒起者：陳蘄艾二斤。焙乾，搗鋪臍上，以絹覆住，熨斗熨之，待口中艾氣出，則痛自止矣。《楊誠經驗方》

BCGM: 15-05-36 Fire eye swelling & pain: Burn mugwort so that the smoke rises. Cover it with a bowl. Wait till the smoke is exhausted. Scrape the soot from the bottom of the bowl and mix it with warm water to turn it into an eyewash. The condition will promptly be cured. Still better, add Huang Lian [Rhizoma Coptidis]. This is especially good. *Constellation Gate Formulas*

火眼腫痛：以艾燒煙起，用碗覆之，候煙盡，碗上刮煤下，以溫水調化洗眼，即瘥。更入黃連尤佳。《斗門方》

BCGM: 15-05-38 Women's facial sores:[15] Called pink flower [*fen hua*] sores. Mix five *qian* of Ding Fen [Lead Carbonate] with mustard seed oil to make a paste inside a bowl. Burn one or two balls of mugwort in this bowl to make smoke. Fume the affected site. Wait for the smoke to be exhausted. Turn the bowl upside down on the ground overnight. Take out the residue, mix it and apply it. You will never have scars. It is also easy to engender flesh to heal the sores. Tan Yeweng's *Tested Formulas*

婦人面瘡，名粉花瘡，以定粉五錢，菜子油調泥碗內，用艾一、二團，燒煙熏之，候煙盡，覆地上一夜，取出調搽，求無瘢痕，亦易生肉。談野翁《試驗方》

BCGM: 15-05-39 Warts on the body and face: Apply

three cones of mugwort fire moxibustion. They will promptly be eliminated. *Sage-like Prescriptions*

身面疣目：艾火灸三壯即除。《聖惠方》

BCGM: 15-05-40 Goose foot wind disease [see glossary]: Boil four or five *liang* of genuine mugwort from Qizhou in four or five bowls of water for five or six boilings.[16] Put the liquid inside a big mouth bottle. Cover the bottle with two layers of sackcloth. Place the palms of the hands over the bottle to fume them. When it gets cold, heat it again. It is like a miracle. *Formulas from Master Lu's Hall of Accumulating Virtue*

鵝掌風病：蘄艾（真者）四、五兩，水四五碗，煮五、六滾，入大口瓶內盛之，用麻布二層縛之，將手心放瓶上熏之，如冷再熱，如神。陸氏《積德堂方》

BCGM: 15-05-41 Fuming method for scab sores: Two *liang* of Qizhou mugwort wool, three *qian* of Mu Bie Zi [Semen Mormordicae], two *qian* of Xiong Huang [Realgar], and one *qian* of Liu Huang [Sulfur]. Make them into a powder. Knead the powder into the mugwort and divide it into four sticks. Each time, place one stick on a yin-yang tile.[17] Place it under a quilt with the patient to bake and fume him. Afterwards, take Tong Sheng San [Free the Sage Powder]. *Summary of Medical Formulas*

蘄艾一兩，木鱉子三錢，雄黃二錢，硫黃一錢，為末，揉入艾中，分作四條。每以一條安陰陽瓦中，置被裹烘熏，後服通聖散。《醫方摘要》

BCGM: 15-05-43 Pediatric erosion sores: Apply the burnt ash of mugwort leaf. It is good. *Secret Record of Mother and Child*

小兒爛瘡：艾葉燒灰，敷之，良。《子母秘錄》

BCGM: 15-05-44 Open shank sores [see glossary] that do not close due to coldness: Fume them with

---

[15] This is probably for treating acne. Today, we are unlikely to use lead compounds applied to the skin.
[16] Five or six boilings: When the water boils, add some cold water, and let it boil again. Do this five or six times.
[17] A yin-yang tile is a U-shaped roof tile. Half of them point up and half point down. Thus they lock into each other.

smoke from burning mugwort wool. *Formulas from Experience*

臁瘡口冷不合：熟艾燒煙熏之。《經驗方》

BCGM: 15-05-46 Clove sores [see glossary] & toxic swellings: Burn one container of mugwort to ashes. Soak the ashes in a bamboo tube and take the liquid. Use one or two *ge*. Mix with limestone to make a paste. First use a needle to prick the sore until there is pain. Then dab on the medicinals. After three times, the root will spontaneously be pulled out. Han Guang from Yushan used this to treat people. It is miraculously effective. At the beginning of Zhenguan's reign [reigned 627-649], Official Xu from Quzhou got this formula. I [Sun Simiao] used it to effectively treat more than 30 people. *True Person Sun's Prescriptions Worth a Thousand Pieces of Gold*

疔瘡腫毒：艾蒿一撮燒灰，于竹筒中淋取汁，以一、二合，和石灰如糊。先以針刺瘡至痛，乃點藥三遍，其根自拔。玉山韓光以此治人神驗。貞觀初，衢州徐使君訪得此方。予用治三十餘人，得效。孫真人《千金方》

BCGM: 15-05-47 Onset of eruptions on the back not yet fully developed: And all hot swellings. Rub damp paper on them. The first place that dries is the head. Apply mugwort moxibustion to it. The number of cones is not discussed [meaning, use as many as it takes]. If there is pain, apply moxibustion until there is no pain. If there is no pain, apply moxibustion until there is pain and then stop. The toxins will promptly scatter. Even if they do not scatter, you will still avoid internal attack [of these toxins]. This is a miraculous formula. Li Jiang's *Handy Collection of Formulas from the Ministry of War*[18]

發背初起未成，及諸熱腫：以濕紙搨上，先乾處是頭，著艾灸之。不論壯數，痛者灸至不痛；不痛者灸至痛乃止。其毒即散，不散亦免內攻，神方也。李絳《兵部手集》

BCGM: 15-05-51 All insect & snake bites: Applying numerous cones of mugwort moxibustion is very good. *Collection of Simple Formulas*

諸蟲蛇傷：艾灸數壯甚良。《集簡方》

BCGM: 15-05-52 Wind worm toothache: Melt a little bit of wax and spread it on paper. Spread mugwort on top. Roll the paper around a chopstick. Burn it to make smoke. In accordance with left or right, fume the nose [inhale the smoke with the nostril that is on the same side as the toothache]. Inhale the smoke to make the mouth full. Exhale the qi [air]. The pain will promptly stop and the swelling will disperse. Jin Jiqian had the disease for over a month. With one try, he promptly recovered. *Prescriptions of Universal Benefit*

風蟲牙痛：化蠟少許，攤紙上，鋪艾，以箸卷成筒，燒煙，隨左右熏鼻，吸煙令滿口，呵氣，即疼止腫消，靳季謙病此月餘，一試即愈。《普濟方》

Yang Jizhou on Mugwort

ZJDC: 9-23 Mugwort Leaf (*Unified Medicine*),[19] (Huang 1996, 990)
《針灸大成・艾葉《醫統》・卷之九》

The *Materia Medica* says: Mugwort has a bitter flavor. Its qi is slightly warm. It is yang within yin. It is nontoxic. It is indicated for the application of moxibustion to treat hundreds of diseases.

---

[18] See also **JYQS: 46-11** and **LJTY: 11-3-23** p. 168.

[19] This whole section came from Gao Wu's *Gatherings*, Part 2, Volume 3 (Huang 1996, 731). It is almost the same, word for word, and we know that Yang passed on many other sections from *Gatherings*. However, in this case, Yang attributes it to the *Great Completion of Unified Ancient and Modern Medicine* by Xu Chunfu 徐春甫《古今醫統大全》, published in 1556 (Ming). Indeed, it is there in Volume 7 (Xu 1991, 470), but Gao Wu does not give this attribution. He could not, as *Unified Medicine* was published 27 years after *Gatherings*. It is strange that Yang attributed it to the later source when he took so many other passages from the earlier source. Perhaps he was confused about the dates of publication or perhaps this attribution was erroneously added by a later editor. It is unclear from which materia medica the first paragraph is taken. The information is fairly standard.

It is picked on the third day of the third lunar month or the fifth day of the fifth lunar month. Dry it in the sun. Aging it is good.

The method to pick mugwort for keeping away malignity and killing ghosts is also on the fifth day of the fifth lunar month; burning mugwort has efficacy.

To process mugwort, first follow the routine method: Dry it, put it in a mortar, and pound it. Use a fine sieve to remove the dust and crumbs. Each time, put it back in the stone mortar and pound it again. Take the clean white floss as superior. It must be baked until it is very dry so that moxibustion will have power and the fire easily ignites. If it is moist, it will not give results.

The *Materia Medica Categorized by Patterns* says:[20] It comes from Mingzhou.

The *Illustrated Classic* says:[21] In the past, they did not record its place of origin, but they said it grows in the fields and open country. Today, every place has it. Only Qizhou mugwort has thick leaves, high branches, and strong qi and flavor of the fruit. Using it is very effective.

Mengzi said:[22] A disease of seven years requires three year-old mugwort.

Zhu Danxi said: The nature of mugwort is extremely hot. When burned as moxibustion, it moves upward. When taken internally as medicine, it moves downward.[23]

《木草》云：艾味苦，氣微溫，陰中之陽，無毒，主灸百病。三月三日，五月五日，採暴乾，陳久者良，避惡殺鬼，又採艾之法，五月五日，灼艾有效。製艾先要如法：令乾燥，入臼搗之，以細篩去塵屑，每入

石臼，搗取潔白為上，須令焙大燥，則灸有力，火易燃，如潤無功。《證類本草》云：出明州。《圖經》云：舊不著所出，但云生田野，今在處有之。惟蘄州葉厚而干高，果氣味之大，用之甚效溪曰：艾性至熱，入火灸則上行，入藥服則下行。

Zhang Jiebin on Mugwort

JYQS: 48-71 Mugwort (71) (Zhang 1995, 1188) 《景岳全書・艾七一・卷之四十八》

The flavor is slightly bitter. The qi is acrid. Used fresh, it is slightly warm. Used as floss, it is slightly hot. It is able to flow freely through the twelve channels, but is especially a medicinal of the liver, spleen, and kidneys.

It is good for warming the center, expelling cold, eliminating damp, moving the qi within the blood and for stagnation of qi. Overall, it is most suitable to use in women with cold blood and stagnant qi. That is why it is able to quiet the fetus, stop pain of the heart region and abdomen, treat vaginal discharge and flooding, warm the lumbar region and knees, stop vomiting of blood and dysentery, repel wind cold or cold damp, miasmic malaria, and cramping from sudden turmoil [*i.e.*, cholera], as well as all cold qi and ghost qi, kill tapeworms and invisible-worm sores on the lower body [see glossary].

Sometimes it is used fresh, pounded to make juice. Sometimes it is used as floss in decoctions. Sometimes it is used to apply moxibustion for hundreds of diseases. Sometimes it is stir-fried hot to apply for ironing as it can flow freely through the channels and network vessels. Sometimes it is put into a bag and wrapped up as it can warm the umbilicus and knees. Exterior or interior, fresh or floss, all of these are suitable for something.

---

[20] By Tang Zhenwei 唐慎微 《證類本草》, published 1108 (Li 1995, 1019).
[21] The *Illustrated Classic Materia Medica* 《圖經本草》 was written by Su Song 蘇頌 (1019-1101, Northern Song). This book has been lost (Li 1995, 708).
[22] The quote from Mengzi 《孟子・離婁》 is from the chapter called *Li Lou*, Part 1 (Mengzi 1997, 124).
[23] For a discussion of Zhu Danxi's statement, see (p. 97-106) below and **BCGM: 15-05** p.101.

味微苦，氣辛，生用微溫，熟用微熱。 能通十二經，
而尤為肝脾腎之藥。 善於溫中逐冷除濕，
行血中之氣，氣中之滯，凡婦人血氣寒滯者，
最宜用之。故能安胎，止心腹痛，治帶下血崩，
煖腰膝，止吐血，下痢，辟風寒寒濕瘴瘧，
霍亂轉筋，及一切冷氣鬼氣，
殺蚘蟲并下部〔虫+匿〕瘡。或生用搗汁，或熟用煎
湯；或用灸百病，或炒熱敷熨，可通經絡；
或袋盛包裹，可溫臍膝，表裏生熟，俱有所宜。

DISCUSSION OF MUGWORT

First, note the wide variety of methods for using mugwort as an external heat treatment: moxibustion (including using a reed tube in the ear, isolated with garlic), ironing, fuming, steam treatment, as ash in the umbilicus, ash mixed with water as a wash, inhalation of the smoke for toothache, and mixed with other substances, such as vinegar, realgar, or sulfur. Today, we have really limited ourselves to a small repertoire of methods using mugwort.

Beyond this, two other areas require some exploration. One is the timing for the gathering of mugwort; however, that will be reserved for Chapter 13 on timing.

The other area is the intriguing analysis attributed to Zhu Danxi (Zhu Zhenheng) regarding the differences between the qi of mugwort when used internally versus its use as moxibustion. This statement is quoted by both Yang and Li. Unfortunately, the citations are not identical and are actually diametrically opposed to each other.

ZJDC: 9-23 says, "Zhu Danxi said: The nature of mugwort is extremely hot. When burned as moxibustion, it moves upward. When taken internally as medicine, it moves downward" (see p. 106).

Li Shizhen cites this statement in **BCGM: 15-05**, "Zhu Zhenheng said: The nature of mugwort is extremely hot. When it enters the patient through the fire of moxibustion, its qi moves downward. When it en-

ters the patient through medicinals, its qi moves upward" (see p. 101).

These two citations disagree on the directions of movement:

DIRECTION OF QI MOVEMENT		
METHOD OF ADMINISTRATION	Yang	Li
mugwort in moxibustion	up	down
mugwort taken internally	down	up

This whole section of the *Great Compendium* came from Gao Wu's *Gatherings*, Part 2, Volume 3 (Huang 1996, 731) and Yang copied it faithfully. Gao Wu and Yang say the same thing. None of these authors, Li, Yang, or Gao, give references for the source of this statement in Zhu Danxi's writings and I am unable to find the original source at this time. In does not seem to be anywhere in *[Zhu] Danxi's Medical Collection* (Zhu 2000).

Which is correct? Yang did not discuss the internal use of mugwort beyond this statement, but Li did. The contents of the discussion in Li's section on mugwort back up his contention that taking mugwort internally makes qi ascend, "On the one hand, they [Su Gong and Su Song] view mugwort as able to check all bleeding, but on the other hand they view it as causing hot qi to surge upward… This is erroneous… The reason there is heat is because taking it internally for a long time sends fire surging upward." Here, Li is arguing that the side effect of hot qi surging upward is due to excessive internal use of mugwort, not because mugwort is inherently unbalanced. In any case, this statement is in agreement with Li's version that "when mugwort enters the patient through the fire of moxibustion, its qi moves downward. When it enters the patient through medicinals, its qi moves upward."

Beyond this, we saw in earlier chapters that moxibustion on points of the lower body, such as Zu San Li (ST 36) descend excessive qi or heat in the upper body (**LJTY: 4-27-4**, **ZJDC: 9-7**, **LJTY: 7-1-35**, and **LJTY: 10-1-6**). However, it is an over-simplification to say "moxibustion descends qi." Otherwise we would not have warnings to avoid a lot of moxibustion on the head (**LJTY: 11-2-3**), we would not need to apply moxibustion above first and below second (**LJTY: 11-2-4**), and we would not need to apply moxibustion to Zu San Li (ST 36) after applying it to Gao Huang Shu (UB 43) (**ZJDC: 9-8, LJTY: 7-1-35**) or points on the head (**LJTY: 4-27-4**). It seems that moxibustion draws heat or fire to the region where it is applied, whether upper or lower body. So, moxibustion draws hot qi down *if it is applied to points on the lower body*.

In any case, these statements show that mugwort used for moxibustion has a different effect from mugwort used internally. We cannot simply read the materia medica for mugwort and understand the mechanisms of moxibustion. It is also likely that the functions of other medicinals, such as garlic, ginger, and aconite, are somewhat changed when used as an isolating substance or mixed in with the mugwort as a powder. We must not regard the functions of moxibustion as identical to the functions of the same substances when taken internally.

GARLIC

Garlic is probably the most common isolating substance for moxibustion. Both Zhang and Li wrote a lot about it. Yang did not seem to use isolating substances very often. Even when he did, he did not mentioned garlic.

Li Shizhen on Garlic

BCGM: 26-09 Garlic [Hu, also Da Suan] (Li 1996, 704)
《本草綱目•菜部第二十六卷•菜之一•葫》

Explanation of the name

Large Suan [*i.e.*, Da Suan] *Tao Hongjing*

Strong-smelling vegetable for meat [Hun Cai] *Tao Hongjing* said: Today people call Hu "large Suan." Suan is small Suan. Their type of qi resembles each other.

Li Shizhen says: Note that Sun Mian's *Tangyun* says: Zhang Qian (Han dynasty) was an envoy to the western cities. That was when we began to obtain garlic and Hu Sui [Fructus Coriandri]. Since small suan is from China, they had it in the past, but garlic comes from a barbarian [*hu*] place. Therefore, the barbarian herb has "barbarian" in its name. Both Suans belong to five strong-smelling vegetables [*hun*]. This led to calling it "strong-smelling vegetable" [Hun Cao].[24]

【釋名】大蒜（弘景）、葷菜。
弘景曰：今人謂葫為大蒜，蒜為小蒜，以其氣類相似也。
時珍曰：按孫《唐韻》云：張騫使西域，始得大蒜、胡荽。則小蒜乃中土舊有，而大蒜出胡地，故有胡名。二蒜皆屬五葷，故通可稱葷。……

Qi & flavor: Acrid, warm, toxic. Long-term consumption harms the eyes...

【氣味】辛，溫，有毒。久食損人目。……

---

[24] Suan refers to Xiao Suan, small Suan, the indigenous Chinese garlic (**BCGM: 26-07**). Da Suan refers to what we call garlic in the West. We are familiar in the West with garlic that has a head consisting of many cloves. Indigenous garlic only has one clove in the head. Therefore, it is also called single-clove garlic [独蒜 Du Suan].

Li's section on small Suan discusses 葷 *hun* (also pronounced *xun*) which are strong-smelling vegetables that are often cooked with meat and are also avoided by certain types of vegetarians. Traditionally, there are five strong-smelling vegetables to avoid. Different books list different sets of five. They include various types of garlic, onions, and leeks. Li said they all cloud the spirit. When eaten fresh, they increase anger. When cooked, they arouse licentiousness. They also harm intelligence.

Indications

Returns the five viscera; scatters abscesses, swellings, and invisible-worm sores; eliminates wind evils, detoxifies qi. *Records of Famous Doctors*

Descends qi, disperses grains, and transforms meat. *Su Gong*

Removes water and maligns itching qi, eliminates wind damp, breaks cold qi, erodes strings and aggregations [*xian pi*], latent evil malignity, perfuses, warms, supplements, cures sores and lichens, kills ghosts, and removes pain. *Chen Cangqi*

Fortifies the spleen and stomach, orders kidney qi, checks sudden turmoil [or cholera] with cramping and abdominal pain, eliminates evil spirits, resolves warm epidemics, eliminates *gu* toxins, cures taxation, malaria, and cold wind. Pound it and apply it to wind harm and cold pain, malign sores, snake and insect bites, stream toxins, and sand lice bites. It is good when processed by soaking it in vinegar for an entire year. *Da Ming's Rihua Bencao*[25]

When pounded and mashed with warm water, it treats summerheat stroke loss of consciousness. Pounded and applied to the soles of the feet, it checks incessant nosebleed. Mixed with fermented soybean and made into pills, it treats sudden onset of bloody stool and frees the water passages. *Kou Zongshi*

Pound it to make juice and drink it to treat vomiting blood and heart pain. Boil the juice and drink it to treat arched-back rigidity. Make it into pills with silver carp to treat diaphragm qi. Make it into pills with clamshell powder to treat water swelling. Make it into pills with Huang Dan [Minium] to treat dysentery complicated with malaria, and dysentery during pregnancy. Make it into pills with Ru Xiang [Olibanum] to treat abdominal pain. When it is

pounded into a paste and applied to the umbilicus, it is able to extend to the lower burner to disperse water and disinhibit urine and feces. When applied to the soles of the feet, it is able to lead heat to move down and treats diarrhea and sudden dysentery, as well as dry or damp sudden turmoil [or cholera], and stops nosebleeds. Inserted into the anus, it is able to unblock the dark gate, and treats block and repulsion blockage. *Li Shizhen*

【主治】歸五臟，散癭腫〔匿+虫〕瘡，除風邪，殺毒氣。《別錄》
下氣，消穀，化肉。蘇恭
去水惡癢氣，除風濕，破冷氣，爛痃癖，伏邪惡，宣通溫補，療瘡癬，殺鬼去痛。藏器
健脾胃，治腎氣，止霍亂轉筋腹痛，除邪祟，解溫疫，去蠱毒，療勞瘧冷風，敷風損冷痛，惡瘡、蛇蟲、溪毒、沙虱、並搗貼之。熟醋浸，經年者良。《日華》
溫水搗爛服，治中暑不醒。搗貼足心，止鼻衄不止。和豆豉丸服，治暴下血，通水道。宗
搗汁飲，治吐血心痛。煮汁飲，治角弓反張。同鯽魚丸，治膈氣。同蛤粉丸，治水腫。同黃丹丸，治痢瘧、孕痢。同乳香丸，治腹痛。搗膏敷臍，能下達下焦，消水，利大小便。貼足心，能引熱下行，治泄瀉暴痢及乾濕霍亂，止衄血。納肛中，能通幽門，治關格不通。時珍

Explanation [abridged]

Chen Cangqi said: In ancient times, there was a person who suffered strings and aggregations. He was instructed in a dream to eat three heads of garlic each day. Initially he took this dose and subsequently had dim vision, dizziness, counterflow vomiting, and his lower regions burned like fire. Later, someone instructed him to take a few slices with the skin still on, cut off the two ends and swallow them. He called it "internal moxibustion." The result was that he reaped great effects.

Su Song said: The classics say garlic scatters abscesses

---

25 大明《日華本草》 [*Da Ming Ri Hua Ben Cao*]

and swellings. Note that Li Jiang's *Handy Collection of Formulas from the Ministry of War* says: For toxic sores and toxic swellings so bad that the patient cries out and is unable to sleep. People are unable to differentiate it. Pound two heads of single-clove garlic into a pulp, mix with sesame oil, and apply a thick layer on the sores. Change it when it is dry. It has been used repeatedly to save people. No one fails to receive miraculous effects. Official Lu Tan developed a sore on his shoulder. Pain radiated to his heart and he felt chest oppression. He used this as a convenient cure. Official Li also suffered from an enduring brain abscess that did not heal. Lu gave him this formula and he also was cured.

Also, Ge Hong said in *Prescriptions to Keep Up One's Sleeve*: Whenever there are swellings on the back, cut single-clove garlic horizontally into slices one fen thick. Place them on the head of the swelling. Apply 100 cones of mugwort the size of Wu [Firmiana] seeds for garlic moxibustion. If the patient does not feel a gradual dispersal of the swelling, more moxibustion is good. Do not make great heat. If the patient feels pain, promptly lift up the garlic. When the garlic becomes scorched replace it with a new one. Do not damage the skin and flesh. Ge Hong once suffered a big swelling on his lower lesser abdomen. He applied moxibustion to it and was also cured. He often used this moxibustion on people. No one failed to respond effectively.

Also, in the in the Ziji palace in Jiangning Fu, a record of this matter was inscribed on a stone, saying: There is a difference in the onset of back eruptions, abscesses, malign sores, and swollen nodes. Nevertheless, moxibustion can be applied to all of them. Do not count the number of cones. The only important thing is to apply moxibustion until there is no pain on a patient who has pain. On a patient without pain, apply moxibustion until the pain is extreme, and then stop. Apply moxibustion to warts and the like. Only then will they become scabs which slough themself off. The effect is like a miracle. From this, we know that the formula books do not have empty words. However, when people are

unable use this idea with careful consideration, they are unable to completely respond.

Li Shizhen says: Note that Li Xun's *Discussion of Garlic "Coin" Moxibustion* said: The method for treating abscesses: Applying moxibustion is superior to using medicinals. The reason is that hot toxins block the center of the sore so what is above and below it does not pass through. You must drain the toxic qi out. Afterwards, it will resolve and scatter.

Within the first day of the initial eruption, slice a big head of single-clove garlic into the thickness of a small coin. Place it on the vertex of the sore and apply moxibustion to it. Change it after three cones. Use roughly 100 cones as a guideline. [It has three effects:] One, it does not allow the sore to become a big opening. Two, it does not allow the flesh inside to decay. Three, the opening of the sore closes easily. With one action, three objectives are obtained. However, on the head, neck, and above, you really cannot use this or it may lead the qi upward and engender a greater disaster.

Also, Shi Yuan recorded the merits of garlic moxibustion, saying: My mother's back and scapula began itching. It had a red half-*cun* "halo" around a white "grain" the size of millet. Two times seven cones of moxibustion were applied, and the redness then dispersed.

Two nights later, there was a red halo two *cun* long flowing down. The whole family laid the blame on moxibustion. An outside doctor used a paste to protect it. Each day, the "halo" increased. In 22 days, it slanted horizontally about six or seven *cun* [like a red-thread boil]. The pain and suffering were unbearable.

Someone said a nun had had this and recovered after receiving moxibustion. I quickly asked her about it. The nun said: When it was severe, she had clouding loss of consciousness [so she did not know what happened], but she heard that Fan Fengyi sat in attendance applying more than 800 cones of moxibustion, about one sieve-full of mugwort. She revived right after this.

I hastily returned and applied moxibustion with more than 10 cones the size of Yin Xing Ke [Semen Gingkonis]. The difference was imperceptible. Then, I applied moxibustion to the four sides of the red site, all painful. As each cone turned to ashes, the redness shrank. After more than 30 cones, the red halo had withdrawn in retreat.

Since the moxibustion was late, the flesh at the site of the initial eruption must have already decayed. Thus, there was no pain. When the moxibustion reached the good flesh, there was pain.

When it reached nighttime, the heat of the fire had filled her back. The sore made a high mound and was hot. That night, she slept peacefully. At dawn, the sore looked like an overturned bowl, three or four *cun* high. There were more than 100 small holes in it, pure black in color. She was nursed back to health and recovered.

The high mound of swollen flesh was probably the toxins exiting. The many small holes meant the toxins were no longer gathered in one location. The pure black color was decay of the skin and flesh. If the mugwort fire had not sent out the toxins from inside the decayed flesh, they would have threatened the five viscera internally and lead to peril. Vulgar healers apply the theory of cool and cold medicinals to disperse and scatter. How can we have confidence in them?[26]

【發明】……藏器曰：昔有患痃癖者，夢人教每日食大蒜三顆。初服遂至眩眩吐逆，下部如火。後有人教取數片，合皮截卻兩頭吞之，名曰內灸，果獲大效也。

頌曰：《經》言葫散癰腫。按李絳《兵部手集方》云：毒瘡腫毒，號叫臥眠不得，人不能別者。取獨頭蒜兩顆搗爛，麻油和，濃敷瘡上，乾即易之。屢用救人

，無不神效。盧坦侍郎肩上瘡作，連心痛悶，用此便瘥。又李僕射患腦癰久不瘥，盧與此方亦瘥。又葛洪《肘後方》云：凡背腫，取獨顆蒜橫截一分，安腫頭上，炷艾如梧子大，灸蒜百壯，不覺漸消，多灸為善。勿令大熱，若覺痛即擎起蒜。蒜焦更換新者，勿令損皮肉。洪嘗苦小腹下患一大腫，灸之亦瘥。數用灸人，無不應效。又江寧府紫極宮刻石記其事云：但是發背及癰疽惡瘡腫核初起有異，皆可灸之，不計壯數。惟腰痛者灸至不痛，不痛者灸至痛極而止。疣贅之類灸之，亦便成痂自脫，其效如神。乃知方書無空言者。但人不能以意詳審，則不得盡應耳。

時珍曰：按李迅《論蒜錢灸法》云：治癰疽之法，著灸勝於用藥。緣熱毒中鬲，上下不通。必得毒氣發泄，然後解散。凡初發一日之內，便用大獨頭蒜切如小錢濃，貼頂上灸之。三壯一易，大概以百壯為率。一使瘡不開大，二使內肉不壞，三瘡口易合，一舉而三得之。但頭及項以上，切不可用此，恐引氣上，更生大禍也。又史源記蒜灸之功云：母氏背胛作癢，有赤暈半寸，白粒如黍。灸二七壯，其赤隨消。信宿，有赤流下長二寸。舉家歸咎於灸。外醫用膏護之，日增一暈，二十二日，橫斜約六、七寸，痛楚不勝。或言一尼病此，得灸而愈。予奔問之。尼云：劇時昏不知人，但聞範奉議坐守灸八百餘壯方蘇，約艾一簁。予亟歸，以炷如銀杏大，灸十數，殊不覺；乃灸四旁赤處，皆痛。每一壯爐則赤暈縮入，三十餘壯，赤暈收退。蓋灸遲則初發處肉已壞，故不痛，直待灸到好肉方痛也。至夜則火燄滿背，瘡高阜而熱，夜得安寢矣。至曉如覆一甌，高三、四寸，上有百數小竅，色正黑，調理而安。蓋高阜者，毒外出也。小竅多，毒不聚也。色正黑，皮肉壞也。非艾火出其毒于壞肉之裡，則內逼五臟而危矣。庸醫敷貼涼冷消散之說，何可信哉？

Appended formulas [abridged] 【附方】

BCGM: 26-29-01 Moxibustion for back sores: Whenever a patient perceives a hard swelling with pain on his back, apply damp paper to search for the head of the sore. Use 10 heads of garlic, half a *ge* of Dan Dou [Semen Praeparatum Sojae] and one *qian* of Ru Xiang [Olibanum]. Finely grind them. Based on the size of the head of the sore, use a slice of bamboo to

---

[26] See also **JYQS: 46-11** for a related discussion of the treatment of abscesses and sores.

make ring to surround it. Fill it two *fen* thick with the medicinals. Apply moxibustion to it with mugwort. If there is pain, apply moxibustion until it itches. If there is itching, apply moxibustion until there is pain. Take 100 cones as the general rule. Giving garlic "coin" moxibustion has the same effect. *Essentials of External Medicine*[27]

背瘡灸法：凡覺背上腫硬疼痛，用濕紙貼尋瘡頭。用大蒜十顆，淡豉半合，乳香一錢，細研。隨瘡頭大小，用竹片作圈固定，填藥于內，二分濃，著艾灸之。痛灸至癢，癢灸至痛，以百壯為率。與蒜錢灸法同功。《外科精要》

BCGM: 26-09-12 Diarrhea & sudden dysentery: Pound garlic and apply it to the soles of the two feet. You can also apply it to the umbilicus. *Prescriptions Worth a Thousand Pieces of Gold*

泄瀉暴痢：大蒜搗貼兩足心。亦可貼臍中。《千金方》

BCGM: 26-09-32 Pediatric umbilical wind: Cut single-clove garlic into slices. Place them on the umbilicus. Use mugwort to apply moxibustion to it. When there is garlic qi [or smell] in the mouth, it will promptly stop. Retired Scholar Li's *Simple and Easy Formulas*

小兒臍風：獨頭蒜切片，安臍上，以艾灸之。口中有蒜氣，即止。黎居士《簡易方論》

BCGM: 26-09-41 *She gong*[28] & stream toxins: Cut single-clove garlic three *fen* thick. Apply it to the affected site and apply moxibustion on it. Make the garlic qi shoot into the affected site. [Garlic is acrid; so it penetrates.] This will promptly cure it. *Teacher Mei's Formulas*

射工溪毒：獨頭蒜切三分濃，貼上灸之，令蒜氣射入即瘥。《梅師方》

Zhang Jiebin on Garlic

Volumes 48 and 49 of *Jingyue's Complete Works* contain a materia medica. Zhang rarely mentioned moxibustion in these volumes, but he did in the section on mugwort (above) and garlic. Volumes 63 and 64 of the *Complete Works* contain two other sections that focus on the use of garlic-isolated moxibustion. These passages are translated here. Zhang also described the use of garlic-isolated moxibustion in **LJTY: 11-3-23** p. 168, and especially **JYQS: 46-11**. Please refer to them as well.

For the most part, Zhang reserved garlic-isolated moxibustion for external ailments such as abscesses, sores, pox, or bites.

JYQS: 49-229 Garlic (229) (Zhang 1995, 1220) 《景岳全書・蒜二二九・卷之四十九》

The flavor is acrid. The nature is warm. It has minor toxins. It is good to rectify the center, warm the stomach, move stagnant qi, repel grease, open the stomach, promote food intake, disperse cold qi and cold phlegm, flour [or noodle] accumulation, food accumulation, all fish accumulations, evil impediment, drum distention, disquieted food stagnation, and it destroys stream toxins, water toxins, *gu* toxins, snake and insect venom. It is very good pounded to a pulp. [In this form,] it can be applied for moxibustion on abscesses, applied topically to clove swellings, and applied to snake and insect sand wind toxins.

味辛，性溫，有小毒。善理中溫胃，行滯氣，辟肥膩，開胃進食，消寒氣寒痰，麵積食積，魚肉諸積，邪痺膨脹，宿滯不安，殺溪毒水毒，蠱毒蛇蟲毒。搗爛可灸癰疽，塗疔腫，傅蛇蟲沙風毒甚良。

---

[27] The same formula is also found in **LJTY: 11-3-23** p. 168.

[28] *She gong* is discussed in **BCGM: 42-15**, where it is also called "ravine ghost insect" [溪鬼蟲]. That passage says its feet are angled like a crossbow and it uses qi as "arrows." It shoots people's shadows and they become ill. It must be that the garlic qi needs to shoot into the affected site to penetrate to the same depth as the *she gong*'s "arrows." Garlic is frequently used on sores or bites to detoxify, with or without moxibustion. It is also applied to the umbilicus or the soles of the feet as heavenly moxibustion.

JYQS: 63-117 Miraculously Effective Moxibustion on Garlic (117) (Zhang 1995, 1714)

《景岳全書・神效隔蒜灸法百十七・卷之六十三》

This method treats pox, clove sores, and toxin qi blazing exuberantly. It does not let any type of pox erupt. Those that have already erupted are unable to fill up with pus. Those that have already filled up with pus are unable to become dimples. Some have great pain or numbness. If there is pain, apply moxibustion until there is no pain. It there is no pain, apply moxibustion until there is pain. The toxins follow the fire and scatter.

This method uses a head of garlic sliced three *fen* thick. Place a slice on the pox or clove sore. Apply moxibustion using small mugwort cones on the garlic. Change the garlic every five cones and apply moxibustion again. You should especially use moxibustion if the sores bleed purple blood but the swelling and pain does not stop. Someone who treats should carefully consider this.

I have seen masters in the capital treat pox and clove sores by using a sewing needle to pick it open and let out toxic blood. All the pox subsequently filled up with pus. If they are picked open and there is no pain or bleeding, they are difficult to treat [meaning the patient may die]. If this method of moxibustion is used on them, the patient will promptly know pain. Further, use a needle to pick them open, so purple blood subsequently comes out. All the pox will subsequently fill up and some patients will still live.

治痘疔毒氣熾盛，使諸痘不能起發，
已起發者不能灌膿，已灌膿者不能收靨，或大痛，
或麻木，痛者灸至不痛，不痛者灸至痛，
其毒隨火而散。 其法用大蒜頭切三分厚，安痘疔上，
用小艾炷於蒜上灸之，每五壯易蒜再灸，若紫血出後，
腫痛不止，尤當用灸，治者審之。 愚在京師，
嘗見治痘疔者，即以線鍼挑破出毒血，
諸痘隨即灌膿。 若挑破不痛，不出血者難治，
若用此法灸之，即知痛，更用鍼挑破，紫血隨出，
諸痘隨灌，亦有生者。

JYQS: 64-115 Method of the Immortals for Moxibustion on Garlic (115),[29] (Zhang 1995, 1745)

《景岳全書・神仙隔蒜灸法・卷之六十四》

Treats all abscesses and sore-toxins with great pain, or without pain, or with numbness, as well as treating toxic qi blazing exuberantly from pox and clove sores. It does not allow any pox or similar patterns to erupt. Those that have already erupted are unable to fill with pus. Those that are already filled with pus are unable to become dimples. If there is pain, apply moxibustion until there is no pain. If there is no pain, apply moxibustion until there is pain. The toxins follow the fire and scatter. This is a co-acting treatment method[30] of attacking and scattering depressed toxins. It has the great effect of returning the patient to life.

This method uses a head of garlic. Remove the skin and cut it into slices three *fen* thick. Place a slice on the head of the sore. Apply moxibustion to it using mugwort cones on the garlic. Change the garlic every five cones and apply moxibustion again. Some use 30 or 50 cones. Some use 100 or 200 cones. The more cones the more wonderful.

Those sores or pox that have not yet developed will promptly be dispersed. In those that have already developed, it will also kill the overall condition. It is unable to cause harm.

If the sores are big, use garlic that has been pounded to a pulp on the affected site. Spread the mugwort on top and burn it. When the garlic is dried out, replace it again.

Sometimes yin toxins have a purple and white color and they do not erupt. They are not painful and do not make pus. It is still appropriate to use a lot of moxibustion. Further, take an internal expulsion prescription. If after moxibustion there is still no pain, or if it does not make pus and does not erupt, this is a case of qi and blood vacuity in the extreme.

---

[29] This passage is very similar to the previous one, **JYQS: 63-117**.
[30] A coacting treatment is using a like thing, instead of the opposite.

治一切癰疽瘡毒大痛，或不痛，或麻木，
及治痘疔毒氣熾盛，使諸痘不能起發，
已起發者不能灌膿，已灌膿者不能收靨等證。
如痛者灸至不痛，不痛者灸至痛，其毒隨火而散，
此攻散鬱毒從治之法也，大有回生之功。
其用法用大蒜頭去皮切三分厚，按瘡頭上，
用艾灸於蒜上灸之，五壯換蒜復灸，或三五十壯，
或一二百壯，愈多愈妙。未成者即消，
已成者亦殺其人勢，不能為害。
如瘡大用蒜搗爛攤患處，將艾鋪上燒之，蒜敗再換。
或陰毒紫白色，不起發，不痛，不作膿者，
尤宜多灸，仍服托裏之劑。如灸後仍不痛，
或不作膿，不起發者不治，此氣血虛極也。

VARIOUS TYPES OF ACONITE

Aconite is also commonly used as an isolating substance, either as a slice or ground into a powder and made into cakes. This section includes Fu Zi, Wu Tou, and Bai Fu Zi.

Li Shizhen on Aconite

BCGM: 17-17-1 Aconite [Fu Zi] (Li 1996, 528)
《本草綱目・草部第十七卷・草之六・附子》

Qi and flavor: Acrid, warm, very toxic...
【氣味】辛，溫，有大毒。……

Indications

Wind cold cough from counterflow evil qi, cold damp sprains and lameness, hypertonic knee pain, and inability to walk. It breaks up concretions, hard accumulations and gatherings, blood conglomerations, and incised wounds. *Shen Nong Ben Cao Jing*

Wind cold of the lumbar region and spine, leg qi with cold and weakness, cold pain of the heart region and abdomen, sudden turmoil [or cholera] with cramping, red and white dysentery. It warms the center, strengthens the yin [*i.e.*, genitals], and hardens the flesh and bones. It also aborts the fetus. It is

the chief of hundreds of medicinals. *Records of Famous Doctors*

Warms the spleen and stomach, eliminates dampness in the spleen and cold in the kidneys, and supplements yang vacuity of the lower burner. *Zhang Yuansu*

Eliminates deep and long-term coldness in the organs, reversal counterflow of the three yang channels, warms abdominal pain from excess [cold evils], and stomach cold with stirring roundworms. It treats menstrual blockage, supplements vacuity and scatters congestion. *Li Gao*[31]

When the governing vessel is diseased, there is rigidity of the spine and reversal. *Wang Haogu*

Treats cold damage of the three yin channels, yin toxins, cold mounting, cold stroke, wind stroke, phlegm reversal, qi reversal, soft tetany, epilepsy, chronic pediatric fright, wind cold paralysis, leg qi with swelling and fullness, head wind, kidney reversal headache, sudden diarrhea with yang desertion, enduring dysentery, spleen diarrhea, cold malaria, miasma qi, enduring disease with retching and vomiting, stomach reflux, dysphagia-occlusion, abscesses that do not close up, enduring fistulas, and sores due to cold. It is used to stop up the ears to treat deafness when combined with scallion juice. *Li Shizhen*

【主治】風寒咳逆邪氣，寒濕踒躄，拘攣膝痛，不能
行步，破癥堅積聚血瘕，金瘡。《本經》
腰脊風寒，腳疼冷弱，心腹冷痛，霍亂轉筋，下痢赤
白，溫中強陰，堅肌骨，又墮胎，為百藥長。《別錄
》
溫暖脾胃，除脾濕腎寒，補下焦之陽虛。元素
除臟腑沉寒，三陽厥逆，濕淫腹痛，胃寒蛔動，治經
閉，補虛散壅。李杲
督脈為病，脊強而厥。好古
治三陰傷寒，陰毒寒疝，中寒中風，痰厥氣厥，柔〔
疒+至〕癲癎，小兒慢驚，風濕麻痹，腫滿腳氣，頭

---

[31] Also known as Li Dongyuan, one of the four great masters of the Jin-Yuan period.

風，腎厥頭痛，暴瀉脫陽，久痢脾泄，寒瘧瘴氣，久
病嘔噦，反胃噎膈，癲疝不斂，久漏冷瘡。合蔥涕，
塞耳治聾。時珍

Appended formulas [abridged] 【附方】

BCGM: 17-17-1-52 Deep-source nasal congestion brain discharge: Mix powdered uncooked Fu Zi [Radix Lateralis Praeparata Aconiti] with scallion juice until it is the consistency of mud and cover Yong Quan [KI 1]. *Prescriptions of Universal Benefit*

鼻淵腦泄：生附子末，蔥涎和如泥，〔八+酉+皿〕涌
泉穴。《普濟方》

BCGM: 17-17-1-54 Sudden deafness & blockage of the ears: Take Fu Zi [Radix Lateralis Praeparata Aconiti] that has been steeped in vinegar and pare it so it is tapered. Insert it into the ear. Or better, apply two times seven cones of moxibustion on top. *Ben Cao Shiyi*

耳卒聾閉：附子醋浸，削尖插之。或更于上灸二七壯
。《本草拾遺》

BCGM: 17-17-1-108 Vacuity fire with heat in the back: Vacuity fire ascends and there is heat inside the back like it was roasted with fire. Apply powdered Fu Zi [Radix Lateralis Praeparata Aconiti] mixed with saliva on Yong Quan [KI 1]. *Zhai Xuan Fang*

虛火背熱，虛火上行，背內熱如火炙者：附子末，津
調，塗涌泉穴。《摘玄方》

BCGM: 17-17-1-110 To terminate delivery and abort the fetus: Powder uncooked Fu Zi [Radix Lateralis Praeparata Aconiti], mix it with thick wine, and apply it to the heart of the sole on the right foot.

The fetus will descend and be removed. *Short Sketches of Formulas*

斷產下胎：生附子為末，淳酒和塗右足心，胎下去之
。《方》

BCGM: 17-17-1-113 Abscesses & enduring fistulas: Cold in the opening of the sores with incessant secretion of watery pus; there is no malign flesh inside. Cut large Fu Zi [Radix Lateralis Praeparata Aconiti] that has been thoroughly soaked in water into large slices, three *fen* thick. Place them on the opening of the sore. Apply moxibustion to it using mugwort. At intervals of a few days, reapply moxibustion five or seven times. The patient can also take internal medicinals to draw out the toxins and pus, and the flesh will naturally grow and fill in. You can also grind it into a powder and make cakes. Xue Ji's *Heart Method of External Medicine*

癲疝久漏，瘡口冷，膿水不絕，內無惡肉：大附子以
水浸透，切作大片，濃三分，安瘡口上，以艾灸之。
隔數日一灸，灸至五七次。仍服內托藥，自然肌肉長
滿。研末作餅子，亦可。薛己《外科心法》

BCGM: 17-17-1-114 Abscess with outcropping [see glossary]: Like an eye that does not close. No medicinals can treat it. This method is very wonderful. Pare Fu Zi [Radix Lateralis Praeparata Aconiti] to the size of a [Chinese] chess piece. Stick it on with spittle.[32] Apply moxibustion to it using mugwort fire. When the Fu Zi becomes scorched, moisten it with spittle again and continue applying moxibustion. Make the hot qi penetrate inside for a prompt cure. *Prescriptions Worth a Thousand Pieces of Gold*

癲疝弩肉，如眼不斂，諸藥不治，此法極妙：附子削
如棋子大，以唾粘貼上，用艾火灸之。附子焦，復唾
濕再灸，令熱氣徹內，即瘥。《千金方》

---

[32] Here and in other writings (such as **LJTY: 11-3-4** p. 144 and **LJTY: 11-3-23** p. 168), Aconite is mixed with spittle. Of course, we would not consider doing this today because of the possibility that it could transmit disease. However, all substances can be used as medicine in the appropriate situation, at least according to the prevailing thought of earlier times. During the Ming dynasty, spittle was included in the materia medica. Remember, spittle is the humor of the kidneys, and as such, it should have a greater medicinal effect than water. Li discusses the properties of spittle in **BCGM: 52-19**, where he said "Spittle is transformed from a person's essence qi." Therefore, it should be a powerful agent to mix with the Aconite.

BCGM: 17-21-1 Wild Aconite [Wu Tou] (Li 1996, 537)

《本草綱目 • 草部第十七卷 • 草之六 • 烏頭》

Qi & flavor: Acrid, warm, very toxic...

【氣味】辛，溫，有大毒。……

Indications

Windstroke, aversion to wind, constant sweating. It eliminates cold damp impediment, ascending qi, counterflow cough, breaks accumulations and gatherings with fever and chills. When the juice is boiled, it is called *she wang* [see glossary] and kills birds and beasts. *Shen Nong Ben Cao Jing*

Disperses phlegm cold in the chest, inability to get food down, cold phlegm in the heart region and abdomen, pain around the umbilicus, cannot bend forward and backward, pain in the eyes, cannot look at things for a long time. Also, abortion. *Records of Famous Doctors*

Governs aversion to wind, abhorrence of cold, cold phlegm enveloping the heart, chronic dull pain of the intestines and abdomen, strings and aggregations [*xuan pi*], qi lumps, and toothache. It boosts yang affairs [*i.e.*, male sexual activity] and strengthens the will. *Zhen Quan*

Treats head wind, throat impediment, toxins from abscesses, swellings, and clove sores. *Li Shizhen*

【主治】中風惡風，洗洗出汗，除寒濕痹，咳逆上氣，破積聚寒熱，其汁煎之名射罔，殺禽獸。《本經》
消胸上痰冷，食不下，心腹冷痰，臍間痛，不可俯仰，目中痛，不可久視。又墮胎。《別錄》
主惡風憎寒，冷痰包心，腸腹〔疒+丂〕痛，痃癖氣塊，齒痛，益陽事，強志。甄權
治頭風喉痹，癰腫疔毒。時珍

Appended formulas [abridged] 【附方】…

BCGM: 17-21-4 Paralysis with stubborn wind & joint pain: The lower origin [*i.e.*, kidney] is cold and vacuous. Also all wind hemorrhoids and fistulas with blood in the stool and all wind sores. Three *qian* of both types of Tou—Cao Wu Tou [Radix Aconiti Kusnezoffi] and Chuan Wu Tou [Radix Praeparata Aconiti]. One *qian* each of Liu Huang [Sulfur], She Xiang [Secretio Moschi], and Ding Xiang [Flos Caryophylli]. Five seeds of Mu Bei Zi [Semen Momordicae]. Make them into a powder. Knead mugwort wool from Qizhou until it is soft and compound it all together in one place. Wrap it in rough paper. Burn it to fume the diseased site. This is called a "thunder pill."[33] Sun Tianren's *Collected Effective Formulas*

癱瘓頑風，骨節疼痛，下元虛冷，諸風痔漏下血，一切風瘡：草烏頭、川烏頭、兩頭尖各三錢，硫黃、麝香、丁香各一錢，木鱉子五個。為末。以熟蘄艾揉軟，合成一處，用鈔紙包裹，燒熏病處。名雷丸。孫天仁《集效方》

BCGM: 17-21-41 Onset of clove sore toxins: Seven pieces of Cao Wu Tou [Radix Aconiti Kusnezoffi], three pieces of Chuan Wu Tou [Radix Praeparata Aconiti], nine pieces of Xing Ren [Semen Armeniacae], one *liang* of very fine wheat flour. Make a powder. Mix it with unrooted water[34] and apply it to the sore. Cover it with paper, but leave the sore-opening uncovered. When it dries out, moisten it with water. Tang Yao's *Formulas from Experience*

疔毒初起：草烏頭七個，川烏頭三個，杏仁九個，飛羅麵一兩，為末。無根水調搽，留口以紙蓋之，乾則以水潤之。唐瑤《經驗方》

---

[33] This recipe is related to that of the moxa roll. See **BCGM: 06-07** p. 129, **ZJDC: 9-18**, and **JYQS: 51-54**.
[34] Unrooted water is flood water, according to **BCGM: 5-2**. It is rain water pouring down, excessive rain water.

BCGM: 17-22 Typhonium [Bai Fu Zi, Rhizoma Typhonii] (Li 1996, 540)
《本草綱目・草部第十七卷・草之六・白附子》

Qi & flavor: Acrid, sweet, very warm, slightly toxic...

【氣味】辛、甘，大溫，有小毒......

Indications

Heart pain, blood impediment, the hundreds of diseases of the face. It moves the influence of medicinals [*i.e.*, guides the other medicinals]. *Records of Famous Doctors*

Windstroke with loss of voice, all cold wind qi, facial spots, scars, and blemishes. *Da Ming*

All wind cold qi, weak feeble legs, scabs and lichens, wind sores, damp itching of the genitals, scars [or marks] of the head and face, used in facial cosmetics. *Li Xun*

Supplements vacuity that has caused liver wind. *Wang Haogu*

Wind phlegm. *Zhu Zhenheng*

【主治】心痛血痹，面上百病，行藥勢。《別錄》
中風失音，一切冷風氣，面䵟瘢疵。大明
諸風冷氣，足弱無力，疥癬風瘡，陰下濕癢，頭面痕，入面脂用。李珣
補肝風虛。好古
風痰。震亨......

Appended formulas [abridged] 【附方】......

BCGM: 17-22-10 One-sided sinking mounting qi [*i.e.*, unilateral descending of the testes]: One piece of Bai Fu Zi [Rhizoma Typhonii], powdered. Mix with saliva and fill up the umbilicus. Apply three or five cones of mugwort moxibustion. The patient will promptly recover. Yang Qi's *Simple and Convenient Formulas*

偏墜疝氣：白附子一個，為末，津調填臍上，以艾灸
三壯或五壯，即愈。楊起《簡便方》......

Zhang Jiebin on Aconite-isolated Moxibustion

JYQS: 64-116 Aconite [Fu Zi] Cakes (116) (Zhang 1995, 1745)
《景岳全書・附子餅・卷之六十四》

Treats ulcerating sores when both qi and blood are vacuous, making the sores unable to close, or wind cold assails them resulting in inability of blood and qi to move. Neither condition allows the sores to close.

Use blast-fried Fu Zi [Radix Lateralis Praeparata Aconiti]. Remove the skin and the "umbilicus." Grind it into a powder. Mix it with spittle to make a cake. Place the cake on the opening of the sore. Put mugwort cones on the cake and apply moxibustion to it. Apply several cones each day. However, just make it slightly hot. Do not cause pain. If the cake becomes dry, mix it with spittle again. Strive to make opening of the sore alive-looking and moist as the measure of success.

治潰瘍氣血俱虛，不能收斂，或風寒襲之，
以致血氣不能運行，皆令不斂。
用炮附子去皮臍研末，以唾津和為餅，置瘡口上，
將艾炷於餅上灸之，每日灸數壯，但令微熱，
勿令痛，如餅乾，再用唾津調和，
務以瘡口活潤為度。

FERMENTED SOYBEANS

Fermented soybeans may be made into cakes for isolating moxibustion. These cakes are used in the treatment of sores.

Li Shizhen on Fermented Soybeans

BCGM: 25-01 Fermented Soybeans [Da Dou Chi, also Dan Dou Chi, Semen Praeparatum Sojae] (Li 1996, 679) 《本草綱目・穀部第二十五卷・穀之四・大豆豉》

Qi & flavor: Bitter, cold, non-toxic...

【氣味】苦，寒，無毒。......

Indications

Cold damage headache with fever and chills, miasma qi, malign toxins, vexation and agitation, fullness and oppression, vacuity taxation panting, pain and coldness of the two legs. Detoxifies all of the six livestock and fetuses. *Records of Famous Doctors*

Treats seasonal febrile disease with sweating. Boiled and powdered, it is able to stop night sweating and eliminate vexation. The fresh is pounded and made into pills to treat fever and chills from wind and sores developing on the chest. Taken boiled, it treats bloody dysentery and abdominal pain. It is finely ground and applied topically for sores developing on the penis. *Nature of Medicinals Materia Medica*

Treats malaria with steaming bones, detoxifies medicinals, *gu* toxin qi, and rabid dog bite. *Da Ming's Rihua Bencao*

Descends qi and harmonizes. Treats cold damage, warm toxin macular eruptions, and vomiting counterflow. *Li Shizhen*

Uses it in *Hei Gao* [Black Ointment] to treat warm toxins. *Prescriptions Worth a Thousand Pieces of Gold*

【主治】傷寒頭痛寒熱，瘴氣惡毒，煩躁滿悶，虛勞喘吸，兩腳疼冷。殺六畜胎子諸毒。《別錄》
治時疾熱病發汗。熬末，能止盜汗，除煩。生搗為丸服，治寒熱風，胸中生瘡。煮服，治血痢腹痛。研塗陰莖生瘡。《藥性》
治瘧疾骨蒸，中毒藥蠱氣，犬咬。大明
下氣調和，治傷寒溫毒發斑嘔逆。時珍。
《千金》治溫毒黑膏用之。

Appended formulas [abridged]　【附方】

BCGM: 25-01-35 Abscesses & swellings erupting on the back: Already ulcerated or not yet ulcerated. Add a small amount of water to three *sheng* of fermented soybeans and pound them to make a paste. Make a cake based on the size of the swollen place, three *fen* thick. If the sore has an opening, do not cover the opening. Spread the bean cake around the sore. Arrange mugwort on top and apply moxibustion to it. However, make mild warmth; do not break the flesh with the heat of moxibustion. If there is hot pain, promptly change the bean cake, and the suffering should be reduced. Quickly apply moxibustion to it two times per day. If it already has an opening, it is wonderful to make fluids come out of it.[35] *Prescriptions Worth a Thousand Pieces of Gold*

發背癰腫，已潰、未潰：用香豉三升，入少水搗成泥，照腫處大小作餅，濃三分。瘡有孔，瘡有孔，勿覆孔上。鋪豉餅，以艾列于上灸之。但使溫溫，勿令破肉。如熱痛，即急易之，患當減。快一日二次灸之。如先有孔，以汁出為妙。

Zhang Jiebin on Fermented Soybean-isolated Moxibustion

JYQS: 64-117 Fermented Soybean [Dou Chi] cakes (117) (Zhang 1995, 1745)
《景岳全書・豆豉餅・卷之六十四》

Treats the swelling and toxins of sores that are hard and do not ulcerate as well as those that ulcerate and do not close, and all stubborn sores and malign sores.

Mix powdered Dou Chi [Semen Praeparatum Sojae] cakes from Jianxi province with spittle to make a cake the size of a coin and as thick as three or six coins. Place it on the affected site. Apply moxibustion on the cake using mugwort cones. When the cake is dry, change it again. If applying moxibustion to sores on the back, cover the affected site with cakes mixed with water that has been used to rinse the mouth. Spread mugwort on the cake and apply moxibustion to it. If the sores have not yet developed, it will promptly disperse them. If they have already developed, it also destroys great toxins. If it is

---

[35] A similar formula is also found in **LJTY: 11-3-23** (see p. 168-75) and **BCGM: 26-29-01** p. 111.

not effective, the patient's qi must be vacuous and the blood must have withered.

治瘡瘍腫毒硬而不潰，及潰而不斂，
並一切頑瘡惡瘡。用江西豆豉餅為末，
唾津和作餅子，如錢大，厚如三六錢，置患處，
以艾炷於餅上灸之，乾則再易。如灸背瘡，
用漱口水調餅覆患處，以艾鋪餅上灸之。如未成者即
消，已成者亦殺其大毒。如有不效，必氣血虛敗也。

SCALLIONS

Scallions are especially used for ironing swellings and pain but are also used in washes and as an isolating substance for moxibustion.

Li Shizhen on Scallions

BCGM: 26-03 Scallion [Cong, Bulbus Fistulosi] (Li 1996, 699)

《本草綱目•菜部第二十六卷•菜之一•蔥》

Qi & flavor: Acrid, balanced. The leaf is warm. The root hairs are balanced. Both are nontoxic.

蔥莖白【氣味】辛，平。葉：溫。根鬚：平。並無毒。

Indications

As a decoction, it treats fever and chills from cold damage, wind stroke, and superficial swelling of the face and eyes. It can make people sweat. *Shen Nong Bencao Jing*

Pain of the bones and flesh like they are breaking due to cold damage, throat impediment blockage. It quiets the fetus, returns and boosts the eyes, eliminates evil qi in the liver, quiets the center, disinhibits the five viscera, and detoxifies the hundred medicinals. The roots treat headache from cold damage. *Records of Famous Doctors*

Governs heaven current seasonal diseases [or epi-

demics], headaches, heat mania, sudden turmoil [or cholera] with cramping, as well as running piglet qi, leg qi, pain of the heart region and abdomen, dizzy vision, and stops confounding oppression of the heart. *Da Ming*

Frees the joints, stops nosebleeds, and disinhibits urine and feces. *Meng Xian*

Treats yang brightness dysentery and bloody diarrhea. *Li Gao*[36]

Reaches the exterior and harmonizes the interior, stops bleeding. *Ning Yuan*

Eliminates wind damp, body pains and paralysis, and worm accumulation pain of the heart region. Stops adult yang desertion and abdominal pain caused by yin toxins, pediatric twisted intestines with internal hooking [see glossary], bloody urine in pregnant females, frees breast milk, and scatters breast abscesses, disinhibits tinnitus, eliminates toxins from rabid dog bites, detoxifies earthworm [*qiu yin*]. *Li Shizhen*

Detoxifies all fish or meats. *Chen Shiliang*

【主治】作湯，治傷寒寒熱，中風面目浮腫，能出汗
。《本經》
傷寒骨肉碎痛，喉痹不通，安胎，歸目益目睛，除肝
中邪氣，安中利五臟，殺百藥毒。根：治傷寒頭痛。
《別錄》
主天行時疾，頭痛熱狂，霍亂轉筋，及奔豚氣、腳氣
，心腹痛，目眩，止心迷悶。大明
通關節，止衄血，利大小便。孟詵
治陽明下痢、下血。李杲
達表和裡，止血。寧原
除風濕，身痛麻痹，蟲積心痛，止大人陽脫，陰毒腹
痛，小兒盤腸內釣，婦人妊娠溺血，通乳汁，散乳癰
，利耳鳴，塗〔犬+折〕犬傷，制蚯蚓毒。時珍
殺一切魚、肉毒。士良

---

[36] Also known as Li Dongyuan, one of the four great masters of the Jin-Yuan period.

Appended formulas [abridged] 【附方】

BCGM: 26-03-1-23 Blockage of urine & stool: Pound scallion whites and mix them with vinegar. Cover the small abdomen with them. Then apply seven cones of moxibustion. *Secret Necessities of a Frontier Official*

大小便閉：搗蔥白和酢，封小腹上。仍灸七壯。《外臺秘要》

BCGM: 26-03-1-26 Acute strangury with genital swelling: Mash a half *jin* of scallions, roast them until hot, and mash them until soft. Apply them on the umbilicus. *Secret Necessities of a Frontier Official*

急淋陰腫：泥蔥半斤，煨熱杵爛，貼臍上。《外臺》

BCGM: 26-03-1-27 Urinary strangury & roughness: Sometimes the urine looks white. Cut off about a *cun* near the red roots of several scallions. Set them in the umbilicus. Apply moxibustion with seven cones of mugwort. *Formulas from Experience*

小便淋澀或有白者：以赤根樓蔥近根截一寸許，安臍中，安臍中，以艾灸七壯。《經驗方》

Zhang Jiebin on Scallions

JYQS: 64-121 Miraculously Effective Ironing with Scallions (121) (Zhang 1995, 1746)
《景岳全書・神效蔥熨法・卷之六十四》

Treats streaming sores, bound nodes, bone abscesses, crane's knee, and swollen lumps in the limbs. Some have pain and some do not have pain. Sometimes there is wind cold assailing the channels and network vessels, streaming sores on the limbs, hypertonicity of the joints, or bone pain. Sometimes there is damage due to knocks and falls. This is a good method to stop pain, scatter blood, and disperse swelling. Sometimes you have used moxibustion on garlic first but the residual swelling has not yet dispersed. Ironing is most appropriate to use in order to reinforce qi and blood and move congestion and stagnation. It is extremely effective.

Use thinly-sliced scallion heads, pounded to a pulp and stir-fried hot. Apply them to the affected site. When they become cold, promptly change them. Some also iron them several times with a hot iron. The swelling and pain promptly stops. The effect is like a miracle. Some use a decoction of scallions to steam or wash the damaged site. This is also wonderful. Some use a big handful of scallions, bind them in several sections and cut them into thin cakes to place on the affected site, ironing them with something hot. Some spread mugwort on it to apply moxibustion. The cakes must be changed often. Ironing is wonderful.

治流注結核，骨癰鶴膝，肢體腫塊，
或痛或不痛。或風寒襲於經絡，流注肢體，
筋攣骨痛。或跌撲損傷，
止痛散血消腫之良法。或先用隔蒜灸法而餘腫未消，
最宜用熨，以助氣血而行壅滯，
其功甚大。用蔥頭細切，杵爛炒熱敷患處，
冷即易之，再或熱熨數次，腫痛即止，
其效如神。或用蔥煎湯，
薰洗傷處亦妙。或用蔥一大把，束其數節，
切為薄餅置患處，用熱物熨之，或鋪艾灸之亦可，
必易餅多熨為妙。

OTHER ADJUNCTS USED FOR MOXIBUSTION

Many other medicinals are used in moxibustion besides mugwort. They are used as isolating substances or powdered and mixed in with the mugwort. A few are used in lieu of mugwort or as other types of external heat treatment. It is impossible to include all medicinals used like this, but a variety of them are translated below. Some are commonly used and others seem quite unusual.

All passages in this section come from the *Great Pharmacopoeia*. Li wrote extensively on the use of medicinals, not just in internal formulas or external washes, but also for other types of external heat treatments. The variety of medicinals and techniques seen below is astonishing.

BCGM: 11-01 Salt [Shi Yan] (Li 1996, 298)

《本草綱目•石部第十一卷•金石之五•食鹽》

Qi & flavor: Sweet, salty, cold, nontoxic.

【氣味】甘、鹹，寒，無毒。

Indications

Bound heat of the stomach and intestines with panting counterflow and diseases in the chest. It makes a person vomit [*i.e.*, ejection]. *Shen Nong Bencao Classic*

Cold damage with fever and chills. It ejects phlegm aggregation from the chest, stops sudden pain in the heart region and abdomen, kills ghost and gu evil infixation [see the glossary] toxic qi, invisible-worm sores of the lower regions, and hardens the flesh and bones. *Records of Famous Doctors*

Eliminates wind evils, ejects and precipitates malign things, kills worms, removes wind toxins from the skin, harmonizes the organs, disperses things that linger, and makes people vigorous and fortified. *Chen Cangqi*

Reinforces the water viscus [or kidneys] and [can be used for] sudden turmoil [*i.e.*, cholera] with pain of the heart region, incised wounds, brightens the eyes, stops evil qi wind tears, all worm damage sores and swellings, sores from fire burns, grows flesh, supplements the skin, unblocks urine and feces, cures mounting qi, and enriches the five flavors. *Da Ming*

Scrub your teeth [with salt] on an empty stomach, and use the spitting water to wash your eyes. This helps you see small characters at night. *Zhen Quan*

Resolves toxins, cools the blood, moistens dryness, settles pain, stops itching, spitting, all seasonal qi wind heat, all phlegm-rheum block and repulsion disease. *Li Shizhen*

【主治】腸胃結熱喘逆，胸中病，令人吐。《本經》
傷寒寒熱，吐胸中痰癖，止心腹卒痛，殺鬼蠱邪疰毒
氣，下部〔匿+虫〕瘡，堅肌骨。《別錄》

除風邪，吐下惡物，殺蟲，去皮膚風毒，調和臟腑，
消宿物，令人壯健。藏器
助水臟，及霍亂心痛，金瘡，明目，止風淚邪氣，一
切蟲傷瘡腫火灼瘡，長肉補皮膚，通大小便，療疝氣
，滋五味。大明
空心揩齒，吐水洗目，夜見小字。甄權
解毒，涼血潤燥，定痛止癢，吐一切時氣風熱、痰飲
關格諸病。時珍

Appended formulas [abridged] 【附方】

BCGM: 11-01-13 Sudden turmoil [or cholera] & cramping: The patient is about to die, [their] qi is expiring, but the abdomen still has warm qi. Use salt to fill in the umbilicus and apply seven cones of moxibustion on the salt. The patient will promptly revive. *Formulas to Rescue the Acute*

霍亂轉筋：欲死氣絕，腹有暖氣者。以鹽填臍中，灸
鹽上七壯，即蘇。《救急方》

BCGM: 11-01-23 Pediatric urinary stoppage: Set salt in the umbilicus. Apply moxibustion to it with mugwort. *Discussion on the Nature of Medicinals*

小兒不尿：安鹽于臍中，以艾灸之。《藥性論》

BCGM: 11-01-26 Urinary & fecal stoppage: Mix salt with vinegar and apply it in the umbilicus. When it dries, change it. *Jiacang Formulas*

二便不通：鹽和苦酒敷臍中，乾即易。仍以鹽汁灌肛
內；並內用紙裹鹽投水中飲之。《家藏方》

BCGM: 11-01-33 Pediatric pursed mouth [or lockjaw]: Pound a piece of salt and put it in the umbilicus. Apply moxibustion to it. *Secret Record of Mother and Child*

小兒撮口：鹽頭搗貼臍上，灸之。《子母秘錄》

BCGM: 11-01-64 Toxic snake bite poisons: Chew salt and smear it on the bite. Apply three cones of moxibustion. Chew more salt and smear it again. *Xu Boyu Formulas*

毒蛇傷螫：嚼鹽塗之，灸三壯，仍嚼鹽塗之。《徐伯玉方》

BCGM: 11-01-67 Poisoned arrow toxin qi: Apply salt on the sore. Apply 30 cones of moxibustion. This is good. *Collection of Effective Formulas*

藥箭毒氣：鹽貼瘡上，灸三十壯，良。《集驗方》

BCGM: 11-01-68 Rescue from water death by drowning: Use a big bench to lie them down. Then place the feet higher. Rub salt in the umbilicus until water spontaneously flows out. Do not by any means turn the person upside-down to get the water out. *Formulas to Rescue the Acute*

救溺水死：以大凳臥之，後足放高，用鹽擦臍中，待水自流出，切勿倒提出水。《救急方》

BCGM: 26-17 Uncooked Ginger [Sheng Jiang, Rhizoma Recens Zingiberis] (Li 1996, 714)
《本草綱目•菜部第二十六卷•菜之一•生薑》

Qi & flavor: Acrid, slightly warm, non-toxic.

【氣味】辛，微溫，無毒。

Indications

Long term consumption removes bad smells and unblocks the spiritual brilliance. *Shen Nong Ben Cao Classic*

Returns the five viscera, eliminates wind evils: fever and chills, cold damage with headache, nasal congestion, cough and ascending counterflow qi. It checks vomiting, removes phlegm, and descends qi. *Records of Famous Doctors*

Removes fullness due to water and qi, cures cough and seasonal disease. It governs acute pain below the heart when mixed with Ban Xia [Rhizoma Pinelliae]. It descends qi repletion with acute pain, heart and chest congestion and blockage, and cold and hot qi when made into a decoction with Xing Ren [Semen Armeniacae]. This is miraculously effective. It treats heat in the center causing retching, counterflow, and inability to get food down when made into a decoction with Xing Ren. *Zhen Quan*

Scatters vexation and oppression and opens up stomach qi. When taken as a decoction made from the juice, it descends all bound repletion and malign qi that surge up to the chest and diaphragm. This is proven miraculous. *Meng Xian*

Breaks blood stasis, regulates the center, and removes cold qi. The juice detoxifies medicinals. *Chen Cangqi*

Eliminates strong heat; treats phlegm with panting, distention, and fullness; cold dysentery with abdominal pain and cramping; fullness of the heart region; removes bad smells in the chest and foxy smell [or armpit odor], and kills long worms inside the abdomen. *Zhang Ding*

Boosts the spleen and stomach and scatters wind cold. *Zhang Yuansu*

Detoxifies all kinds of mushrooms and fungus. *Wu Rui*

The fresh is used to effuse and scatter. The cooked is used to harmonize the center. It resolves toxins which becomes throat impediment from eating wild fowl. Take the juice from soaking it in water and dab it on red eyes. Pound it to make juice and boil it with *Huang Ming Jiao* [Gelatinum Corii Bovis, ox hide glue]. Apply this for wind damp pain. It is very wonderful. *Li Shizhen*

【主治】久服去臭氣，通神明。《本經》
歸五臟，除風邪寒熱，傷寒頭痛鼻塞，咳逆上氣，止嘔吐，去痰下氣。《別錄》
去水氣滿，療咳嗽時疾。和半夏，主心下急痛。和杏仁作煎，下急痛氣實，心胸擁隔冷熱氣，神效。搗汁和蜜服，治中熱嘔逆不能下食。甄權
散煩悶，開胃氣。汁作煎服，下一切結實，沖胸膈惡氣，神驗。孟詵

破血調中，去冷氣。汁，解藥毒。藏器
除壯熱，治痰喘脹滿，冷痢腹痛，轉筋心滿，去胸中
臭氣、狐臭，殺腹內長蟲。張鼎
益脾胃，散風寒。元素
解菌蕈諸物毒。吳瑞
生用發散，熟用和中。解食野禽中毒成喉痹。浸汁，
點赤眼。搗汁和黃明膠熬，貼風濕痛甚妙。時珍

Appended formulas [abridged][37] 【附方】

BCGM: 26-17-1-37 Spider bite: It is good to cut a slice of blast-fried ginger and apply it. *Prescriptions Worth a Thousand Pieces of Gold*

蜘蛛咬人：炮姜切片貼之，良。《千金》

BCGM: 26-17-1-45 Onset of eruptions on the back: Broil a piece of fresh ginger on a charcoal fire. Scrape off the charred layer, and make it into a powder. Mix it with pig bile and apply it. *Formulas on the Sea*

發背初起：生姜一塊，炭火炙一層，刮一層，為末，
以豬膽汁調塗。《海上方》

BCGM: 27-07 Chinese Chives [Suan or Xiao Suan][38] (Li 1996, 703)
《本草綱目•菜部第二十六卷•菜之一•蒜》

Qi & flavor: Acrid, warm, slightly toxic...
【氣味】辛，溫，有小毒。

Indications

Returns the spleen and stomach, governs sudden turmoil [or cholera] and disquieted abdomen, disperses grains, rectifies the stomach and warms the center, eliminates evil impediment and toxic qi. *Records of Famous Doctors*

Governs stream toxins. *Tao Hongjing*

Descends qi, treats gu toxins. Apply it to snake, worm, and sand lice sores. *Da Ming's Ri Hua Ben Cao*

Su Gong said: These Chinese chives and garlic are used together. They govern malign *ci* toxins, sand lice in mountain streams, and water toxins. They are very effective. Mountain people, the Li and Lao, sometimes use them.[39]

Very good when applied to clove sores and swellings. *Meng Xian*

【主治】歸脾腎，主霍亂，腹中不安，消穀，理胃溫
中，除邪痹毒氣。《別錄》
主溪毒。弘景
下氣，治蠱毒，敷蛇、蠱、沙虱瘡。《日華》
恭曰：此蒜與胡蔥相得。主惡螫毒、山溪中沙虱、水
毒，大效。山人、狸獠時用之。
塗疔腫甚良。孟詵

Appended formulas [abridged] 【附方】

BCGM: 27-01-3 Sudden turmoil [cholera] with cramping: Entering the abdomen and killing the person. Pound one *liang* each of Chinese chives and salt and put them into the umbilicus. Apply seven cones of moxibustion and it will immediately stop. *Record of Sage-like Benefits*

霍亂轉筋，入腹殺人：以小蒜、鹽各一兩，搗敷臍中
，灸七壯，立止。《聖濟錄》

BCGM: 27-07-6 A person struck by *she gong* [see the glossary]: Making sores. Cut Chinese chives into slices. Place on the sore and apply seven cones of moxibustion. *Prescriptions Worth a Thousand Pieces of Gold*

射工中人成瘡者：取蒜切片，貼瘡上，灸七壯。《千
金》

---

[37] Surprisingly, none of the appended formulas involve mugwort moxibustion.
[38] Li Jingwei (1995, 126) says this medicinal is the same as 薤白 *Xie Bai*, Bulbus Allii.
[39] *Ci* is some kind of insect or worm. It is discussed in **BCGM: 39-15**. The Lao are a minority people in Guizhou and Yunnan. The Li are another minority group, perhaps on Hainan Island.

BCGM: 22-08 Buckwheat [Qiao Mai] (Li 1996, 651)

《本草綱目・穀部第二十二卷・穀之一・蕎麥》

Qi & flavor: Sweet, balanced, cold, non-toxic.

【氣味】甘，平，寒，無毒。

Indications

Fills the intestines and stomach, boosts qi and bodily strength, prolongs essence-spirit. It able to condense the filth of the five viscera. *Meng Xian*

Eaten as a grain, it suppresses toxins from elixir minerals. It is very good. *Xiao Bing*

Mix vinegar with the flour and apply it to pediatric cinnabar toxins and red swollen heat sores. *Wu Rui*

Downbears qi and loosens the intestines, grinds up accumulations and fullness, disperses hot swellings and wind pain, eliminates white turbid urine, white vaginal discharge, and spleen accumulation diarrhea. Mix-fry granulated sugar water with two *qian* of the flour and take this to treat dysentery. When taken scorch-fried and then drenched with hot water, it treats pain from intestine-gripping sand [i.e., dry cholera]. *Li Shizhen*

【主治】實腸胃，益氣力，續精神，能煉五臟滓穢。
孟詵
作飯食，壓丹石毒，甚良。蕭炳
以醋調粉，塗小兒丹毒赤腫熱瘡。吳瑞
降氣寬腸，磨積滯，消熱腫風痛，除白濁白帶，脾積

泄瀉。以沙糖水調炒麵二錢服，治痢疾。炒焦，熱水
沖服，治絞腸沙痛。時珍

Appended formulas [abridged] 【附方】

BCGM: 22-08-13 Head wind & wind eye: Make buckwheat cakes the size of a coin. Stick them on the four corners of the eyes. Apply moxibustion with mugwort cones the size of a grain of rice on the buckwheat cakes. This is promptly effective like a miracle.[40]

頭風風眼：蕎麥作錢大餅，貼眼四角，以米大艾炷灸
之，即效如神。

BCGM: 29-06-08 Stems and White Bark of Peach Tree [Tao Shu Jing Ji Bai Pi][41] (Li 1996, 769)

《本草綱目・果部第二十九卷・果之一・桃莖及白皮》

Qi & flavor: Bitter, balanced, non-toxic.

【氣味】苦，平，無毒。

Indications

Eliminates evil ghost malignity stroke with abdominal pain and removes heat in the stomach. *Records of Famous Doctors*

Treats demonic influx [see glossary] and visiting hostility [see glossary], pain of the heart region and abdomen, resolves gu toxins, prevents epidemic pestilence, cures jaundiced body and eyes that are the color of gold, kills all worms in sores. *Li Shizhen*

---

[40] This formula had no attribution, unusual for the *Great Pharmacopoeia*.

[41] **BCGM: 29-06** discusses various parts of the peach tree. Li often specified an east-growing branch for decoctions that are used as a wash. In **BCGM: 06-07** p. 129, an east-growing peach branch is used like a moxa stick. This is translated below. In **29-06-8-6**, Li quoted the recommendation from Sun's *Prescriptions* to carve such a branch into a human figure and attach it to the patient's clothes for amnesia due to a debilitated heart.

East-growing peach branches were used in magical remedies in the Mawangdui manuscripts (Harper 1998, pages 268 and 302 for example), so this type of usage has been passed down for a long time.

Peach was thought to have special properties. It had the ability to protect against ghosts and demons, so talismans were often made of peach wood (a practice which continues to the present). The fruit also symbolizes long life, and therefore may have a protective effect on health. Peach corresponds to the third month of the year, the time around the vernal equinox, and a time associated with the east when yang is growing (Eberhard 1986, 227-9).

【主治】除邪鬼中惡腹痛，去胃中熱。《別錄》
治疰忤心腹痛，解蠱毒，辟疫癘，療黃癉身目如金，
殺諸瘡蟲。時珍

Appended formulas [abridged] 【附方】

BCGM: 29-06-8-11 Suddenly suffering scrofula: No
pain. Put the white bark of the peach tree on the
sores. Applying two times seven cones of moxibustion on it is good. *True Person Sun's formula*

卒患瘰癧，不痛者：取桃樹白皮貼瘡上，灸二七壯良
。孫真人

BCGM: 35-21 Gleditsia Pod [Zao Jiao, Fructus Gleditsiae] (Li 1996, 886)
《本草綱目•木部第三十五卷•木之二•皂莢》

Qi & flavor: Acrid, salty, warm, slightly toxic.

【氣味】辛、鹹，溫，有小毒。

Indications

Wind impediment, eliminates dead flesh and evil qi,
head wind with tearing, disinhibits the nine orifices,
kills goblins, cures abdominal distention and fullness, disperses grains, eliminates cough, nodes in the
neck, retention of placenta, brightens the eyes and
boosts essence. It can be used as a medicinal wash.
Do not put it in a decoction [do not take orally].
Shen Nong Bencao Classic

Frees the joints, head wind, disperses phlegm, kills
worms, treats steaming bones, opens the stomach,
wind stroke with clenched jaw. *Da Ming*

Breaks hard concretions, pain in the abdomen, and
is able to descend the fetus. Also, soak it in wine to
completely get its essence. Decoct it to make a paste,
smear it on cloth, and apply it to all swelling and
pain. *Zhen Quan*

During the sweltering summer and enduring rainy
season, combine it with Cang Zhu [Rhizoma Atracty-
lodis]. Burn them to make smoke in order to avoid
scourge epidemic evil damp qi. *Kou Zongshi*

Burn it to make smoke to fumigate the anal region
for enduring dysentery and prolapse of the anus.
Wang Ji

Tracks down liver wind; drains liver qi. *Wang Haogu*

Frees lung and large intestine qi, treats throat impediment blockage, phlegm or qi panting and cough,
wind scrofula, scabs and lichens. *Li Shizhen*

【主治】風痹死肌邪氣，風頭淚出，利九竅，殺精物
。《本經》
療腹脹滿，消穀，除咳嗽囊結，婦人胞不落，明目益
精。可為沐藥，不入湯。《別錄》
通關節，頭風，消痰殺蟲，治骨蒸，開胃，中風口噤
。大明
破堅癥，腹中痛，能墮胎。又將浸酒中，取盡其精，
煎成膏塗帛，貼一切腫痛。甄權
溽暑久雨時，合蒼朮燒煙，辟瘟疫邪濕氣。
通肺及大腸氣，治咽喉痹塞，痰氣喘咳，風癩疥癬。
時珍

Appended formulas [abridged] 【附方】

BCGM: 35-21-1-56 Resolving nine-*li* wasp toxins:[42]
Drill a hole through a gleditsia pod and apply it with
the hole directly on the site of the sting. Apply three
times five cones of mugwort moxibustion on the
hole in the gleditsia pod. It will promptly quiet
down. *Formulas to Rescue the Acute*

九里蜂毒：皂莢鑽孔，貼叮處，艾灸孔上三五壯即安
。《救急方》

---

[42] Nine-*li* wasp: Nine *li* is about three miles. This must be some kind of wasp that flies far.

BCGM: 35-47 Croton Seed [Ba Dou, Semen Crotonis] (Li 1996, 902)
《本草綱目•木部第三十五卷•木之二•巴豆》

Appended formulas [abridged] 【附方】

BCGM: 35-47-1-14 Urinary & fecal stoppage: Crush a half *liang* each of Ba Dou [Semen Crotonis] (including the oil) and Huang Lian [Rhizoma Coptidis] with a mortar and make it into cakes. First drop scallion juice and brine into the umbilicus. Place a cake on top and apply two times seven cones of moxibustion. The measure of success is when urine and stool flow freely. *Collection of Formulas from the Yang Family*[43]

二便不通：巴豆（連油）、黃連各半兩，搗作餅子。先滴蔥、鹽汁在臍內，安餅于上，灸二七壯，取利為度。《楊氏家藏方》

BCGM: 35-47-1-17 Yin toxin cold damage: The heart region is bound up and pressing it is extremely painful, urination and defecation are blocked, but exhalation has a little warmth. Quickly grind 10 Ba Dou [Semen Crotonis] seeds finely and mix them with one *qian* of flour. Pinch them into cakes and place one inside the umbilicus. Apply five small mugwort cones of moxibustion. When qi extends, there is free passage. This is a formula from Grand Preceptor Chen Beishan. *Renzhai Zhizhi Fang*[44]

陰毒傷寒：心結，按之極痛，大小便閉，但出氣稍暖者。急取巴豆十粒研，入麵一錢，捻作餅，安臍內，以小艾炷灸五壯，氣達即通。此太師陳北山方也。《仁齋直指方》

BCGM: 38-42 Arrow Shaft and Head [Jian Ke Ji Cu] (Li 1996, 962)
《本草綱目•服器部第三十八卷•服器之一•箭（竹+可）及鏃》

Indications

For itching in the abdomen after childbirth, secretly put it under the mat where she sleeps. *Chen Cangqi*

For damage by a splinter [or thorn] with superficial swelling [literally, "wind water"], scrape an arrow below the coat of lacquer and apply it. It also governs clove sores and malign swellings. Scrape arrow shaft shavings and make cones. Apply two times seven cones of moxibustion. *Li Shizhen*

【主治】婦人產後腹中癢，密安所臥席下，勿令婦知。藏器

刺傷風水，刮箭下漆塗之。時珍

BCGM: 38-58 Axle Grease of Carts and Wagons [Che Zhi] (Li 1996, 964)
《本草綱目•服器部第三十八卷•服器之一•車脂》

Qi & flavor: Acrid, non-toxic.

【氣味】辛，無毒。

Appended formulas 【附方】

BCGM: 38-58-3 Sudden turmoil [or cholera] with cramping & abdominal pain: Apply grease from inside the hub of a cart to the heart of the foot. *Prescriptions Worth a Thousand Pieces of Gold*

霍亂轉筋：入腹痛。車轂中脂塗足心。《千金方》

BCGM: 38-58-14 Moxa sores that do not recover: It is good to apply grease from the hub of a wheel to them. *Prescriptions Worth a Thousand Pieces of Gold*

灸瘡不瘥：車缸脂塗之，良。《千金方》

---

[43] See also **ZJDC: 9-16**.
[44] See also **ZJDC: 9-17**.

BCGM: 40-5 Jujube Cat [Zao Mao, Purpuricenus Temmickii, a.k.a. Jujube Longicorn] (Li 1996, 988)
《本草綱目・蟲部第四十卷・蟲之二・棗貓》

Explanation

Li Shizhen says: The ancient formula books did not investigate Zao Mao. In formulas from recent generations, it was included in Fang Guang's *Danxi's Heart Methods Appended Remnants*,[45] where it was used in pediatric formulas. The notes say: They are flying insects that grow on Jujube date trees. They are as big as the Jujube dates, green [*qing*] and grey, and have two horns. Gather them on days with yin stems.

【集解】時珍曰：棗貓，古方無考，近世方廣《丹溪心法附餘》，治小兒方用之。注云：生棗樹上飛蟲也。大如棗子，青灰色，兩角。采得，陰乾用之。

Indications

Pediatric umbilical wind: Li Shizhen says: Note that Fang Guang said: In newborn infants, use silk floss to bind the umbilical cord securely five or six *cun* away from the umbilicus, and bite it apart. Use a goose quill to deliver one or two *fen* of medicinals into the big opening of the umbilical cord, rubbing the powder in very gently. Apply three cones of mugwort moxibustion to the end of the umbilicus. Once it has coagulated, do not touch it, [but] wait for it to drop off by itself. The patient will never suffer umbilical wind. You will not lose one in 10,000. Use it when the umbilicus is hard. If it is soft, there is no disease and you must not use it. This method uses three Jujube cats gathered on yin stem days (ground to a powder) and 49 grains of Zhen Zhu [Margaritia] (beat them to grind them). Stir-fry until yellow and use five *fen*, plus stir-fried Huang Dan [Minium], Bai Ku Fan [Alum], Ge Fen [Concha Mere-

tricis], Xue Jie [Sanguis Draconis], five *fen* each. Grind them evenly. Use the method described above. The umbilical cord has three openings; one is big and two are small.

【主治】小兒臍風。
時珍曰：按方廣云：小兒初生，以綿裹臍帶，離臍五、六寸扎定，咬斷。以鵝翎筒送藥一、二分，入臍大孔，輕輕揉散。以艾炷灸臍頭三壯。結住勿打動，候其自落，永無臍風之患，萬不失一。臍硬者用之，軟者無病，不必用也。其法用陰乾棗貓兒（研末）三個，珍珠（捶研）四十九粒，炒黃用五分、白枯礬、蛤粉、血竭各五分，研勻，如上法用。臍有三孔，一大二小也。

DISCUSSION

It seems that the only limitation to the use of medicinals for moxibustion is the imagination of the practitioner. The next chapter will contain some even more unusual methods. A few additional substances will be seen in the chapters on treatment.

Historically, there have been some authors such as Wang Tao or Zhu Danxi that were primarily known as herbalists but also wrote about the use of moxibustion. This type of doctor rarely used the fine needle for acupuncture. Wang Tao actually wrote, "The *Classic* says, 'Acupuncture is able to kill living people,' but it is unable to raise dead people. If you want to employ it, I fear it will damage life. Today, do not employ acupuncture on the channels; only apply moxibustion."

In view of the relationship between the materia medica and moxibustion, it is easy to see why herbal doctors might favor this modality. It is not restricted to mugwort and it can use many of the materials familiar to them.

---

[45] Fang Guang was a Ming dynasty author (16th century). He had great respect for Zhu Danxi and wrote *Appended Remnants of Danxi's Heart Methods* (Li 1995, 327-8).

CHAPTER 9
SPECIAL METHODS & FORMULAS

MIRACULOUS NEEDLES: MOXA ROLLS & OTHER TYPES OF MOXA STICKS

Li Shizhen was the first to publish a recipe for a moxa roll that had other medicinals mixed in with the mugwort. A few years later, Yang Jizhou published his own recipe.

Zhang Jiebin did not include this type of formula in the *Illustrated Supplement* (published in 1624), but he did 12 years later in his *Complete Works* (1636). An unanswered question is this: Was Zhang unaware of the moxa roll when he published the *Illustrated Supplement* or did he know about it but want to keep it secret? Perhaps when he was near the end of his life he was ready to let this special technique out into the world. Or perhaps in 1624, he had not had the chance to see the *Great Compendium* and the *Great Pharmacopoeia*. Once Zhang knew that these secret recipes had been published, he may have decided to contribute his own.

Li and Zhang also gave directions for using peach twigs and mulberry twigs as moxa sticks.

BCGM: 06-07 Fire from a Miraculous Needle [Shen Zhen Huo] (Li 1996, 203)
《本草綱目・火部第六卷・火之一・神針火》

Indications

Cold pain affecting the heart region and abdomen, wind cold damp impediment, yin abscesses attached to the bone. Whenever there is dull pain in the sinews and bones, use the miraculous needle on it. The fire qi will directly extend into the diseased site. It is extremely effective. *Li Shizhen*

【主治】心腹冷痛，風寒濕痹，附骨陰疽，凡在筋骨隱痛者，針之，火氣直達病所，甚效。時珍

Explanation

Li Shizhen says:

Miraculous needle fire: On the fifth day of the fifth lunar month, take a peach twig that is growing eastward. Pare it to make a wooden needle the size of a chicken egg, five or six *cun* long, and dry it. At the time of use, take three or five layers of cotton paper to cover the affected site. Dip the needle in sesame oil, light it, blow it out, and take advantage of the hot needle.[1]

There is also the thunder-fire miraculous needle method: Use one *liang* of powdered mugwort floss from Qizhou, one *qian* each of powdered Ru Xiang [Olibanum], Mo Yao [Myrrha], Chuan Shan Jia [Squama Manitis], Liu Huang [Sulfur], Xiong Huang [Realgar], Cao Wu Tou [Radix Aconiti Kusnezofii], Chuan Wu Tou [Radix Praeparata Aconiti], and Tao Shu Pi [peach tree bark] and five *fen* of She Xiang [Secretio Moschi]. Powder them and mix them with the mugwort. Cut thick paper into long narrow pieces. Spread the medicinals and the mugwort inside. Roll it firmly so it is the size of a finger, three or four *cun* long. Put it away and store it inside a jar. Bury it in the earth for seven times seven days and then take it out. At the time of use, light it in a lamp and blow it out. Place 10 layers of paper to isolate the affected site and take advantage of the hot needle. The hot qi enters directly into the diseased site. The effect is quicker [than with the previous item, the peach branch]. With both, avoid cold water.

【發明】時珍曰：神針火者，五月五日取束引桃枝，削為木針，如雞子大，長五、六寸，干之。用時以綿紙三、五層襯于患處，將針蘸麻油點著，吹滅，乘熱針之。
又有雷火神針法，用熟蘄艾末一兩，乳香、沒藥、穿山甲、硫黃、雄黃、草烏頭、川烏頭、桃樹皮末各一錢，麝香五分，為末，拌艾，以濃紙裁成條，鋪藥艾于內，緊卷如指大，長三、四寸，收貯瓶內，埋地中七七日，取出。用時，于燈上點著，吹滅，隔紙十層，乘熱針于患處，熱氣直入病處，其效更速。并忌冷水。

ZJDC: 9-18 Thunder-fire Needle Method (Huang 1996, 990)
《針灸大成 • 雷火針法 • 卷之九》

Treats wrenching and contusion, all pain within the bones, as well as cold damp qi, but the patient is afraid of acupuncture. Use three *qian* each of Chen Xiang [Lignum Aquilariae], Mu Xiang [Radix Auklandiae], Ru Xiang [Olibani], Yin Chen [Herba Artemisiae Scopariae], Qiang Huo [Radix Et Rhizoma Notopterygii], Gan Jiang [dry Rhizoma Zingiberis], and Chuan Shan Jia [Squama Manitis]; add a little She Xiang [Secretio Moschi] and two *liang* of mugwort from Qizhou. Take half a *chi* of calligraphy paper.[2] First spread the mugwort and Yin Chen on top. Next, mix in the medicinal powder and roll it up very tightly. Store it for later use.

Palpate to determine the painful point and mark it with a brush. Outside, use six or seven layers of paper to isolate the point. Take the roll of mugwort and medicinals, which is named "thunder-fire needle," and apply greater yang true fire.[3] You can use either a round bead or a fire mirror to light it.[4] When it is burning red, press it onto the point for a good while. Raise it back up and cut it with scissors to remove the ash. Light it again and press again for a total of nine times. The patient will promptly recover.

Chant this incantation once each time you apply moxibustion. First, with the burning fire in your hands, chant the incantation, saying, "Thunderbolt official general, gentleman of the stars with the virtue and power of fire, this medicine must perform with extraordinary results. Right now enable the spirits of the three worlds and the six mansions. This needle conceals blazing flames with which the

---

[1] See **BCGM: 29-06-08** p. 124 for a discussion of other uses of peach. The fifth day of the fifth lunar month is quite near the summer solstice and increases the yang in the twig, as does selecting it from the east side of the tree. Zhang also discusses this use of the peach twig in **JYQS: 51-54**, p. 131.
[2] This paper is soft but strong.
[3] Fire from the sun.
[4] See also **BCGM: 06-06**. A fire mirror is a concave metal reflecting device to focus the sun's rays and start a fire. The round bead resembles a crystal and also focuses the sun's rays to start a fire, like we might use a magnifying glass. Lighting it with fire from the sun makes it more yang.

process of tempering by fire is completed, and allows entry into the capital of the immortals through the nine gates of transformation. It removes pain and suffering; it clears away and sweeps off goblin airs. I serve the six stars of the southern constellation and the uppermost old gentleman.[5] Quickly, quickly, this is a lawful order."[6] When the incantation is completed, promptly press the thunder-fire needle on the point to apply moxibustion to it.[7]

True Person Sun created the thunder-fire needle, and it is still effective today. While engaged in this, it is important that you are sincere and respectful. Do not let women, chickens, or dogs see. This formula is completely genuine and has often been self-kept as a secret because people have not followed the principles of the ancients. If your heart is not united with the Dao, the treatment will not easily bring about a cure. Here I have expressed it out into the world.[8]

治閃挫諸骨間痛，及寒濕氣而畏刺者。用沉香、木香、乳香、茵陳、羌活、乾薑、川山甲各三錢，麝少許，蘄艾二兩，以綿紙半尺，先鋪艾茵於上，次將藥末摻捲極緊，收用。按定痛穴，筆點記，外用紙六七層隔穴，將捲艾藥，名雷火針也。
取太陽真火，用圓珠、火鏡皆可，燃紅按穴上，良久取起，剪去灰，再燒再按，九次即愈。灸一火，念咒一遍，先燃火在手，念咒曰：：雷霆官將，火德星君，藥奏奇功，方得三界六府之神，針藏烈焰煉成，於仙都九轉之門，蠲除痛患，掃蕩妖氛，吾奉南斗六星，太上老君，急急如律令。咒畢，即以雷火針按穴灸之，迺孫真人所製，今用亦驗。務要誠敬，毋令婦女雞犬見，此方全真多自秘，緣人不古，若心不合道，治不易療也。茲故表而出之。

JYQS: 51-54 Thunder-fire needle (54) (Zhang 1995, 1290)
《景岳全書・雷火鍼五四・卷之五十一》

Treats wind, cold, damp, or toxic qi lingering and stagnant in the channels and network vessels that makes pain or swelling which is unable to be scattered.

On the fifth day of the fifth lunar month, take an east-growing peach twig[9] and remove the skin. Carve the two ends into the shape of the tip of an egg, about one or two *cun* long. At the time of needling, put the needle over a lamp to ignite it. Then take three or five layers of paper; cloth can also be used. Cover the affected site with it. Take the hot needle and press it into the paper. Then chant this incantation three times: "Fire of heaven, fire of earth, the three hidden true fires: When heaven is needled, heaven opens. When the earth is needled, the earth splits open. When ghosts are needled, the ghosts are destroyed. When a person is needled, the person gains long life, the hundred diseases are dispersed and eliminated, and the tens of thousands of diseases are dispersed and destroyed. I serve the uppermost old gentleman.[10] Quickly, quickly, this is a lawful order."

治風寒濕毒之氣留滯經絡，而為痛為腫不能散者。
五月五日取束引桃枝，去皮，兩頭削如雞子尖樣，長一，二寸許。 鍼時以鍼向燈上點著，隨用紙三，五層，或布亦可，貼蓋患處，將熱鍼按於紙上，隨即念咒三遍，病深者再燃再刺之，立愈。 咒曰：
天火地火，三昧真火，鍼天天開，鍼地地裂，
鍼鬼鬼滅，鍼人人得長生，百病消除，萬病消滅。
吾奉太上老君急急如律令。

---

[5] This may refer to Laozi.
[6] *Lei2 ting2 guan1 jiang, huo3 de2 xing1 jun1, yao4 zou4 qi2 gong, fang1 de2 san1 jie liu fu zhi1 shen2, zhen1 cang2 lie4 yan4, lian4 cheng2 yu2 xian1 dou1 jiu3 zhuan zhi1 men2, juan1 Chu2 tong4 huan, sao3 dang4 yao1 fen1. Wu2 feng4 nan2 dou liu4 xing1, tai4 shang4 lao3 jun1, ji ji ru2 lu4 ling4.*
[7] The moxa stick is pressed nine times into the patient and the incantation, repeated each time, mentions nine gates of transformation, so each pressing should take the patient through one gate.
[8] True Person Sun refers to Sun Simiao. Yang thought this formula came from Sun. So he must have received it from an earlier source. None of the extant writings of Sun contain it. It is an unlikely claim, although Yang must have believed it. Yang's source could have been through his family tradition.
   In **BCGM: 29-06-8-2**, Li repeats a formula for jaundice using peach. In it, he said, "Do not let chickens, women, and dogs see." This is the same admonition here, so it must have been a standard statement for special techniques.
[9] Li also discusses this use of the peach twig in **BCGM: 06-07**, p. 129.
[10] This may refer to Laozi.

Another new formula for thunder-fire needle uses medicinals as the needle. This method is more wonderful.

Bai Zhi [Radix Angelicae Dahuricae], Du Huo [Radix Angelicae Pubescentis], Chuan Xiong [Rhizoma Chuanxiong], Xi Xin [Herba Asari], Ya Zao [small Fructus Gledistsiae], Chuan Shan Jia [Squama Manitis] (blast-fried and stone-baked), Ding Xiang [Flos Caryophylli], Zhi Ke [Fructus Aurantii], Song Xiang [Resina Pini], Xiong Huang [Realgar], Ru Xiang [Olibanum], Mo Yao [Myrrha], Du Zhong [Cortex Eucommiae], Gui Zhi [Ramulus Cinnamomi] (each 1 *qian*), Liu Huang [Sulfur] (2 *qian*), She Xiang [Secretio Moschi] (no limit), mugwort floss (2-3 *liang*)

Pound the above to make a coarse powder. Mix it evenly. Take the mugwort and spread it at the bottom. Mix the medicinals on top. Use the best quality heavy wrapping paper to roll it into a tube. You must first sew up the two ends with thread to prevent the medicinals from extending out. Next, add more paper to protect it. Try hard to pack it very solid and roughly the shape of the tip of an egg. This is the measure of success. Then use egg white to thoroughly brush the outer layer [as glue]. Roll it up and bind it. Dry it in the shade. Use this method in the same way as the earlier one.

One formula includes eight *fen* of Ba Dou Ren [Semen Crotonis] and three *qian* of Ban Mao [Mylabris]. Remove the head, feet, and wings to use.

又雷火鍼新方，乃以藥為鍼者，其法更妙。 白芷，獨活，川芎，細辛，牙皂，穿山甲，炮，倍 ¹¹ 用，丁香，枳殼，松香，雄黃，乳香，沒藥，杜仲，桂枝，各一錢。 硫黃，二錢。 麝香，不拘，熟艾，二三兩。 右搗為粗末，和勻，取艾鋪底，摻藥於上，用上好皮紙捲筒，先須用線絆約兩頭，防其伸長，然後加紙再掉，務令極實，粗如雞子尖樣，是其度也。 乃用雞子清盡刷外層，捲而裹之，

陰乾。 用法如前。 一方有巴豆仁八分，斑蝥三錢，去頭，足，翅用。

BCGM: 06-03 Fire from Mulberry Twigs (Li 1996, 202)
《本草綱目•火部第六卷•火之一•桑柴火》

Indications

For abscesses erupting on the back that do not develop, with stasis in the flesh so it does not putrefy, and genital sores, streaming scrofula sores, shank sores, and stubborn sores: light the fire, blow it out, and apply moxibustion twice daily. If it has not ulcerated, this dispels toxins and stops pain. If it has already ulcerated, it supplements and welcomes yang qi, removes the putrid and engenders flesh.

All supplementing medicinals and pastes should be decocted on this fire [from mulberry wood]. However, you cannot light mugwort with it as it will damage the flesh. *Li Shizhen*

【主治】癰疽發背不起，瘀肉不腐，及陰瘡瘰癧流注，臁瘡頑瘡，然火吹滅，日灸二次，未潰拔毒止痛，已潰補接陽氣，去腐生肌。凡一切補藥諸膏，宜此火煎之。但不可點艾，傷肌。時珍

Explanation

Zhu Zhenheng[12] said: This fire is used to extend without inhibition, and to dispel and conduct depressed toxins out. This is a method of coacting treatment.[13]

Li Shizhen says: Mulberry wood is able to disinhibit the joints and nourish body fluids. When it is used to make fire, it dispels and conducts toxic qi out, dispels wind and expels cold, so it is able to remove the putrid and engender the new.

Baopuzi[14] said: Medicinals used for becoming immortal cannot be taken internally if they are not decocted

---

[11] 倍 should be 焙, but this is what is in the original text.
[12] Also known as Zhu Danxi, one of the four great masters of the Jin-Yuan period.
[13] Also called paradoxical treatment, using like to treat like.
[14] Baopuzi was a nickname for Ge Hong 葛洪, and also the title of a book attributed to him.

with fire from mulberry. Mulberry is the essence of the winnowing basket constellation.[15] It is able to reinforce the potency of the medicinals. It eliminates all wind cold impediment pain because whoever takes it over a long period of time will not suffer wind disease their entire life.

【發明】震亨曰：火以暢達拔引郁毒，此從治之法也。
時珍曰：桑木能利關節，養津液。得火則拔引毒氣，
而祛逐風寒，所以能去腐生新。
《抱朴子》云：一切仙藥，不得桑煎不服。桑乃箕星
之精，能助藥力，除風寒痹諸痛，久服終身不患風疾
故也。

JYQS: 64-120 Miraculously Effective Mulberry Twig Moxibustion (120) (Zhang 1995, 1746)
《景岳全書・神效桑枝灸・卷之六十四》

Treats eruptions on the back that do not develop or stasis in the flesh that does not ulcerate. This is due to vacuous and weak yang qi.

Use an ignited Sang Zhi [Ramulus Mori, mulberry twig]. Blow on it to extinguish the flames. Use fire moxibustion on the affected site for a short while, three or five times per day, in order to assist the swelling to ulcerate. If the putrid flesh has already been removed, and new flesh is slowly being engendered, it is appropriate to apply moxibustion to the four sides. It is also appropriate to use it for yin sores, scrofula, streaming sores [see glossary], shank sores, and malign sores that are enduring and do not recover.

The general idea of this method is that when the sores have not yet ulcerated, it resolves heat toxins, stops pain, and disperses stasis swelling. When the sores have already ulcerated, it supplements yang qi, scatters residual toxins, and engenders flesh. This method can be used for the initial arising of yang patterns with swelling and pain that are severe or serious and the sore feels like it is carrying a stone. They will exude toxic fluids and promptly disperse internally. Use it on someone with sores that have endured for days. Even though the sores have ulcerated, they are also shallow, and will be without suffering. Pity the patient who does not know about this because those who treat them are unwilling to use this.[16]

治發背不起，或瘀肉不潰，此陽氣虛弱。
用桑枝燃著，吹熄其焰，用火灸患處片時，
日三五次，以助腫潰。 若腐肉已去，新肉生遲，
宜灸四畔。 其陰瘡瘰癧，流注臁瘡，惡瘡久不愈者，
亦宜用之。 大抵此法，未潰則解熱毒，止疼痛，
消瘀腫，已潰則補陽氣，散餘毒，生肌肉。
若陽證腫痛，甚或重如負石，初起則用此法，
出毒水即內消；其日久者用之，雖潰亦淺，
且無苦楚。 惜患者不知有此，治者亦不肯用此也。

DISCUSSION OF MOXA ROLLS

The earliest record of the moxa roll was written in the beginning of the Ming dynasty (although the use of peach or mulberry twigs predates the moxa roll). A doctor named Zhu Quan (dates unknown) wrote *Miraculous Formulas from Longevity Land*.[17] His roll contained pure mugwort with no additives. He described the technique for its use as pressing the lighted roll into the affected site or acupuncture point which was covered with layers of cloth or paper. This method is still described today in Chinese books on moxibustion and is also mentioned in *Chinese Acupuncture and Moxibustion* (Cheng 1987, 345). However, most practitioners in the West hold

---

[15] The winnowing basket (*Ji Xing*) is one of the 28 constellations. These constellations were discussed at least as far back as the *Huainanzi* (Major 1993, 69). The winnowing basket was mentioned in the *Book of Odes* (*Shi Jing*). It is associated with the water phase and is considered a lucky portent (Walters 1992, 97-8). The winnowing basket is located in the northeast, in the direction corresponding to the beginning of spring.

[16] Mulberry twigs are used as moxa sticks for sores and ulcers. Even so, mulberry wood cannot be used to light moxa cones, as it is said that the moxa will damage the flesh. However, it is good to cook medicinals over a fire made with mulberry wood. See also **ZJDC: 9-26** and **BCGM: 06-06** in Chapter 5 on general guidelines.

[17] Shoucheng Shenfang

the moxa roll over a point and do not allow it to touch the patient.

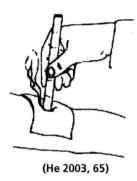

(He 2003, 65)

In **JYQS: 64-122 Formula of the immortals for fuming and radiating** below, Zhang describes a hand technique for using a different type of roll that does not include mugwort. In this case, it is circled around the affected area much the way people are taught to handle a moxa roll today.

These doctors held the "miraculous" moxa rolls in very high esteem. Moxa rolls were an important innovation at the time and were treated with great respect. Doctors gave them special names like "miraculous needle" or "thunder-fire miraculous needle." They included incantations to be chanted during treatment. Yang Jizhou instructed us to be respectful while we make the rolls. We should not let yin influences be present (women, chickens, and dogs).[18]

These rolls were called "needles" because of their long thin shape and because it was felt that their effects could penetrate deeply, like a needle. In addition, the early method of application, pressing the burning roll into the site, resembled the insertion of an acupuncture needle.

Ming and Qing dynasty doctors experimented with recipes, trying to find the most effective medicinals. They made different formulas based on the type of

illness to be treated. Since these doctors often had their own stock of medicinals, they could easily concoct new formulas and test them on their patients.

Because it is generally agreed that moxibustion warms coldness, dispels wind, dries dampness, and moves qi and blood, recipes include medicinals with these functions. In addition, medicinals such as *She Xiang* (Secdretio Moschi) were added to help the effects penetrate more deeply.

Moxa rolls were not used solely because of their convenience. Doctors in the Ming and Qing dynasties felt that this application technique improved the ability of the mugwort qi to penetrate into the body, and also enabled them to enhance or modify the effects of moxibustion by varying the medicinals included in the formula.

In contemporary times, moxa rolls seem to be more often used because they are the easiest way to apply moxibustion. It is rare that a doctor will design a formula today. The common practice is to buy moxa rolls in bulk from a distributor, with little thought given to the ingredients. Perhaps it is time to re-examine the moxa roll and stop taking it for granted.

STEAMING AND FUMING

JYQS: 64-122 Formula of the Immortals for Fuming & Radiating (122) (Zhang 1995, 1746) 《景岳全書・神仙薰照方・卷之六十四》

Xiong Huang [Realgar]
Zhu Sha [Cinnabar]
Xue Jie [Sanguis Draconis] (the genuine)
Mo Yao [Myrrha] (each one *qian*)
She Xiang [Secretio Moschi] (two *fen*)[19]

Grind the above five medicinals into a fine powder. Use a roll of thin soft paper, about a *chi* long, and

---

[18] I hope Yang can understand that times have changed and that my writing about it (being female) is not making him uncomfortable in his grave.
[19] This exact recipe is also in Chen Shigong's *Correct Model of External Medicine*, 陳實功《外科正宗》 published in 1617 (Ming).

make rough pinches in it. Put three *fen* of the medic-inals securely inside each twist. Use true sesame oil to moisten it thoroughly. Light it and burn it over the sores. It must be about a half *cun* away from the sores. Circle it around from outside the sore's red halo, slowly irradiating it in order to gradually send [the heat and qi] of the pinched section of the roll into the opening of the sore. This is called "from the outside inward." Further, you must suddenly lift the twisted section towards the outside in order to con-duct the toxic qi out. This is the manipulation. The qi of the medicinals effuses upward from the fire end of the twist. [Thus,] when it penetrates into the sore, the toxins follow the qi and scatter, and so they do not spontaneously invade the organs internally. Ini-tially use three sticks. Gradually increase to five or seven sticks. The power of the sores will gradually disperse. It can gradually reduce them. When the fuming is finished, follow it with an external appli-cation of medicinals.[20]

雄黃，硃砂，血竭真者，沒藥，各一錢。 麝，
二分。右五味，研細末，用棉紙捲為粗撚，
約長尺許，每撚中入藥三分裹定，以真麻油潤透，
點灼瘡上。 須離瘡半寸許，
自紅暈外圈周圍徐徐照之，以漸將撚收入瘡口上，
所謂自外而內也。 更須將撚猛向外提，以引毒氣，
此是手法。此藥氣從火頭上出，內透瘡中，
則毒隨氣散，自不內侵臟腑。 初用三條，
漸加至五七條，瘡勢漸消，可漸減之，
薰罷隨用後敷藥。

Li Du from Guangling said: For those who suffer sores on the back, there is only internal attack and external ulceration. The pattern belongs to fire tox-ins brewing and developing into this. If you are un-able to scatter it externally, the condition will attack internally. If you are unable to make it exit from the center, the condition will ulcerate on the sides. Doc-tors often use cooling medicinals topically all around to resolve the toxins, so the patient is often stricken by these two types of sufferings.

Also, for yin sores that do not erupt, there is only one method: moxibustion on garlic. When it is like this, you also are never able to acquire efficacy with certainty.

廣陵李杜云：背瘡所患，惟內攻與外潰耳。
證屬火毒，醞釀斯成，不能外散，勢必內攻，
不能中出，勢必旁潰。 醫者往往以涼藥圖解，
多罹此二患。 又陰瘡不起發者，止有隔蒜灸一法，
然亦未見鑿鑿取效。

This formula first uses the medicinal twist to fume and radiate; it uses fire to draw out the fire. The toxic qi will scatter outwardly. Afterwards, apply medicinals all around the sore to expel pus and stop pain. The toxins exit through the opening in the vertex of the sore so you can avoid ulceration on the sides. As soon as you radiate yin sores, a red halo ap-pearing like a steamed cake will promptly arise and it will mutate into a yang pattern. You can safeguard without mishap; this is the general idea.

此方初用藥撚薰照，以火引火，毒氣外散，
後用藥敷圍，追膿止痛，毒從孔竅及瘡頂中出，
可免旁潰矣。 陰瘡一照，即起紅暈，狀如蒸餅，
變為陽證，可保無虞，此其奇中大略也。

The radiation method: Once per day. At the initial time, use the length of three or four pinches. The next day, use four or five pieces. Each time gradually increase up to six or seven pieces, and then stop. Generally, look at the seriousness of the sores to de-termine the number of pinches. The serious case will not exceed six or seven days. The putrid flesh will completely transform into pus, continuously gush-ing out from the opening of the sore. New flesh will grow strung together like pomegranate seeds. At this time you must not radiate the sore again.

照法日每一次，初次用撚三根或四根，
次日用四根或五根，再次漸至六七根止，
大率看瘡輕重，酌撚多寡。重者不過六七日，
腐肉盡化為膿，從瘡口中陸續湧出，
新肉如石榴子纍纍而生，此時不必再照… …

---

[20] This method is similar to using a moxa roll, but there is no mugwort in the formula and the hand technique is different than for the moxa rolls above.

ZJDC: 9-19 Method of Steaming the Umbilicus to Treat Disease (Huang 1996, 990)
《針灸大成 • 蒸臍治病法 • 卷之九》

Wu Ling Zhi [Faeces Trogopterori] (eight *qian*, use fresh)

rough pieces of Qing Yan [Halitum] (five *qian*, use fresh)

Ru Xiang [Olibanum] (one *qian*)

Mo Yao [Myrrha] (one *qian*)

Tian Shu Fen [Heaven Mouse Droppings], (meaning bat droppings [Ye Ming Sha, Faeces Vespertilionis], two *qian*, slightly stir-fried)

Di Shu Fen [hamster droppings[21] (three *qian*, slightly stir-fried)

Cong Tou [Scallion head, Bulbus Allii Fistulosi] (dried, two *qian*)

Mu Tong [Caulis Akebiae], (three *qian*)

She Xiang [Secretio Moschi] (a little)

Make the above into a fine powder. Mix water with buckwheat flour and make a ring. Place it on the umbilicus. Take the previously made medicinal powder and put two *qian* inside the umbilicus. Cut Huai Pi [Sophora bark] into the shape of a coin and place it on top of the medicinals. Apply one cone of mugwort moxibustion to it for each year of age. Frequently replenish and change the medicinals and the "coins" of Sophora bark.

When used on an open day, it takes the right qi of heaven and earth, yin and yang, and brings it into the five viscera so that no evils can invade, the hundred diseases cannot enter, long life can withstand aging, and the spleen and stomach are strong.

Spring begins: *si* hour [9-11 am];
Spring equinox: *wei* hour [1-3 pm];
Summer begins: *chen* hour [7-9 am];

Summer solstice: *you* hour [5-7 pm];
Autumn begins: *xu* hour [7-9 pm];
Autumnal equinox: *wu* hour [11 am-1 pm];
Winter begins: *hai* hour [9-11 pm];
Winter solstice: *yin* hour [3-5 am].

This combines the right qi of the four seasons and completes the creation of heaven and earth. This method of moxibustion is never ineffective.[22]

五靈脂八錢，生用，斗子青鹽五錢，生用，乳香一錢，沒藥一錢，天鼠糞即夜明沙，二錢微炒，地鼠糞三錢，微炒，蔥頭乾者，二錢，木通三錢，麝香少許。右為細末，水和菜麵作圓圈，置臍上，將前藥末，以二錢放於臍內，用槐皮剪錢，放於藥上，以艾灸之，每歲一壯，藥與錢不時添換。依後開日，取天地陰陽正氣，納入五臟，諸邪不侵，百病不入，長生耐老，脾胃強壯。立春巳時，春分未時，立夏辰時，夏至酉時，立秋戌時，秋分午時，立冬亥時，冬至寅時，此乃合四時之正氣，全天地之造化，灸無不驗。

INHALING SMOKE

Zhang includes two treatments that involve inhaling smoke. These formulas all contain mugwort but not in large quantity. The additional medicinals in the two formulas are similar. Both treat cough or asthma. The idea would be to treat the lungs directly with the smoke, but this is unlikely to be used today for fear of toxicity.

JYQS: 60-266 Smoke Tube for Coughing (266) (Zhang 1995, 1625)
《景岳全書 • 嗽煙筒二六六 • 卷之六十》

Treats all cough that occurs as soon as winter arrives due to invasion by cold.

Kuan Dong Rui [Stamen Tussilaginis]

---

[21] According to **BCGM: 51-39**, this animal is like a mouse but smaller. It is also called } 鼩 *qu2jing1*.

[22] Li Chan has a similar passage in *Entering the Gate*, Volume 1 (Li Y. 1999, 283-5). Li has a larger number of ingredients, but there is a lot of overlap in the medicinals used. Yang gives two options in choosing a day: open days, or at special times on the eight main solar divisions of the year. Li Chan recommends this treatment four times a year, once per season. We know Yang studied *Entering the Gate*, but we cannot be sure whether he found this recipe in another book, developed it himself, or learned it from his family tradition. The day selection (open days or the eight times in a year) from this passage will be discussed in Chapter 13 on timing.

E Guan Shi [Stalactitum]

Xiong Huang [Realgar]

Ai Ye [Folium Artemisiae Argyi] (each equal *fen*)

Make the above into a powder and spread it on mugwort. Use paper to roll it into a tube. Burn it and inhale the smoke into the mouth, swallowing it down. Promptly gulp a mouthful of tea or boiled water to push it down. The patient will spontaneously recover. One formula has Fo Er Cao [Herba Gnaphalii, marsh cudweed] without the mugwort leaf. Use paper to roll it into a stick. Cut it into sections, each about three or five *fen* long. Burn it in a stove. Inhale the smoke and gulp it down.

治一切犯寒欬嗽，遇冬便作。 款冬蕊，鵝管石，
雄黃，艾葉，各等分。 右為末，鋪艾上，用紙捲筒，
燒煙吸入口內吞下， 即嚥茶水一口壓之， 自效。
一方有佛耳草， 無艾葉， 用紙捲成條， 每切一節，
約長三五分許， 焚爐中， 吸煙嚥之。

JYQS: 60-267 Magic Gem Smoke Tube (267) (Zhang 1995, 1625)

《景岳全書 • 靈寶煙筒二六七 • 卷之六十》

Treats all cold panting and cough.

Huang La [Yellow Wax]

Xiong Huang [Realgar] (each three *qian*)

Fo Er Cao [Herba Gnaphalii]

Kuan Dong Rui [Stamen Tussilaginis] (each one *qian*)

Ai Ye [Folium Artemisiae Argyi] (three *fen*)

First, melt the wax. Apply it to the paper. Next, spread the mugwort on it. Grind the three medicinals evenly into a fine powder, mix them and roll it into a tube. Use fire to light one end. Inhale the smoke and swallow it. Drink green tea to send it down.

治一切寒喘欬嗽。 黃蠟，雄黃，各三錢。 佛耳草，
款冬蕊，各一錢。 艾葉，三分。 先將蠟溶化，
塗紙上， 次以艾鋪之， 將三味細研勻， 摻捲成筒。
用火點一頭， 吸煙吞之， 清茶送下。

IRONING MEDICINAL CAKES

We have already seen many instances of ironing using mugwort, scallions, or other medicinals. Here are a few additional recipes.

JYQS: 64-118 Mu Xiang [Auklandia] Cakes (118) (Zhang 1995, 1746)

《景岳全書 • 木香餅 • 卷之六十四》

It is equally effective to treat all qi stagnation bindings and swellings, sometimes with pain, sometimes a wrenching sprain, as well as damage by wind cold that causes pain.

Mu Xiang [Radix Auklandiae] (five *qian*)

Sheng Di Huang [uncooked Radix Rehmanniae] (one *liang*)

Powder the Mu Xiang and pound the Sheng Di Huang into a paste. Mix them evenly. Measure the size of the affected site and make a cake. Place it on the swollen site and iron it with a hot iron.

治一切氣滯結腫或痛， 或閃肭， 及風寒所傷作痛，
並效。 木香，五錢。 生地黃，一兩。
右以木香為末， 生地黃杵膏和勻， 量患處大小作餅，
置腫處， 以熱熨斗熨之。

JYQS: 64-119 Xiang Fu [Cyperus] Cakes (119) (Zhang 1995, 1746)

《景岳全書 • 香附餅 • 卷之六十四》

Treats scrofula, streaming sores [see glossary], and swellings, sometimes with wind cold assailing the channels and network vessels; bindings and swellings, sometimes with pain.

Use powdered Xiang Fu [Rhizoma Cyperi] mixed with wine. Measure the size of the sore-toxin and make a cake. Cover the affected site. Iron it with a hot iron. If the sores have not yet developed, it will disperse them internally. If they have already developed, they will spontaneously ulcerate. If it is due to wind, cold, or damp toxins, it is appropriate to use ginger juice to make the cakes.

治療瘰癧流注腫塊，或風寒襲於經絡，結腫或痛。
用香附為末，酒和量瘡毒大小作餅，覆患處，
以熱熨斗熨之。 未成者內消，已成者自潰。
若風寒濕毒，宜用薑汁作餅。

JUNCUS MOXIBUSTION

BCGM: 06-09 Lamp Fire (Li 1996, 203)
《本草綱目・火部第六卷・火之一一・燈火》

Indications

All pediatric fright-wind diseases with stupor, con-
vulsions, clenching fists, staring eyes, and squinting.

It also treats distending pain from head wind: Look
for a site of exuberance in the greater yang network
vessels on the forehead. Use Deng Xin [Medulla
Junci] dipped in sesame oil, light it in a lamp, and
touch it to the site. This is good.

For the swelling and pain of external hemorrhoids,
also touch them.

The sesame oil is able to eliminate wind and resolve
toxins. Fire is able to unblock the channels... *Li Shizhen*

【主治】小兒驚風、昏迷、搐搦、竄視諸病。又治頭
風脹痛，視頭額太陽絡脈盛處，以燈心蘸麻油點燈淬
之，良。外痔腫痛者，亦淬之。油能去風解毒，火能
通經也。……時珍

Appended formulas [abridged]

06-09-1 Agitated intestinal sand pain: Yin and yang
abdominal pain, cold hands and feet, but there are
red spots on the body. Dip Deng Cao [Medulla Junci]
in oil, light it, and touch it on the spots.[23] *Formulas
to Set the Acute in Order [Qi Ji Fang]*

年深疥癬，遍身延蔓者：硫黄、艾葉研匀作捻，浸油
點燈，于被中熏之。以油塗口鼻耳目，露之。《集玄
方》

06-09-7 Scabs & lichens that have lasted for years:
Extending like a vine all over the body. Pound Liu
Huang [Sulfur] and mugwort in a mortar and mix
them evenly. Take a pinch, soak it in oil, and light
the "lamp." Fumigate the patient with it under a
quilt. Smear oil on his mouth, nose, ears, and eyes,
and expose him to the smoke. *Collection of Profound
Formulas [Ji Xuan Fang]*

攪腸沙痛：陰陽腹痛，手足冷，但身上有紅點。以燈
草蘸油點火，淬于點上。《濟急方》

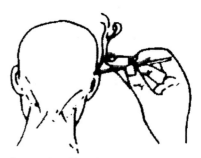

Juncus Moxibustion (He 2003, 74)

DISCUSSION OF JUNCUS MOXIBUSTION

Juncus moxibustion on Jiao Sun (SJ 20) is still recommended today for treating mumps in *Chinese
Acupuncture and Moxibustion* (Cheng 1987, 472). The
last formula does not use Juncus, but Li called the
entry *Lamp Fire* and included various types in his discussion. Deng Xin Cao means "lamp wick herb" and
can be used as the wick of a candle or lamp. That is
why it is included under the heading *Lamp Fire*.

MOXIBUSTION IN THE EAR

JYQS: 60-63 Moxibustion for Sudden Deaf-ness (63) (Zhang 1995, 1592)
《景岳全書・暴聾灸法六三・卷之六十》

Use a small piece of Cang Zhu [Rhizoma Atractylodis]

---

[23] Intestinal sand is the same as dry cholera (Wiseman 1998, 152). "Yin and yang abdominal pain" was translated into English by
others as "acute and dull abdominal pain" (Li 2004). It could also mean abdominal pain accompanied by yin symptoms such as
cold legs and yang symptoms such as red spots.

seven *fen* long. Pare one end into a point and cut one end flat. Insert the pointed end into the ear with the flat end up. Apply moxibustion with mugwort cones the size of the end of a chopstick on the flat end. If the case is mild, use seven cones. If severe, use 14 cones. When the inner ear feels hot, it will be effective.

Another formula: Use Bin Lang [Semen Arecae] that is shaped like a chicken heart. Inside its "umbilicus," scoop out a "nest" the size of the eye of a coin. Fill it with She Xiang [Secretio Moschi] and set it inside the affected ear. Apply moxibustion with mugwort cones on top. The patient will promptly recover after no more than two or three times.

用小蒼朮一塊長七分，一頭削尖，一頭截平，
將尖頭插入耳內，平頭上用箸頭大艾炷灸之，
輕者七壯，重者十四壯，覺耳內有熱氣則效。　又方：
用雞心檳榔一個，將臍內剜一窩如錢眼大，
實以麝香，坐於患耳內，上以艾炷灸之，
不過二三次即效。

CONCLUSION

In addition, many unusual techniques are included in other sections of this book. While some of these cannot be used today, it is quite possible that others are effective and safe. The scope of moxibustion techniques has become quite narrow today. Clinical research on the efficacy of some of the more unusual techniques may prove fruitful.

CHAPTER 10

ZHANG JIEBIN'S TREATMENT FORMULARY IN THE *ILLUSTRATED SUPPLEMENT*

Chapter Contents

Zhang Jiebin must have favored moxibustion over acupuncture since he wrote this section describing moxibustion treatments for 24 categories of disease but did not write a similar section on the treatment of disease using acupuncture.[1]

This section comes immediately after one of Zhang's sets of guidelines for treating with moxibustion: **LJTY: 11-2** *Important Points Used for Applying Moxibustion to All Patterns*. This passage was presented above.

Sometimes the points listed for a condition are a prescription. More often, they are a selection from which to choose. For example, under **LJTY: 11-3-7** (see p. 138) *Accumulations, Gatherings, and Glomus Lumps*, Zhang said, "Apply moxibustion to any of the above points for accumulation lumps. You can select the function according to the pattern."

Moxibustion treatment protocols prescribed by Li

and Yang, as well as Zhang's prescriptions for moxibustion from his *Complete Works* are included in the next chapter.

ZHANG'S TREATMENT FORMULARY

LJTY: 11-3-1 Wind Stroke[2] [中風 Zhong Feng] (Zhang 1991, 931)

Visceral stroke with qi blockage, phlegm ascending, critical clouding, and loss of consciousness:

- Bai Hui [Du 20], Feng Chi [GB 20], Da Zhui [Du 14], Jian Jing [GB 21], Jian Shi [PC 5], Qu Chi [LI 11], Zu San Li [ST 36].
  Whenever someone feels hypertonic impediment in his hands and feet and his heart spirit is clouded and deranged, he is about to have the symptoms of wind stroke. Do not discuss wind

---

[1] However, note that when Zhang did recommend acupuncture, he frequently wrote to "prick" (刺 *ci*) the point when we would usually say "needle" today. It does not mean prick to bleed unless this is specifically stated.

[2] Historically, many doctors have felt moxibustion was effective for wind stroke. Zhang must be among them as he placed this entry first and it is relatively long.

and qi. If you can apply moxibustion to these seven points successively, he will recover.[3]

中臟氣塞痰上，昏危不省人事：百會、風池、大椎、肩井、間使、曲池、足三里。凡覺手足攣痺，心神昏亂，將有中風之候，不論是風與氣，可依次灸此七穴則愈。

• He Gu [LI 4], Feng Shi [GB 31], Shou San Li [LI 10], Kun Lun [UB 60], Shen Mai [UB 62].

合谷、風市、手三里、崑崙、申脈

• Shen Que [Ren 8]: Whenever someone has sudden wind stroke, Shen Que is the best. Luo Tianyi said: In windstroke, taking medicinals can only help sustain the patient. If you want to receive full results, mugwort fire is good. It not only expels and scatters wind evils and perfuses the blood vessels, but it also has the result of returning yang and boosting qi. Truly, no one is able to tell the complete story. For details see this point.[4]

神闕：凡卒中風者，神闕最佳。羅天益曰：中風服藥，只可扶持，要收全功，艾火為良。蓋不惟逐散風邪，宜通血脈，其於回陽益氣之功，真其有莫能盡述者。詳見本穴。

Hemilateral wind paralysis: If the left is affected, apply moxibustion to the right. If the right is affected, apply moxibustion to the left. Jian Yu [LI 15], Bai Hui [Du 20], Jian Jing [GB 21], Ke Zhu Ren [GB 3] (governs wry mouth), Lie Que [LU 7], Shou San Li [LI 10], Feng Shi [GB 31], Qu Chi [LI 11], Yang Ling Quan [GB 34], Huan Tiao [GB 30], Zu San Li [ST 36], Jue Gu [GB 39], Kun Lun [UB 60], Shen Mai [UB 62].

偏風半身不遂：左患灸右，右患灸左。肩髃、百會、

肩井、客主人主口歪、列缺、手三里、風市、曲池、陽陵泉、環跳、足三里、絕骨、崑崙、申脈

Deviated eyes and mouth: Jia Che [ST 6], Di Cang [ST 4], Shui Gou [Du 26], Cheng Jiang [Ren 24] (hemilateral wind, deviated mouth), Ting Hui [GB 2], He Gu [LI 4].

Whenever the mouth is deviated towards the right, the vessels on the left have been struck by wind and are slack. It is appropriate to apply two times seven cones of moxibustion to the deviated depression on the left. If deviated toward the left, the vessels on the right have been struck by wind and are slack. It is appropriate to apply two times seven cones of moxibustion to the deviated depression on the right. You can use mugwort cones the size of a grain of wheat.

口眼〔口+㖞〕斜：頰車、地倉、水溝、承漿偏風口〔口+㖞〕、聽會、合谷。凡口口+㖞〕向右者，是左脈中風而緩也，宜灸左〔口+㖞〕陷中，二七壯；〔口+㖞〕向左者，是右脈中風而緩也，宜灸右〔口+㖞〕陷中，二七壯。艾炷如麥粒可灸。

Jaw clenched and will not open: Jia Che [ST 6], Cheng Jiang [Ren 24], He Gu [LI 4].

口〔口+禁〕不開：頰車、承漿、合谷

Mutism: Tian Tu [Ren 22], Ling Dao [HT 4], Yin Gu [KI 10], Fu Liu [KI 7], Feng Long [ST 40], Ran Gu [KI 2].

瘖瘂：天突、靈道、陰谷、復溜、豐隆、然谷

Upcast eyes: Shen Ting [Du 24]. Apply moxibustion to the spine on the third and fifth vertebra, each

---

[3] This point prescription came from Sun's *Supplement* (Sun 1993, b151). It was later included in Zhu Quan's *Vitality of Qian and Kun* and Volume 8 of the *Great Compendium of Acupuncture and Moxibustion*. The phrase "do not discuss wind and qi..." means that it doesn't matter what the cause is. Just use these seven points as quickly as possible and the patient will recover.

[4] Zhang discussed Shen Que Ren 8 in **LJTY: 8-3-8**, above. Luo Tianyi (1220-1290, Yuan) was the author of *Precious Mirror of Protecting Life*.

fives times seven cones.[5] Together, they descend fire. They are immediately effective.

戴眼：神庭。脊骨三椎、五椎，各灸五七壯，齊下火，立效。

Paralysis: Jian Jing [GB 21], Jian Yu [LI 15], Qu Chi [LI 11], Zhong Zhu [SJ 3], He Gu [LI 4], Yang Fu [GB 38], Yang Xi [LI 5], Zu San Li [ST 36], Kun Lun [UB 60].

癱瘓：肩井、肩髃、曲池、中渚、合谷、陽輔、陽谿、足三里、崑崙

Arched-back rigidity: Bai Hui [Du 20], Shen Men [HT 7], Jian Shi [PC 5], Pu Can [UB 61] (seven cones), Ming Men [Du 4], Tai Chong [LV 3].

角弓反張：百會、神門、間使、僕參七壯、命門、太衝

Wind impediment and numbness: Tian Jing [SJ 10], Chi Ze [LU 5], Shao Hai [HT 3], Yang Fu [GB 38], Zhong Zhu [SJ 3], Huan Tiao [GB 30], Tai Chong [LV 3].

風痺不仁：天井、尺澤、少海、陽輔、中渚、環跳、太衝

LJTY: 11-3-2 Reverse Flow [厥逆 Jue Ni] [see glossary] (Zhang 1991, 933)

Ren Zhong [Du 26] (apply seven cones of moxibustion or insert a needle to reach the teeth. Wonderful!), Dan Zhong [Ren 17] (21 cones), Bai Hui [Du 20] (fulminant reverse flow cold), Qi Hai [Ren 6].[6]

人中灸七壯，或鍼入至齒，妙、膻中二十一壯、百會暴厥冷、氣海

One method uses a rope to measure around the left wrist on males, the right wrist on females. Use the rope to measure down the spine from Da Zhui [Du 14]. Apply 21 cones of moxibustion to the site at the end of the rope.[7]

一法以繩圍，男左女右，臂腕為則，將繩從大椎向下，度至脊中，繩頭盡處是穴，灸二十一壯。

Deathlike reversal, sudden collapse, qi desertion: Bai Hui [Du 20], Ren Zhong [Du 26], He Gu [LI 4], Jian Shi [PC 5], Qi Hai [Ren 6], Guan Yuan [Ren 4].

屍厥卒倒氣脫：百會、人中、合谷、間使、氣海、關元

Sudden hostility [see glossary]: Jian Jing [GB 21], Ju Que [Ren 14].

卒忤：氣海、巨闕

LJTY: 11-3-3 Cold Damage [傷寒 Shang Han] (Zhang 1991, 933)

Headache and generalized fever: Er Jian [LI 2], He Gu [LI 4], Shen Dao [Du 11], Feng Chi [GB 20], Qi Men [LV 14], Jian Shi [PC 5], Zu San Li [ST 36].

頭疼身熱：二間、合谷、神道、風池、期門、間使、足三里

No sweating: He Gu [LI 4], Wan Gu [SI 4], Tong Li [HT 5], Qi Men [LV 14], Zu San Li [ST 36], Fu Liu [KI 7].

汗不出：合谷、腕骨、通里、期門、足三里、復溜

With mania: Bai Hui [Du 20], Jian Shi [PC 5], Fu Liu [KI 7], Yin Gu [KI 10],[8] Zu San Li [ST36].

---

5 The third and fifth vertebra may refer to Shen Zhu (Du 12) and Shen Dao (Du 11), respectively, or Zhang may have meant right on the vertebra.

6 The directions for Ren Zhong (Du 26) come from Ge Hong's *Emergency Prescriptions to Keep Up Your Sleeve*, which also recommends moxibustion on Dan Zhong (Ren 17) and needling on Bai Hui (Du 20) (Ge 1996, 4-5).

7 This is from the same section of Ge Hong's *Emergency Prescriptions* as the previous entry. Ge attributes it to Bian Que (Ge 1996, 4-5).

8 Yin Gu is the primary name for KI 10 and an alternate name for Yong Quan (KI 1). KI 1 may have been intended here.

發狂：百會、間使、復溜、陰谷、足三里

Yin patterns: Qi Men [LV 14], Jian Shi [PC 5], Qi Hai [Ren 6], Guan Yuan [Ren 4].

陰證：期門、間使、氣海、關元

Mute voice: Tian Tu [Ren 22], Qi Men [LV 14], Jian Shi [PC 5], He Gu [LI 4] (prick), Tai Chong [LV 3] (prick). He Gu and Tai Chong are what are called "opening the four bars."

聲啞：天突、期門、間使、合谷刺、太衝刺。所謂開四關者，即合谷、太衝也。

Deafness: Shen Shu [UB 23], Pian Li [LI 6], Ting Hui [GB 2].

耳聾：腎俞、偏歷、聽會

Urinary blockage: Yin Gu [KI 10],[9] Guan Yuan [Ren 4], Yin Ling Quan [SP 9].

小便閉：陰谷、關元、陰陵泉

Curled tongue, retracted scrotum: Tian Tu [Ren 22], Lian Quan [Ren 23], He Gu [LI 4], Shen Shu [UB 23], Fu Liu [KI 7], Ran Gu [KI 2], Xue Hai [SP 10].

舌捲囊〔足+卷〕：天突、廉泉、合谷、腎俞、復溜、然谷、血海

Abdominal distention: Tai Bai [SP 3], Fu Liu [KI 7], Zu San Li [ST 36].

腹脹：太白、復溜、足三里

Residual heat: Qu Chi [LI 11], Jian Shi [PC 5], Hou Xi [SI 3]. (Residual heat refers to incompletely eliminated heat evils in the aftermath of a warm disease.)

餘熱：曲池、間使、後谿

LJTY: 11-3-4 Vacuity Consumption [虛癆 *Xu Lao*] (Zhang 1991, 934)

Vacuity detriment, summer influx [see glossary], getting thinner:

- Da Zhui [Du 14], Fei Shu [UB 13], Ge Shu [UB 17], Wei Shu [UB 21], San Jiao Shu [UB 22], Shen Shu [UB 23], Zhong Wan [Ren 12], Tian Shu [ST 25], Qi Hai [Ren 6] (true qi insufficiency), Zu San Li [ST 36], San Yin Jiao [SP 6], Chang Qiang [Du 1], the Four Flowers and six points of Master Cui.[10]

虛損注夏羸瘦：大椎、肺俞、膈俞、胃俞、三焦俞、腎俞、中脘、天樞、氣海真氣不足、足三里、三陰交、長強、崔氏四花六穴

- **A treatment:** Apply treatment to the root of the thumb on the palms, a little in front of the fleshy fish area [Yu Ji LU 10 region], about a half a finger from the inner side of the big crease. He Gu [LI 4] of the hand yang brightness is in the opposite place on the outside. When you press this point, it is extremely sore. Apply seven cones of moxibustion each to it and to Chang Qiang [Du 1]. It is very wonderful.

一法：取手掌中大指根稍前肉魚間近內側大紋半指許，外於手陽明合谷相對處，按之極痠者是穴，此同長強，各灸七壯甚妙。

Corpse-transmitted consumption:

- First, worms have damaged the heart. So it is appropriate to apply moxibustion to Xin Shu [UB 15] as well as above and below in the style of the Four Flowers. Second, apply moxibustion to four points of Fei Shu [UB 13] as before. Third, apply moxibustion to four points of Gan Shu [UB 18] as before. Fourth, apply moxibustion to four points of Jue Yin Shu [UB 14] as before. Fifth, apply moxibustion to four points

---

9   Yin Gu is the primary name for KI 10 and an alternate name for Yong Quan (KI 1). KI 1 may have been intended here.

10 The Four Flowers and six points of Master Cui are discussed in **LJTY: 10-1-6**, above.

of Shen Shu [UB 23] as before. Sixth, apply moxibustion to four points of San Jiao Shu [UB 22] as before.

• This pattern has five mild days and five severe days. During the mild days, the worms are very drunk. Right at that point, you can apply moxibustion. You also must seek the assistance of the Lotus Sutra and chant the Pu'an mantra to suppress it.[11]

第一代蟲傷心，宜灸心俞穴，並上下如四花樣。○
第二代灸肺俞四穴如前。○第三代灸肝俞四穴如前
。○第四代灸厥陰俞四穴如前。○第五代灸腎俞四
穴如前。○第六代灸三焦俞四穴如前。此證五日輕
，五日重，輕日其蟲大醉，方可灸，又須請《蓮經
》並普庵咒鎮念之。

• **A treatment:** Apply moxibustion to lumbar eyes [Yao Yan, non-channel] (the method is in the tenth volume of the *Illustrated Supplement*).[12]

一法：灸腰眼穴法在《圖翼・十卷》

• **A treatment:** Whenever applying treatment for consumption worms, you can apply seven cones of moxibustion each to a point on the third vertebrae and Gao Huang [UB 43] bilaterally.[13] Afterwards, use drink and food to regulate the patient, and then medicinals such as those to precipitate and to treat the worms.

一法：凡取癆蟲，可於三椎骨上一穴，並膏肓二穴，
各灸七壯，然後以飲食調理，方下取蟲等藥。

Steaming bones, cold and heat, nighttime fevers: Bai Lao [non-channel], Gao Huang [UB 43], Fei Shu [UB 13], Po Hu [UB 42], Pi Shu [UB 20], Shen Shu [UB 23], the Four Flowers points, Jian Shi [PC 5], Zu San Li [ST 36].

骨蒸寒熱夜熱：百勞、膏肓、肺俞、魄戶、脾俞、腎
俞、四花穴、間使、足三里

Vacuity timidity, non-transformation of drink and food: Ge Shu [UB 17], Pi Shu [UB 20], Wei Shu [UB 21], Zhong Wan [Ren 12], Liang Men [ST 21], Nei Guan [PC 6], Tian Shu [ST 25], Zu San Li [ST 36].

虛怯飲食不化：膈俞、脾俞、胃俞、中脘、梁門、內
關、天樞、足三里

Profuse sweating, diminished strength: Da Heng [SP 15].

多汗少力：大橫

Night sweating: Fei Shu [UB 13], Fu Liu [KI 7], Yi Xi [UB 45] (profuse sweating in malaria).

盜汗：肺俞、復溜、譩譆瘧多汗

Intractible cold of the lower origin: This is kidney and urinary bladder vacuity cold. If you use a lot of moxibustion, recovery will be wonderful.

Shen Shu [UB 23], Shen Que [Ren 8], Guan Yuan [Ren 4], Qi Hai [Ren 6] (yang desertion), San Yin Jiao [SP 6].

下元瘤冷：此腎與膀胱虛寒也，多灸愈妙。腎俞、神
闕、關元、氣海陽脫、三陰交

---

[11] In Zhang's version of the Four Flowers, two points are bilateral to the spine and two points are on the spine, diamond-shaped, not square. Zhang is instructing the same type of arrangement here, with the listed back transport points as the two bilateral points.

Corpse-transmitted consumption is another name for consumption which was often transmitted from family member to family member. Since the Song dynasty, consumption was attributed to worms (Wiseman 1998, 96). The worms are also mentioned in **LJTY: 10-1-2-20** on lumbar eyes [Yao Yan], above.

Because this case is so serious, Zhang felt help was needed from the *Lotus Sutra* and a Buddhist mantra. This last sentence was censored from the modern edition (Zhang 1996, 319).

[12] For lumbar eyes [Yao Yan], see **LJTY: 10-1-2-20**, above.

[13] For Gao Huang (UB 43), see **LJTY: 7-1-35**, above. The point on the third vertebrae may be Shen Zhu (Du 12). If not, it is nearby.

Cold genitals, abdominal pain, desire to die: After a person has excessive sexual activity or his way of life transgresses coldness, it results in extreme, frequent, and critical pain in the umbilical region. Quickly mix a powder of Da Fu Zi [Radix Lateralis Praeparata Aconiti] with spittle and make cakes the thickness of a big coin. Place one on the umbilicus and apply big cones of mugwort moxibustion on top. If it is difficult to obtain the Da Fu [Radix Lateralis Praeparata Aconiti] in a hurry, you can also just use slices of fresh ginger or scallion whites to take its place. If the medicinal cake becomes scorching hot, use spittle to mix with it or change it for another. Continue the moxibustion until sweating occurs and the patient's body is warm and then stop. Some add moxibustion on Qi Hai [Ren 6], Dan Tian [Cinnabar Field], or Guan Yuan [Ren 4]: two times seven cones of moxibustion on each. This frees yang qi on the inside and drives the cold to go outside. When the hands and feet are warm and the pulse and breathing rise, yin is dispersed and yang will recover.[14]

陰寒腹痛欲死：人有房事之後，或起居犯寒，以致臍腹痛極頻危者，急用大附子為末，唾和作餅如大錢厚，置臍上，以大艾炷灸之。如倉卒難得大附，只用生薑，或蔥白頭切片代之亦可。若藥餅焦熱，或以津唾和之，或另換之，直待灸至汗出體溫爲止。或更於氣海、丹田、關元各灸二七壯，使陽氣内通，逼寒外出，手足溫煖，脈息起發，則陰消而陽復灸。

LJTY: 11-3-5 Bleeding Patterns [血證 *Xue Zheng*] (Zhang 1991, 935)

Vomiting blood: Bai Lao [non-channel], Fei Shu [UB 13], Xin Shu [UB 15] (stop at five cones in the summer), Ge Shu [UB 17], Gan Shu [UB 18], Pi Shu [UB 20], Shen Shu [UB 23], Ji Gu [Spine Bone, non-channel] (see the details below under bloody stool),[15] Zhong Wan [Ren 12] (vacuity taxation vomiting blood), Tian Shu [ST 25], Tai Yuan [LU 9], Tong Li [HT 5], Jian Shi [PC 5], Da Ling [PC 7], Wai Guan [SJ 5] (prick), Zu San Li [ST 36].

吐血：百勞、肺俞、心俞夏止五壯、膈俞、肝俞、脾俞、腎俞、脊骨詳後便血、中脘虛勞吐血、天樞、太淵、通里、間使、大陵、外關刺、足三里

Anger qi damages the liver, vomiting blood: Ge Shu [UB 17], Gan Shu [UB 18], Pi Shu [UB 20], Shen Shu [UB 23], Jian Shi [PC 5], Zu San Li [ST 36].

怒氣傷肝吐血：膈俞、肝俞、脾俞、腎俞、間使、足三里

Nosebleed:

• Shang Xing [Du 23] (apply one cone of moxibustion and it will promptly stop. Someone said seven times seven cones must be applied. When fewer, it is unable to break the root), Xin Hui [Du 22] (like Shang Xing, Du 23), Bai Lao [non-channel], Feng Men [UB 12], Ge Shu [UB 17], Ji Gu [Spine Bon, non-channel] (see the details p. 147, under bloody stool), He Gu [LI 4], Yong Quan [KI 1].

衄血：上星灸一壯即止。一曰須七七壯，少則不能斷根、顖會亦如上星、百勞、風門、膈俞、脊骨詳後便血、合谷、涌泉

• **A treatment:** Apply three cones of moxibustion to the point behind the nape, in the hairline, in the depression between the two sinews. It is likely that blood from this area enters the brain and pours into the nose. That is why it immediately stops when you apply moxibustion there.[16]

---

[14] In a number of recipes from Zhang and Li Shizhen, Aconite power is made into a cake with spittle. Spittle is the humor of the kidneys, and, as such, it theoretically would have a greater medicinal effect than water. See also **BCGM 17-17-1** on aconite, above.
   The Cinnabar Field (Dan Tian) could be Shi Men (Ren 5) or Yin Jiao (Ren 7), both of which have "cinnabar field" as a secondary name. However, Zhang could also be referring to the whole region below the umbilicus.

[15] Ji Gu (Spine Bone, non-channel) is located on the spine at the same level as the umbilicus. For details, see the second item under bloody stool p. 147.

[16] This may be referring to Ya Men (Du 15) which treats nosebleed that does not stop (Deadman 1998, 547).

一法：於項後髮際兩筋間宛中穴，灸三壯。蓋血自此入腦注鼻中，故灸此立止。

Bloody stool:

• Zhong Wan [Ren 12], Qi Hai [Ren 6]. Apply moxibustion to the above two points for blood desertion, white complexion, soggy weak pulse, cold hands and feet, little thought of drink and food, vomiting if forced to eat. It is appropriate to apply moxibustion; its efficacy is miraculous.

便血：中脘、氣海。上二穴灸脫血色白，脈濡弱，手足冷，飲食少思，強食即嘔，宜灸之，其效如神。

• Overall, no treatment for bloody stool is effective except applying treatment on Ji Gu [Spine Bone, non-channel] which is level with the umbilicus. You must press the site of the high protuberance of the spine bone [in this location]. If the patient feels aching pain, it is this point. Right then, you can apply moxibustion to it. If it is not painful, then it is not the point. Apply seven cones of moxibustion and the bloody stool will promptly stop. If the condition re-emerges, promptly apply seven cones of moxibustion again, and you can eliminate the root once and for all.[17]

As for vomiting blood, nosebleed, and all bleeding diseases, the hundreds of other treatments are not effective, but these conditions will never re-emerge after undergoing moxibustion.

凡大便下血，諸治不效者，但取脊骨中與臍相平，須按脊骨高突之處，覺痠疼者是穴，方可於上灸之，不疼者非也，灸七壯即止。如再發即再灸七壯，永可除根。至於吐血衄血一切血病，百治不效者，經灸永不再發。

• **A treatment:** Apply moxibustion on the spine below the 20th vertebra [S3]. The number of cones is based on the years of age.[18]

一法：於脊中第二十椎下，隨年壯灸之。

Blood in the urine: Ge Shu [UB 17], Pi Shu [UB 20], San Jiao Shu [UB 22], Shen Shu [UB 23], Lie Que [LU 7], Zhang Men [LV 13], Da Dun [LV 1].

尿血：膈俞、脾俞、三焦俞、腎俞、列缺、章門、大敦

LJTY: 11-3-6 Drum Distention [鼓脹 *Gu Zhang*] (Zhang 1991, 936)

(Generally speaking, when water swelling is extreme, acupuncture is contraindicated. 大抵水腫極禁鍼刺。) Drum distention commonly corresponds to ascites.

You must first know the 10 kinds of drum swelling.
Be sure to avoid the umbilicus when it is protruding highly all around.
When there are veins on the abdomen, cease using medicinals.
When the scrotum is without a seam, he cannot sustain a cure.
When the back is as flat as a board, it is terminal and difficult to treat.
When the palms have no lines, he has a limited time.
When the five grains are not dispersed for 10 days, he will die.
When the belly is as smooth as a drum,[19] treatment responds slowly.
There are no medicinals for both profuse phlegm and shortness of breath.
You should know that 9 out of 10 are critical.
Even for a god-like physician, this is difficult to treat.
Advise a gentleman to always remember this document.[20]

---

[17] Sun's *Supplement* mentions Ji Gu (Spine Bone, non-channel) for bloody stool in Volume 27 (Sun 1993, b255).
[18] This treatment is also found in Sun's *Prescriptions* (Sun 1993, a178).
[19] Smooth as a drum because the skin is tight from the swelling.
[20] This is a 12-line memorization poem of seven characters per line.

Also:

Since ancient times, qi swelling could never be cured. The belly is smooth as a drum. It is extremely strange. It is like pressing a stone and it echoes if it is flicked. It is rare that formulas to discharge qi are able to see effect.[21]

又：
氣腫從來不可醫，肚光如鼓甚蹺蹊，
按之如石彈之響，泄氣方能見效奇。

Shui Gou [Du 26] (three cones), Shui Fen [Ren 9] (very good to apply moxibustion to it), Shen Que [Ren 8] (three cones; governs water drum distention, quite wonderful), Ge Shu [UB 17], Gan Shu [UB 18], Pi Shu [UB 20], Wei Shu [UB 21], Shen Shu [UB 23], Zhong Wan [Ren 12], Qi Hai [Ren 6] (qi distention, water drum distention, yellow swelling), Yin Jiao [Ren 7] (water swelling), Shi Men [Ren 5] (water swelling, seven cones), Zhong Ji [Ren 3] (water distention), Qu Gu [Ren 2] (water swelling), Zhang Men [LV 13] (stone water), Nei Guan [PC 6], Yin Shi [ST 33] (water swelling), Yin Ling Quan [SP 9] (water swelling), Zu San Li [ST 36], Fu Liu [KI 7], Jie Xi [ST 41] (vacuity swelling), Zhong Feng [LV 4], Tai Chong [LV 3], Xian Gu [ST 43] (water swelling), Ran Gu [KI 2] (stone water), Zhao Hai [KI 6], Gong Sun [SP 4]. Take all the above points, select the appropriate ones, and use them.

水溝三壯、水分灸之大良、神闕三壯，主水鼓、甚妙、膈俞、肝俞、脾俞、胃俞、腎俞、中脘、氣海氣脹、水鼓、黃腫、陰交水腫、石門水腫、七壯、中極水脹、曲骨水腫、章門石水、內關、陰市水腫、陰陵泉水腫、足三里、復溜、解谿虛腫、中封、太衝、陷谷水腫、然谷石水、照海、公孫。已上諸穴，擇宜用之。

Blood drum distention: Ge Shu [UB 17], Pi Shu [UB 20], Shen Shu [UB 23], Jian Shi [PC 5], Zu San Li [ST 36], Fu Liu [KI 7], Xing Jian [LV 2]. This is drum distention due to blood stasis.

血鼓：膈俞、脾俞、腎俞、間使、足三里、復溜、行間

Simple abdominal distention:[22] Gan Shu [UB 18], Pi Shu [UB 20], San Jiao Shu [UB 22], Shui Fen [Ren 9], Gong Sun [SP 4], Da Dun [LV 1].

單腹脹：肝俞、脾俞、三焦俞、水分、公孫、大敦

Vacuity taxation puffy swelling: Tai Chong [LV 3].

虛勞浮腫：太衝

LJTY: 11-3-7 Accumulations, Gatherings, and Glomus Lumps [積聚痞塊 Ji Ju Pi Kuai] (Zhang 1991, 937)

Enduring glomus:

• On the back and spine, you can apply moxibustion to the point about four fingers lateral to Ming Men [Du 4]. If the glomus is on the left, apply moxibustion to the right. If it is on the right, apply moxibustion to the left.

久痞：灸背脊中命門穴兩旁各四指許是穴，痞在左灸右，在右灸左。

• **A treatment says:** Whenever treating glomus, you must treat Pi Gen [Glomus Root, non-channel]. It will not be effective without this. The method is: Below the 13th vertebrae [L1], right on the center of the spine, mark a spot with ink. Use the fingers to palpate on both sides, 3.5 *cun* lateral to the ink spot. There must be a moving place.[23] Promptly select this point and apply moxibustion to it. The point is approximately level with the umbilicus. Apply a lot of moxibustion to the left side or apply moxibustion to both the left and right. This is Pi Gen [Glomus Root]. Or, if the left side is

---

[21] This is another memorization poem of seven characters per line, four lines.
[22] Simple abdominal distention is distention only, without water swelling.
[23] Volume 23 of *Jingyue's Complete Works* says 'moving pulse.'

affected, apply moxibustion to the right. If the right side is affected, apply moxibustion to the left. This is also effective.[24]

一法曰：凡治痞者，須治痞根，無不獲效。其法於十三椎下，當脊中點墨為記，墨之兩旁，各開三寸半，以指揣摸，自有動處，即點穴灸之，大約穴與臍平，多灸左邊，或左右俱灸，此痞根也。或患左灸右，患右灸左，亦效。

• Shang Wan [Ren 13], Zhong Wan [Ren 12], You Men [KI 21], Tong Gu [KI 20] (bound up accumulations, lodged rheum), Liang Men [ST 21], Tian Shu [ST 25], Qi Men [LV 14] (100 cones; treats an accumulation of qi running upward, very urgent desire to expire), Zhang Men [LV 13] (all accumulations, gatherings, and glomus lumps), Qi Hai [Ren 6] (100 cones; treats all qi lumps), Guan Yuan [Ren 4] (100 cones; treats running piglet qi counterflow, unendurable pain), Pi Shu [UB 20], San Jiao Shu [UB 22]. Apply moxibustion to any of the above points for accumulation lumps. You can select the function according to the pattern.

上脘、中脘、幽門、通谷結積留飲、梁門、天樞、期門百壯，治積氣上奔甚急欲絕、章門一切積聚痞塊、氣海百壯，治一切氣塊、關元百壯，治奔豚氣逆，痛不可忍、脾俞、三焦俞。右穴皆灸積塊，可按證選用。

Lung accumulation: Called rushing respiration, located below the right rib-side. Chi Ze [LU 5], Zhang Men [LV 13], Zu San Li [ST 36]. This is one of the five accumulations for various types of abdominal masses.

肺積：名息奔，在右脅下。尺澤、章門、足三里

Heart accumulation: Called deep-lying bean, arises above the umbilicus, ascending to reach the region below the heart. Shen Men [HT 7], Hou Xi [SI 3], Ju Que [Ren 14], Zu San Li [ST 36].

心積：名伏梁，起臍上，上至心下。神門、後谿、巨闕、足三里

Liver accumulation: Called fat qi, located below the left rib-side. Gan Shu [UB 18] (seven cones), Zhang Men [LV 13] (three times seven cones), Xing Jian [LV 2] (seven cones).

肝積：名肥氣，在左脅下。肝俞七壯、章門三七壯、行間七壯

Spleen accumulation: Called glomus qi, located horizontally two *cun* above the umbilicus. Pi Shu [UB 20], Wei Shu [UB 21], Shen Shu [UB 23], Tong Gu [KI 20], Zhang Men [LV 13] (two times seven cones), Zu San Li [ST 36] (seven cones on each of the above points).

脾積：名痞氣，橫在臍上二寸。脾俞、胃俞、腎俞、通谷、章門二七壯、足三里上俱七壯

Kidney accumulation: Called running piglet, generated below the umbilicus, or running up and down constantly. Shen Shu [UB 23], Guan Yuan [Ren 4] (conglomerations and aggregations), Zhong Ji [Ren 3] (painful accumulations and gatherings below the umbilicus), Yong Quan [KI 1] (you cannot exceed four times five cones the size of a grain of wheat).[25]

腎積：名奔豚，生臍下，或上下無時。腎俞、關元瘕癖、中極臍下積聚疼痛、湧泉四五壯，不可太過，炷如麥粒

Qi lumps: Pi Shu [UB 20], Wei Shu [UB 21], Shen Shu [UB 23], Liang Men [ST 21] (pain), Tian Shu [ST 25].

氣塊：脾俞、胃俞、腎俞、梁門疼痛、天樞

---

[24] For Pi Gen [Glomus Root, non-channel], see also **ZJDC: 9-6-5**, above. The left, being the yang side, is favorable to disperse an accumulation of yin.

[25] The five patterns above are the five accumulations. They were discussed as a group and systematized in the 56th Difficulty.

Changsang Jun[26] needled accumulations, lumps, concretions, and conglomerations. First, needle into the lump. If it is severe, insert another needle into the head of the lump and another into the tail of the lump. When the needles are in, apply moxibustion to it. It will immediately respond.

長桑君鍼積塊癥瘕，先於塊上鍼之，甚者又於塊頭一鍼，塊尾一鍼，鍼訖灸之立應。

LJTY: 11-3-8 Pain & Distention of the Heart Region, Abdomen, Chest, and Rib-sides [心腹胸脅痛脹 *Xin Fu Xiong Xie Tong Zhang*] (Zhang 1991, 938)

Lung-type heart pain: Sleeps face-down like a turtle. Tai Yuan [LU 9] (five cones), Chi Ze [LU 5] (five cones), Shang Wan [Ren 13], Dan Zhong [Ren 17] (chest impediment pain).[27]

肺心痛：臥者伏龜。太淵五壯、尺澤五壯、膻中胸痹痛

Spleen-type heart pain: Needle-like pain. Nei Guan [PC 6], Da Du [SP 2] (five cones), Tai Bai [SP 3] (five cones), Zu San Li [ST 36] (connected to Cheng Shan [UB 57]),[28] Gong Sun [SP 4].

脾心痛：痛如鍼刺。內關、大都五壯、太白五壯、足三里連承山、公孫

Liver-type heart pain: Grey complexion, death-like appearance, cannot rest at the end of day. Xing Jian [LV 2] (seven cones), Tai Chong [LV 3] (seven cones).

肝心痛：色蒼蒼如死狀，終日不得休息。行間七壯、太衝七壯

Kidney-type heart pain: Sorrow and dread gripping each other. Tai Xi [KI 3], Ran Gu [KI 2] (each seven cones).

腎心痛：悲懼相控。太谿、然谷各七壯

Stomach-type heart pain: Abdominal distention, chest fullness, or severe pain from bound-up roundworms, roundworm heart pain. Ju Que [Ren 14] (two times seven cones), Da Du [SP 2], Tai Bai [SP 3], Zu San Li [ST 36] (connected to Cheng Shan [UB 57]).

胃心痛：腹脹胸滿，或蚘結痛甚蚘心痛也。巨闕二七壯、大都、太白、足三里連承山

Stomach duct pain:[29] Ge Shu [UB 17], Pi Shu [UB 20], Wei Shu [UB 21], Nei Guan [PC 6], Yang Fu [GB 38], Shang Qiu [SP 5].

胃脘痛：膈俞、脾俞、胃俞、內關、陽輔、商丘

Abdominal pain, abdominal distention: Ge Shu [UB 17], Pi Shu [UB 20], Wei Shu [UB 21], Shen Shu [UB 23], Da Chang Shu [UB 25], Zhong Wan [Ren 12] (cold spleen), Shui Fen [Ren 9], Tian Shu [ST 25], Shi Men [Ren 5] (hardness and fullness below the heart), Nei Guan [PC 6], Zu San Li [ST 36], Shang Qiu [SP 5] (spleen vacuity abdominal distention), Gong Sun [SP 4].

腹痛腹脹：膈俞、脾俞、胃俞、腎俞、大腸俞、中脘脾寒、水分、天樞、石門心下堅滿、內關、足三里、商丘脾虛腹脹、公孫

Lesser abdomen distention and pain: San Jiao Shu [UB 22], Zhang Men [LV 13], Yin Jiao [Ren 7] (cold pain below the umbilicus), Zu San Li [ST 36], Qi Hai [Ren 6] (treats the 36 diseases below the umbilicus, smaller abdominal pain, and desire to die. Apply moxibustion to it. There will promptly be life.), Qiu Xu [GB 40], Tai Bai [SP 3], Xing Jian [LV 2] (cold damp).

少腹脹痛：三焦俞、章門、陰交臍下冷疼、足三里、氣海治臍下三十六疾，小腹痛欲死者，灸之即生、坵墟、太白、行間寒濕

---

[26] Changsang Jun was Bian Que's teacher, according to the *Historical Records*.

[27] This and the other four types of heart pain listed below are based on *Magic Pivot*, Chapter 24.

[28] Acupuncture is applied to Zu San Li ST 36, threading it through to Cheng Shan UB 57. This technique is also suggested for stomach-type heart pain.

[29] Stomach duct pain is more commonly translated as epigastric pain (Deng 1999, 82).

Ascending qi, chest and back fullness and pain: Fei Shu [UB 13], Gan Shu [UB 18], Yun Men [LU 2], Ru Gen [ST 18], Ju Que [Ren 14], Qi Men [LV 14], Liang Men [ST 21], Nei Guan [PC 6], Chi Ze [LU 5].

上氣胸背滿痛：肺俞、肝俞、雲門、乳根、巨闕、期門、梁門、內關、尺澤

All qi pain, qi occlusion, qi ascending and not descending: Tian Tu [Ren 22], Dan Zhong [Ren 17], Zhong Fu [LU 1], Ge Shu [UB 17].

諸氣痛氣膈上氣不下：天突、膻中、中府、膈俞

Pain around the abdomen: Large intestine disease. Shui Fen [Ren 9], Tian Shu [ST 25], Yin Jiao [Ren 7], Zu San Li [ST 36].

繞氣痛：大腸病也。水分、天樞、陰交、足三里

Rib-side distention and pain: Ge Shu [UB 17], Zhang Men [LV 13] (seven cones), Yang Ling Quan [GB 34], Qiu Xu [GB 40] (three cones).

脅肋脹痛：膈俞、章門七壯、陽陵泉、坵墟三壯

LJTY: 11-3-9 Dysphagia-Occlusion [噎隔 *Ye Ge*] [see glossary] (Zhang 1991, 939)

All occlusion patterns: Xin Shu [UB 15] (seven cones), Ge Shu [UB 17] (seven cones), Gao Huang [UB 43] (100 cones, using many is good), Pi Shu [UB 20], Dan Zhong [Ren 17] (seven cones), Ru Gen [ST 18] (seven cones), Zhong Wan [Ren 12] (seven cones), Tian Fu [LU 3] (seven cones), Zu San Li [ST 36] (three times seven cones).

諸隔證：心俞七壯、膈俞七壯、膏肓百壯，多為佳、脾俞、膻中七壯、乳根七壯、中脘七壯、天府七壯、足三里三七壯

Qi dysphagia: Tian Tu [Ren 22], Ge Shu [UB 17], Pi Shu [UB 20], Shen Shu [UB 23], Ru Gen [ST 18], Guan Chong [SJ 1] (three times five cones), Zu San

Li [ST 36], Jie Xi [ST 41] (qi counterflow dysphagia, about to die), Da Zhong [KI 4].

氣噎：天突、膈俞、脾俞、腎俞、乳根、關衝三五壯、足三里、解谿氣逆噎將死、大鍾

Taxation dysphagia: Lao Gong [PC 8].　勞噎：勞宮

Thought and preoccupation dysphagia: Shen Men [HT 7], Pi Shu [UB 20].

思慮噎：神門、脾俞

LJTY: 11-3-10 All Cough, Panting, Retching, Vomiting & Qi Counterflow [諸咳喘嘔噦氣逆 *Zhu Ke Chuan Ou Yue Qi Ni*] (Zhang 1991, 939)

Cough: Tian Tu [Ren 22] (seven cones), Shu Fu [KI 27] (seven cones), Hua Gai [Ren 20], Ru Gen [ST 18] (three cones), Feng Men [UB 12] (seven cones), Fei Shu [UB 13], Shen Zhu [Du 12], Zhi Yang [Du 9] (14 cones), Lie Que [LU 7].

咳嗽：天突七壯、俞府七壯、華蓋、乳根三壯、風門七壯、肺俞、身柱、至陽十四壯、列缺

Cold phlegm cough: Fei Shu [UB 13], Gao Huang [UB 43], Ling Tai [Du 10] (nine cones; you cannot use more), Zhi Yang [Du 9], He Gu [LI 4], Lie Que [LU 7].

寒痰嗽：肺俞、膏肓、靈臺九壯，不可多、至陽、合谷、列缺

Hot phlegm cough: Fei Shu [UB 13], Dan Zhong [Ren 17], Chi Ze [LU 5], Tai Xi [KI 3].

熱痰嗽：肺俞、膻中、尺澤、太谿

All panting and rapid breathing: Tian Tu [Ren 22], Xuan Ji [Ren 21], Hua Gai [Ren 20], Dan Zhong [Ren 17], Ru Gen [ST 18], Qi Men [LV 14], Qi Hai [Ren 6]. Apply three cones of moxibustion to the point on the spine below the seventh vertebrae.[30] It is miraculously effective.

---

[30] This should be Zhi Yang (Du 9).

諸喘氣急：天突、璇璣、華蓋、膻中、乳根、期門、
氣海。背脊中第七椎骨節下穴，灸三壯神效。

Wheezing and panting: Of the five wheezings, only
water wheezing, breast wheezing, and wine wheez-
ing are difficult to treat.[31] Xuan Ji [Ren 21], Hua Gai
[Ren 20], Shu Fu [KI 27], Dan Zhong [Ren 17], Jian
Jing [GB 21] (wonderful for cold wind wheezing; if
pregnant do not apply moxibustion), Jian Zhong
Shu [SI 15] (wonderful for wind wheezing), Tai Yuan
[LU 9], Zu San Li [ST 36].

哮喘：五哮中，惟水哮、乳哮、酒哮爲難治。璇璣、
華蓋、俞府、膻中、肩井冷風哮妙，有孕勿灸、肩中
俞風哮妙、太淵、足三里

Childhood salt wheezing:[32] In males use the left,
while in females use the right tip of the little finger.
Apply seven small mugwort cones of moxibustion.
There is no one in whom the root is not eliminated.
If it is not yet eliminated, apply moxibustion again.

小兒鹽哮：於男左女右手小指尖上，用小艾炷灸七壯
。無不除根，未除再灸。

Vomiting, qi counterflow: Ge Shu [UB 17], San Jiao
Shu [UB 22], Ju Que [Ren 14] (inability to get down
food), Shang Wan [Ren 13], Zhong Wan [Ren 12]
(three times seven cones; treats vomiting, no
thought of food and drink), Qi Hai [Ren 6], Zhang
Men [LV 13], Da Ling [PC 7] (retching counterflow),
Jian Shi [PC 5] (dry retching, vomiting food), Hou Xi
[SI 3] (vomiting food), Chi Ze [LU 5], Tai Chong [LV
3] (cold qi retching counterflow, inability to eat).

嘔吐氣逆：膈俞、三焦俞、巨闕不下食、上脘、中脘三
七壯，治嘔吐不思飲食、氣海、章門、大陵嘔逆、間使
乾嘔、吐食、後谿吐食、尺澤、太衝冷氣嘔逆不食

Dry retching counterflow:[33] Ru Gen [ST 18] (three
cones. When the fire reaches the flesh, it is immediately settled. If it is not settled, this method will not
be effective.), Cheng Jiang [Ren 24], Zhong Fu [LU
1], Feng Men [UB 12], Jian Jing [GB 21], Dan Zhong
[Ren 17], Zhong Wan [Ren 12], Qi Men [LV 14], Qi
Hai [Ren 6], Zu San Li [ST 36], San Yin Jiao [SP 6].

噦逆：乳根三壯，大到肌即定；其不定者，不可救也
、承漿、中府、風門、肩井、膻中、中脘、期門、氣
海、足三里、三陰交

Cholera [sudden turmoil]:

- Ju Que [Ren 14], Zhong Wan [Ren 12], Jian Li
  [Ren 11], Shui Fen [Ren 9] (most effective),
  Cheng Jin [UB 56] (cramping), Cheng Shan [UB
  57], San Yin Jiao [SP 6] (counterflow cold), Zhao
  Hai [KI 6], Da Du [SP 2], Yong Quan [KI 1].

霍亂：巨闕、中脘、建里、水分最效、承筋轉筋、
承山、三陰交逆冷、照海、大都、湧泉

- For cramping and hypertonicity of the ten
  fingers, inability to bend and stretch: Apply
  seven cones of moxibustion above the lateral tip
  of the ankle.[34]

轉筋十指拘攣，不能屈伸，灸足外踝骨間上七壯。

- Whenever a cholera patient is about to die, use
  salt to fill in the navel and apply seven cones of
  moxibustion. The patient will immediately
  recover.

凡霍亂將死者，用鹽填臍中，灸七壯，立愈。

- Whenever a cholera patient has unceasing

---

[31] At this point, I am unable to find the names or the origin of the five wheezings, although three are listed here. Water wheezing is
due to phlegm and fluids in the lungs (Li 1995, 352). Wine wheezing is due to wine damage (Li 1995, 1300). Breast wheezing is
likely to be a type of pediatric asthma.

[32] Salt wheezing is wheezing made worse by consumption of salty or sour foods in a long-term vacuity condition (Wiseman 1998,
511).

[33] 噦逆 *yue ni* has a few possible translations. It can refer to dry retching, hiccoughs, or belching. It is unclear which Zhang had in
mind when he wrote it.

[34] See **LJTY: 10-1-4-22**, above.

vomiting and diarrhea, apply moxibustion to the four points of Zhong Wan [Ren 12], Tian Shu [ST 25], and Qi Hai [Ren 6]. The patient will immediately recover.

凡霍亂吐瀉不止，灸中脘、天樞、氣海四穴，立愈。

Dry cholera: The common name is "agitated intestinal sand."[35] Quickly use brine and mechanical ejection [*i.e.*, induce vomiting] and take fine, white, dry salt to fill in the umbilicus. When you use two times seven cones of mugwort moxibustion, the patient can immediately revive.

乾霍亂：即俗名攪腸沙也。急用鹽湯探吐，并以細白乾鹽填滿臍中，以艾灸二七壯，則可立甦。

Stomach reflux: Pi Shu [UB 20], Wei Shu [UB 21], Dan Zhong [Ren 17], Ru Gen [ST 18], Shang Wan [Ren 13] (two times seven cones), Zhong Wan [Ren 12] (two times seven cones), Xia Wan [Ren 10] (two times seven cones), Shui Fen [Ren 9], Tian Shu [ST 25] (three times seven cones), Da Ling [PC 7], Zu San Li [ST 36].

翻胃：脾俞、胃俞、膻中、乳根、上脘二七壯、中脘二七壯、下脘二七壯、水分、天樞三七壯、大陵、足三里

Acid regurgitation vomiting with untransformed food: Ri Yue [GB 24], Zhong Wan [Ren 12], Pi Shu [UB 20], Wei Shu [UB 21].

吞酸嘔吐食不化：日月、中脘、脾俞、胃俞

Belching: Zhong Wan [Ren 12]. The *Classic* says: When the foot greater yin vessel moves, the disease of abdominal distention and frequent belching occurs. Observe for exuberance or vacuity, heat or cold, and depressions [in the channel]. Apply treatment [based on the diagnosis].[36] It will promptly stop.

噯氣：中脘。《經》曰：足太陰之脈，是動則病腹脹善噫，視其盛虛熱寒陷下者取之，即止。

Frequent sighing: Zhong Feng [LV 4], Shang Qiu [SP 5], Gong Sun [SP 4].

善太息：中封、商丘、公孫

Tendency toward sorrow: Xin Shu [UB 15], Da Ling [PC 7], Da Dun [LV 1], Yu Ying [Ren 18], Dan Zhong [Ren 17].

The *Classic* says: Reverting yin is the closing. If the closing breaks, it means that qi will expire and there will be joy and sorrow. In sorrow, apply treatment to the reverting yin. Observe for surplus or insufficiency. The root of reverting yin is in Da Dun [LV 1]. The binding is in Yu Ying [Ren 18]. It networks to Dan Zhong [Ren 17].[37]

善悲：心俞、大陵、大敦、玉英、膻中。《經》曰：厥陰為闔，闔折即氣絕而善悲，悲者，取之厥陰，視有餘不足。厥陰根於大敦，結於玉英，絡於膻中也。

Shortness of breath: Da Zhui [Du 14] (inability to speak), Fei Shu [UB 13] (inability to speak), Gan Shu [UB 18] (inability to speak), Tian Tu [Ren 22], Jian Jing [GB 21], Qi Hai [Ren 6] (shortness of breath, yang desertion), Nei Guan [PC 6], Chi Ze [LU 5] (shortness of breath, inability to speak), Zu San Li [ST 36], Tai Chong [LV 3].

氣短：大椎不語、肺俞不語、肝俞不語、天突、肩井、氣海氣短陽脫、內關、尺澤氣短不語、足三里、太衝

LJTY: 11-3-11 Malaria [瘧疾 *Nüe Ji*] (Zhang 1991, 941)

Da Zhui [Du 14] (three cones for prompt recovery. Someone said 100 cones), San Zhui [Third Vertebra, non-channel] (moxibustion on the joint can cure it),

---

[35] Agitated intestinal sand is a synonym for dry cholera (Li 1995, 1487).
[36] Paraphrased from *Magic Pivot*, Chapter 10.
[37] Paraphrased from *Magic Pivot*, Chapter 5.

Yi Xi [UB 45] (profuse sweating), Zhang Men [LV 13], Jian Shi [PC 5], Hou Xi [SI 3] (first cold then hot), Huan Tiao [GB 30], Cheng Shan [UB 57], Fei Yang [UB 58], Kun Lun [UB 60], Tai Xi [KI 3] (cold malaria), Gong Sun [SP 4] (governs treatment), Zhi Yin [UB 67] (cold malaria without sweating), He Gu [LI 4].

大椎三壯，立愈。一曰百壯、三椎骨節上灸，亦可愈、譩譆多汗、章門、間使、後谿先寒後熱、環跳、承山、飛陽、崑崙、太谿寒瘧、公孫爲主治、至陰寒瘧無汗、合谷

For enduring malaria that does not recover accompanied by yellow emaciation and weakness: Apply seven cones of moxibustion to Pi Shu [UB 20] and it will promptly stop. Malaria is due to cold damp drinks and food damaging the spleen. That is why this point is extremely effective.

久瘧不愈黃瘦無力者，灸脾俞七壯即止。蓋瘧由寒濕飲食傷脾而然，故此穴甚效。

LJTY: 11-3-12 Jaundice [黃疸 *Huang Dan*] (Zhang 1991, 941)

Gong Sun [SP 4]. 公孫

LJTY: 11-3-13 Wasting-thirst [消渴 *Xiao Ke*] (Zhang 1991, 941)[38]

Shen Shu [UB 23], Xiao Chang Shu [UB 27].
腎俞、小腸俞

LJTY: 11-3-14 Diarrhea [瀉痢 *Xie Li*] (Zhang 1991, 941)

Bai Hui [Du 20] (enduring diarrhea, efflux desertion downward fall; apply three cones of moxibustion),

Pi Shu [UB 20], Shen Shu [UB 23] (unceasing throughflux diarrhea;[39] five cones), Ming Men [Du 4], Chang Qiang [Du 1] (red and white mixed), Cheng Man [ST 20] (borborygmus), Liang Men [ST 21], Zhong Wan [Ren 12], Shen Que [Ren 8] (very wonderful for central qi vacuity cold, abdominal pain, and diarrhea), Tian Shu [ST 25] (abdominal pain), Qi Hai [Ren 6], Shi Men [Ren 5] (abdominal pain), Guan Yuan [Ren 4] (enduring dysentery and cold dysentery abdominal pain), San Yin Jiao [SP 6] (abdominal fullness and diarrhea).

百會久瀉滑脫下陷者、灸三壯、脾俞、腎俞洞泄不止、五壯、命門、長強赤白雜者、承滿腸鳴者、梁門、中脘、神闕中氣虛寒、腹痛瀉痢甚妙、天樞腹痛、氣海、石門腹痛、關元久痢冷痢腹痛、三陰交腹滿泄瀉

Spleen diarrhea: Black colored [stool]. Pi Shu [UB 20]. 脾泄：色黑。脾俞

Stomach diarrhea: Yellow colored [stool]. Wei Shu [UB 21], Tian Shu [ST 25].

胃泄：色黃。胃俞、天樞

Large intestine diarrhea: White colored [stool]. Da Chang Shu [UB 25].

大腸泄：色白。大腸俞

Small intestine diarrhea: Red colored [stool]. Xiao Chang Shu [UB 27].

小腸泄：色赤。小腸俞

Great conglomeration diarrhea: Abdominal urgency and rectal heaviness [*i.e.*, tenesmus]. Tian Shu [ST 25], Shui Fen [Ren 9] (three times seven cones on each of the above).[40]

---

[38] These last two sections list very few treatment options. Perhaps Zhang felt that moxibustion was not the best modality for these conditions or perhaps part of the text was lost.

[39] Efflux desertion is incontinence of stool from qi falling. This can cause desertion. (Wiseman 1998, 167-8) Throughflux diarrhea has undigested food in the stool and often occurs right after eating (Wiseman 1998, 612).

[40] This and the previous four entries are the five kinds of diarrhea from the *Classic of Difficulties*. For a more detailed description of the signs and symptoms, see the 57th Difficulty.

大瘕泄：裏急後重。天樞、水分上各三七壯

Kidney diarrhea: Diarrhea between midnight and the yin and mao hours [3-7 AM]. Ming Men [Du 4], Tian Shu [ST 25], Qi Hai [Ren 6], Guan Yuan [Ren 4].

腎泄：夜半後及寅卯之間泄者。命門、天樞、氣海、關元

LJTY: 11-3-15 Mania & Epilepsy [狂癇 *Kuang Xian*] (Zhang 1991, 942)

Withdrawal and mania:

- Bai Hui [Du 20], Ren Zhong [Du 26], Tian Chuang [SI 16] (mania evil ghost talk), Shen Zhu [Du 12], Shen Dao [Du 11], Xin Shu [UB 15], Jin Suo [Du 8], Gu Di [Du 1] (20 cones), Zhang Men [LV 13], Tian Shu [ST 25], Shao Chong [HT 9] (apply moxibustion to this point on females), Lao Gong [PC 8], Nei Guan [PC 6], Shen Men [HT 7], Yang Xi [LI 5], Zu San Li [ST 36], Xia Ju Xu [ST 39], Feng Long [ST 40] (two times seven cones), Chong Yang [ST 42] (apply moxibustion to this on males), Tai Chong [LV 3], Shen Mai [UB 62], Zhao Hai [KI 6], Li Dui [ST 45] (apply moxibustion to this point on males).

癲狂：百會、人中、天竅狂邪鬼語、身柱、神道、心俞、筋縮、骨骶二十壯、章門、天樞、少衝女灸此、勞宮、內關、神門、陽谿、足三里、下巨虛、豐隆二七壯、衝陽男灸此、太衝、申脈、照海、厲兌男灸此

- The corner of the nails on the thumbs and big toes:[41] In this treatment, bind the two fingers and two toes side by side in one place. You must apply fire to the nail and flesh in these four places; seven cones.

兩手足拇指甲角：其法以二指並縛一處，須甲肉四處者火，七壯。

Feeble-mindedness: Xin Shu [UB 15], Shen Men [HT 7]. 癡：心俞、神門

Wind epilepsy: Bai Hui [Du 20], Shang Xing [Du 23], Shen Zhu [Du 12], Xin Shu [UB 15], Jin Suo [Du 8], Zhang Men [LV 13], Shen Men [HT 7], Tian Jing [SJ 10], Yang Xi [LI 5] (if applying moxibustion on this point, you must not on He Gu [LI 4]; if applying moxibustion on He Gu, you must not apply moxibustion on Yang Xi [LI 5]), He Gu [LI 4], Zu San Li [ST 36], Tai Chong [LV 3].

風癇：百會、上星、身柱、心俞、筋縮、章門、神門、天井、陽谿灸此不必合谷，灸合谷不必陽谿、合谷、足三里、太衝

LJTY: 11-3-16 Diseases of the Head, Face & Seven Orifices [頭面七竅病 *Tou Mian Qi Qiao Bing*] (Zhang 1991, 942)

Head wind, headache: Bai Hui [Du 20] (head wind), Shang Xing [Du 23] (three cones), Xin Hui [Du 22], Shen Ting [Du 24] (three cones), Qu Cha [UB 4], Hou Ding [Du 19], Shuai Gu [GB 8], Feng Chi [GB 20], Tian Zhu [UB 10] (Select one of the above points for moxibustion. The patient can promptly recover.), Feng Men [UB 12], Tong Li [HT 5], Lie Que [LU 7] (hemilateral head wind), Yang Xi [LI 5], Feng Long [ST 40], Jie Xi [ST 41].

頭風頭痛：百會頭風、上星三壯、顖會、神庭三壯、曲差、後頂、率谷、風池、天柱上穴擇灸一處即可愈、風門、通里、列缺偏頭痛、陽谿、豐隆、解谿

Facial diseases: Jia Che [ST 6] (you can use acupuncture and moxibustion for swollen painful jaw and mouth so tense that it cannot chew), Di Cang [ST 4] (sores and swellings on the face and chin), He Gu [LI 4], Lie Que [LU 7], Xian Gu [ST 43] (Prick to bleed for congested swollen face and eyes; there will be immediate recovery.).

---

41 These points are called the "hand ghost eye" and the "foot ghost eye." For more details, see **LJTY: 10-1-4-32** and **ZJDC: 9-6-2**, above.

面疾：頰車面頰腫痛，口急不能嚼，鍼灸皆可、地倉面頷痏腫、合谷、列缺、陷谿面目壅腫，刺出血立愈

Eye pain: He Gu [LI 4] (pain and dim vision), Wai Guan [SJ 5], Hou Xi [SI 3] (head and eye pain).

眼目疼痛：合谷痛而不明、外關、後谿頭目痛

Green blindness:[42] Gan Shu [UB 18], Dan Shu [UB 19], Shen Shu [UB 23], Yang Lao [SI 6] (seven cones), Shang Yang [LI 1] (five cones), Guang Ming [GB 37].

青肓眼：肝俞、膽俞、腎俞、養老七壯、商陽五壯、光明

Clouded or dim vision: Zu San Li [ST 36].
目昏不明：足三里

Dizzy vision: Tong Li [HT 5], Jie Xi [ST 41].
目眩：通里、解谿

Wind ulceration of the eyes: Gan Shu [UB 18], Dan Shu [UB 19], Shen Shu [UB 23], Wan Gu [SI 4], Guang Ming [GB 37].

風爛眼：肝俞、膽俞、腎俞、腕骨、光明

Deafness: Shang Xing [Du 23] (treats wind deafness; two times seven cones), Yi Feng [SJ 17] (for earache and deafness; apply seven cones of moxibustion), Ting Gong [SI 19], Shen Shu [UB 23], Wai Guan [SJ 5], Pian Li [LI 6], He Gu [LI 4].

耳聾：上星治風聾，二七壯、翳風耳痛而聾，灸七壯、聽宮、腎俞、外關、偏歷、合谷

Purulent ear: Ting Gong [SI 19], Jia Che [ST 6], He Gu [LI 4].

停耳：聽宮、頰車、合谷

Nasal polyps: Shang Xing [Du 23] (clear and turbid snivel flow), Qu Cha [UB 4], Ying Xiang [LI 20] (prick), Xin Hui [Du 22] (seven cones; nasal welling-abscess or polyps), Tong Tian [UB 7] (seven cones; there will be prompt recovery when a lump of malodorous accumulation is removed from the nose),[43] Bai Hui [Du 20], Feng Chi [GB 20], Feng Fu [Du 16], Ren Zhong [Du 26], Da Zhui [Du 14]. (All the above points also treat purulent ear, the previous pattern.)

鼻瘜鼻痔：上星流清濁涕、迎香刺、顖會七壯、鼻癰鼻痔、通天七壯，鼻中去臭積一塊即愈、百會、風池、風府、人中、大椎上穴皆治前證

Deep source nasal congestion: Shang Xing [Du 23], Qu Cha [UB 4], Yin Tang [Seal Hall, non-channel], Feng Men [UB 12], He Gu [LI 4].

鼻淵：上星、曲差、印堂、風門、合谷

Nasal congestion with loss of ability to smell the fragrant and the malodorous: Xin Hui [Du 22] (From seven cones up to seven times seven cones. Apply moxibustion for up to four days and the condition will gradually abate. After seven days, the condition will be cured.), Shang Xing [Du 23], Ying Xiang [LI 20] (prick), Tian Zhu [UB 10], Feng Men [UB 12].

鼻塞不聞香臭：顖會自七壯至七七壯，灸至四日漸退，七日頓愈、上星、迎香刺、天柱、風門

Bitter taste in the mouth, toothache, erosion, and consuming gan:[44] Jia Che [ST 6], Di Cang [ST 4], Lian Quan [Ren 23], Cheng Jiang [Ren 24], Tian Tu [Ren 22], Jin Jin [Gold Fluid, non-channel], Yu Ye [Jade

---

[42] Wiseman (1998, 64) calls this "clear-eye blindness." It is "gradual blindness that in severe cases can be total." In Western medicine, this is often due to optic atrophy.

[43] See the cases of Zhu Danxi in the section *Can Moxibustion be Applied in Heat Patterns?* in Chapter 3. The comments on Tong Tian (UB 7) must come from that source.

[44] Two other editions write the title of this sub-section as "mouth and tongue sores and pain, erosion, and consuming *gan*" (口舌瘡痛糜爛疳蝕) (Zhang 1996, 330 and Zhang 1982, 226).
   There are two types of gan. One is a childhood syndrome. The other meaning, used by Zhang here, is various types of ulcerations and sores. These can affect the nose, teeth, or gums, as well as other parts of the body (Wiseman 1998, 236-8).

Fluid, non-channel] (prick to bleed the above two points), He Gu [LI 4], Yang Ling Quan [GB 34] (treats gallbladder heat, bitter taste in the mouth, frequent sighing).

口苦牙痛糜爛疳蝕：頰車、地倉、廉泉、承漿、天突、金津、玉液上二穴刺出血、合谷、陽陵泉治膽熱口苦善太息

Toothache: Cheng Jiang [Ren 24], Jia Che [ST 6], the point below the earlobes and above the end of the bone (three cones; [works] like a miracle), Jian Yu [LI 15] (seven cones; apply moxibustion on the same side), Lie Que [LU 7] (seven cones; it will immediately stop), Tai Yuan [LU 9] (wind toothache), Yu Ji [LU 10], Yang Gu [SI 5] (upper teeth), He Gu [LI 4], San Jian [LI 3] (lower teeth; seven cones), Zu San Li [ST 36] (upper toothache; seven times seven cones for recovery), Tai Xi [KI 3], Nei Ting [ST 44] (lower teeth).

齒牙痛：承漿、頰車、耳垂下盡骨上穴三壯，如神、肩髃七壯，隨左右灸之、列缺七壯、立止、太淵風牙痛、魚際、陽谷上牙、合谷、三間下齒，七壯、足三里上齒痛者，七七壯愈、太谿、內庭下牙

Kidney vacuity toothache, unceasing bleeding: Jia Che [ST 6], He Gu [LI 4], Zu San Li [ST 36], Tai Xi [KI 3].

腎虛牙痛出血不止：頰車、合谷、足三里、太谿

Throat impediment, throat lichen:[45] Tian Zhu [UB 10], Lian Quan [Ren 23], Tian Tu [Ren 22], Yang Gu [SI 5], He Gu [LI 4] (prick to a depth of five *fen* for prompt recovery), Hou Xi [SI 3] (nipple moth), San Jian [LI 3], Shao Shang [LI 11], Guan Chong [SJ 1], Zu San Li [ST 36], Feng Long [ST 40], San Yin Jiao [SP 6], Xing Jian [LV 2].

喉痹喉癬：天柱、廉泉、天突、陽谷、合谷刺五分，立愈、後谿乳蛾、三間、少商、關衝、足三里、豐隆、三陰交、行間

LJTY: 11-3-17 Diseases of the Chest, Back, Lumbus & Knees [胸背腰膝病 *Xiong Bei Yao Xi Bing*] (Zhang 1991, 944)

Tortoise back:[46] Jian Zhong Shu [SI 15], Gao Huang [UB 43], Xin Shu [UB 15], Shen Shu [UB 23], Qu Chi [LI 11], He Gu [LI 4].

龜背：肩中俞、膏肓、心俞、腎俞、曲池、合谷

Chicken breast:[47] Zhong Fu [LU 1], Dan Zhong [Ren 17], Ling Dao [HT 4] (two times seven cones), Zu San Li [ST 36].

雞胸：中府、膻中、靈道二七壯、足三里

Chest and back pain: Feng Men [UB 12].
胸背痛：風門

Pain from lumbar contusion and wrenching; getting up and resting is difficult: Ji Zhong [Du 6], Shen Shu [UB 23] (three or seven cones), Ming Men [Du 4], Zhong Lu Nei Shu [UB 29], Yao Shu [Du 2] (all, seven cones).

腰挫閃疼起止艱難：脊中、腎俞三壯，七壯、命門、中膂內俞、腰俞俱七壯

Severe pain of the lumbar region and back, difficulty walking:

- Zhang Men [LV 13] (cold pain of the lumbar region and back), Yao Shu [Du 2], Wei Zhong [UB 40] (swelling and pain of the lumbar region and legs; prick to bleed), Kun Lun [UB 60] (seven cones).

---

[45] In throat lichen, the throat appears to have moss or lichen growing in it (Wiseman 1998, 611). Nipple moth means red swollen tonsils with a yellow-white discharge (Wiseman 1998, 14).
[46] Tortoise back is the same as hunchback. It is a rounded back, like a turtle shell and is a congenital defect.
[47] This is a puffed-out chest like a chicken's. It is also a congenital defect.

腰背重痛難行：章門腰脊冷痛、腰俞、委中腰腳腫痛，刺出血、崑崙七壯

- To apply moxibustion for lumbar pain when the patient cannot bend forward and backward, make the patient stand up straight. Use a bamboo pole to measure from the ground to the center of the umbilicus. Mark the pole with an ink spot. Then, use it to measure on the spine. Apply moxibustion to the site [at the level] of the ink spot. The number of cones is based on the years of age. Conceal the bamboo pole and apply moxibustion to the end. Do not let people know.[48]

灸腰痛不可俯仰，令患人正立，以竹杖柱地，量至臍中，用墨點記，乃用度脊中，即於點處隨年壯灸之。灸訖藏竹勿令人知。

Aching pain of the lumbar region and knees: Yang Lao [SI 6], Huan Tiao [GB 30], Yang Ling Quan [GB 34] (treats cold impediment and numbness of the legs and knees), Kun Lun [UB 60], Shen Mai [UB 62].

腰膝痠痛：養老、環跳、陽陵泉治腳膝冷痹不仁、崑崙、申脈

Hypertonicity and pain of the sinews and bones: San Yin Jiao [SP 6].

筋骨攣痛：三陰交

LJTY: 11-3-18 Diseases of the Limbs [手足病 *Shou Zu Bing*] (Zhang 1991, 945)

Cold pain of the shoulder and arms: Overall, everyone with cold shoulders and arm pain has met with wind cold. When the shoulders have a lot of coldness, on some days the patient must heat his hands by rubbing them. At night, he has to cover himself up with lots of quilts and can bear many covers.

Take this as insufficient yang qi, debilitated and diminished qi-blood, and so on. If this treatment is not performed in advance, it is likely that it can develop from this into patterns such as wind stroke and paralysis.

You must apply moxibustion to Jian Yu [LI 15] bilaterally right away to avoid this suffering. It seems that Jian Yu relates to the state of health or disease in the two arms and Huan Tiao [GB 30] relates to the state of health or disease in the two legs. You cannot neglect the application of moxibustion to these points. If the condition is mild, use seven cones. If wind cold is exuberant, 14 cones is the usual dose, or divide the treatment into two or three sessions. However, you cannot exceed this amount by much or the arms may become thin. If you use moxibustion on Huan Tiao, then there is no harm in 40 or 50 cones.

肩臂冷痛：凡人肩冷臂痛者，每遇風寒，肩上多冷，或日須熱手撫摩，夜須多被擁蓋，度可支持，此以陽氣不足，氣血衰少而然，若不預為之治，恐中風不隨等證，由此而成也。須灸肩髃二穴，方免此患，蓋肩髃係兩手之安否，環跳係兩足之安否，此不可不灸之，輕者七壯，風寒盛者十四壯為率，或分二三次報之，但不可過多，恐臂細也。若灸環跳，則四五十壯無害。

Pain and inability to raise the arms: Jian Jing [GB 21], Jian Yu [LI 15], Yuan Ye [GB 22], Qu Chi [LI 11], Qu Ze [PC 3], Hou Xi [SI 3] (stiff neck, elbow pain), Tai Yuan [LU 9] (wrist pain).

臂痛不舉：肩井、肩髃、淵腋、曲池、曲澤、後谿項強肘痛、太淵手腕痛

Contraction of dampness, hypertonicity of the limbs: Qu Chi [LI 11], Chi Ze [LU 5], Wan Gu [SI 4], Wai Guan [SJ 5], Zhong Zhu [KI 15].

受濕手足拘攣：曲池、尺澤、腕骨、外關、中渚

---

[48] The last two sentences were censored from a modern edition (Zhang, J.Y. 1996, 331). This passage originally came from Sun's *Prescriptions* (Sun 1994, a275). See also **LJTY: 11-3-17** p. 157 and Chapter 14: Magical Moxibustion.

The five impediments:[49] Qu Chi [LI 11], Wai Guan [SJ 5], He Gu [LI 4], Zhong Zhu [KI 15].

五痹：曲池、外關、合谷、中渚

Foot fork wind:[50] Shen Shu [UB 23], Huan Tiao [GB 30], Yang Ling Quan [GB 34], Xuan Zhong [GB 39], Kun Lun [UB 60].

腿叉風：腎俞、環跳、陽陵泉、懸鍾、崑崙

Knee wind, swelling and pain: Tian Shu [ST 25], Liang Qiu [ST 34], Xi Yan [Eye of the Knee, non-channel] (can prick; for details, see the category on non-channel points),[51] Xi Guan [LV 7], Zu San Li [ST 36], Yang Ling Quan [GB 34], Yin Ling Quan [SP 9], Tai Chong [LV 3] (cold-damp).

膝風腫痛：天樞、梁邱、膝眼可刺，詳奇俞類、膝關、足三里、陽陵泉、陰陵泉、太衝寒濕

Leg qi: Jian Jing [GB 21], Zu San Li [ST 36], Yang Ling Quan [GB 34], Yang Fu [GB 38], Kun Lun [UB 60], Zhao Hai [KI 6], Tai Chong [LV 3].

腳氣：肩井、足三里、陽陵泉、陽輔、崑崙、照海、太衝

White tiger joint running wind:[52] Xi Guan [LV 7].
白虎歷節風：膝關

Cramping: Zhao Hai [KI 6].　　轉筋：照海

Inner aspect of the legs swollen and painful: Jian Jing [GB 21], San Yin Jiao [SP 6] (three times seven cones), Da Dun [LV 1].

足内廉腫痛：肩井、三陰交三七壯、大敦

Ankles swollen and painful: Jie Xi [ST 41], Qiu Xu [GB 40].

足腕腫痛：解谿、坵墟

Cold-damp leg sores: Apply treatment to the point that is about two *cun* above the dorsum of the foot in the depression right in the center of the ankle. Apply seven cones of moxibustion. It is miraculously effective. This point should be Jie Xi [ST 41]. Zhao Hai [KI 6].

風濕腳瘡：取足跗上二寸許足腕正中陷處是穴，灸七壯，神效，此穴當即解谿也。照海

LJTY: 11-3-19 Diseases of the Two Yin [二陰病　er yin bing] (Zhang 1991, 946)

Dream emission, seminal efflux, and ghost intercourse:[53] (You can apply moxibustion in the spring, autumn, and winter.) Xin Shu [UB 15] (it is not appropriate to use much moxibustion), Gao Huang [UB 43], Shen Shu [UB 23] (the number of cones for moxibustion is based on years of age; you can immediately see the effects), Ming Men [Du 4] (incontinence of semen; five cones; immediately effective), Bai Huan Shu [UB 30] (50 cones), Zhong Ji [Ren 3] (the number of cones is based on years of age), San Yin Jiao [SP 6], Zhong Feng [LV 4], Ran Gu [KI 2].

夢遺精滑鬼交：春秋冬可灸。心俞灸不宜多、膏肓、腎俞灸隨年壯，其效立見、命門遺精不禁者，五壯、立效、白環俞五十壯、中極隨年壯、三陰交、中封、然谷

---

[49] The five impediments refer to sinew, vessel, flesh, skin, and bone according to *Elementary Questions*, Chapter 43. According to the *Central Treasury Canon* (*Zhong Zang Jing*), it is sinew, bone, blood, flesh, and qi; or wind, cold, damp, heat, and qi (Wiseman 1998, 205). It is likely that Zhang meant these points were good for most any kind of impediment.

[50] "Foot fork" must refer to the spaces between the toes. A related term, 足叉發, is described as heat toxins gathering in the spaces between the toes (Li 1995, 753). Perhaps these conditions are similar and today would be called athlete's foot.

[51] For details on *Xi Yan* (Eye of the Knee, non-channel), see **LJTY: 10-1-4-14**, above.

[52] "White tiger joint running wind" is an impediment pattern with acute pain, but no fixed location (Wiseman 1998, 426).

[53] Seminal efflux is involuntary loss of semen without dreams, whether waking or asleep (Wiseman 1998, 524). Ghost intercourse refers to dreaming of intercourse with ghosts (夜夢鬼交) or other unnatural beings (Wiseman 1998, 148).

Seminal loss, cold pain of the knees and lower legs: Qu Quan [LV 8].

失精膝脛冷疼：曲泉

White turbidity:[54] Pi Shu [UB 20], Xiao Chang Shu [UB 27], Zhang Men [LV 13], Qi Hai [Ren 6] (five cones), Guan Yuan [Ren 4], Zhong Ji [Ren 3], Zhong Feng [LV 4].

白濁：脾俞、小腸俞、章門、氣海五壯、關元、中極、中封

The five stranguries:[55] Ge Shu [UB 17], Gan Shu [UB 18], Pi Shu [UB 20], Shen Shu [UB 23], Qi Hai [Ren 6], Shi Men [Ren 5] (blood strangury), Guan Yuan [Ren 4], Jian Shi [PC 5] (it is able to contain the blood of the pericardium), Xue Hai [SP 10], San Yin Jiao [SP 6] (taxation strangury), Fu Liu [KI 7] (blood strangury), Ran Gu [KI 2], Da Dun [LV 1].

五淋：膈俞、肝俞、脾俞、腎俞、氣海、石門血淋、關元、間使能攝心包之血、血海、三陰交勞淋、復溜血淋、然谷、大敦

Inhibited urination or stoppage: San Jiao Shu [UB 22], Xiao Chang Shu [UB 27], Yin Jiao [Ren 7], Zhong Ji [Ren 3] (along with abdominal pain), Zhong Feng [LV 4], Tai Chong [LV 3], Zhi Yin [UB 67].

小便不利不通：三焦俞、小腸俞、陰交、中極兼腹痛、中封、太衝、至陰

Urinary incontinence: Qi Hai [Ren 6] (also treats pediatric enuresis), Guan Yuan [Ren 4], Yin Ling Quan [SP 9], Da Dun [LV 1], Xing Jian [LV 2] (treats incontinence).

小便不禁：氣海兼治小兒遺尿、關元、陰陵泉、大敦、行間治失尿

Constipation: Zhang Men [LV 13] (two times seven

cones), Yin Jiao [Ren 7], Qi Hai [Ren 6] (prick), Shi Men [Ren 5], Zu San Li [ST 36], San Yin Jiao [SP 6], Zhao Hai [KI 6] (prick), Tai Bai [SP 3] (prick), Da Dun [LV 1], Da Du [SP 2].

大便秘結：章門二七壯、陰交、氣海刺、石門、足三里、三陰交、照海刺、太白刺、大敦、大都

Mounting qi: Generally if the pain is severe, it is liver mounting [*i.e., shan*].
疝氣：大都痛甚者，為肝疝。

- Jian Jing [GB 21] (bulging mounting), Zhang Men [LV 13], Qi Hai [Ren 6], Gui Lai [ST 29], Guan Yuan [Ren 4] (governs large bulging mounting on one side; apply 100 cones of moxibustion), Chong Men [SP 12], Ji Mai [LV 12], Hui Yin [Ren 1], San Yin Jiao [SP 6] (liver, spleen), Tai Xi [KI 3] (cold mounting), Tai Chong [LV 3], Da Dun [LV 1], Yin Bai [SP 1] (spleen mounting).

肩井〔疒+頹〕疝、章門、氣海、歸來、關元主〔疒+頹〕疝偏大，灸百壯、衝門、急脈、會陰、三陰交肝脾、太谿寒疝、太衝、大敦、隱白脾疝

- Lan Men [Screen Gate, non-channel]: This point is located three *cun* lateral to the root of the penis on both sides. Needle to a depth of 1.5 *cun* and apply two times seven cones of moxibustion. This treats wooden kidney with unilateral sagging [of a testicle].[56]

闌門：在陰莖根兩旁，各開三寸是穴，鍼一寸半，灸二七壯，治木腎偏墜。

A treatment: Apply seven cones of moxibustion on the vein three *cun* bilateral to Guan Yuan [Ren 4] for prompt recovery.

一法：於關元兩旁，相去各三寸青脈上，灸七壯即愈。

---

[54] White turbidity is cloudy white urine. It can also mean a white discharge from the urethra (Wiseman 1998, 677).

[55] The five stranguries (*lin*) are stone, qi, unctuous, taxation, and blood strangury (Wiseman 1998, 207).

[56] The external kidneys are the male genitals. Wooden kidney is a condition where the scrotum is swollen, enlarged, hard, and numb, caused by cold and damp in the lower burner (Li 1995, 183).

• **A treatment:** Make the patient close his mouth. Use a piece of straw to horizontally measure the length between the two corners of the mouth. This is one fold of the straw. Following this pattern, add two more folds. Altogether there are three folds. Bend it to make the three corners into the shape of a triangle. Place the upper corner in the center of the umbilicus. Place the other two corners below the umbilicus on the two sides. The points are right at the site of the two corners. If the left is affected, apply moxibustion to the right. If the right is affected, apply moxibustion to the left. If both the left and right are affected, apply moxibustion to both of the points. Use mugwort cones the size of a grain of wheat. Apply 14 or 21 cones of moxibustion for immediate relief.[57]

一法：令病者合口以草橫量兩口角為一摺。照此再加二摺，共為三摺，屈成三角如△樣，以上角按臍中心兩角按臍下兩旁當兩角處是穴，左患灸右，右患灸左，左右俱患即兩穴俱灸，艾炷如麥粒，灸十四壯或二十一壯，即安。

Impotence: Ming Men [Du 4], Shen Shu [UB 23], Qi Hai [Ren 6], Ran Gu [KI 2].

陽不起：命門、腎俞、氣海、然谷

Persistent erection: Qu Quan [LV 8], Tai Chong [LV 3], Ran Gu [KI 2], Zhao Hai [KI 6].

陰挺：曲泉、太衝、然谷、照海

Pain in the penis: Lie Que [LU 7] (genital pain, bloody urine), Xing Jian [LV 2].

莖中痛：列缺陰痛尿血、行間

Hemorrhoids & fistulas: Ming Men [Du 4], Shen Shu [UB 23], Chang Qiang [Du 1] (most effective for the five types of hemorrhoids[58] and bloody stool. Apply moxibustion to it. The number of cones is based on years of age.), San Yin Jiao [SP 6] (bleeding hemorrhoids), Cheng Shan [UB 57] (enduring hemorrhoids).

痔漏：命門、腎俞、長強五痔便血最效，隨年壯灸之、三陰交痔血、承山久痔

• Whenever there is hemorrhoidal disease with swelling and the prevailing situation is severe, first use Huai Liu Zhi Jian Tang [Sophora & Willow Branch Decoction]. Take advantage of the heat by steam-washing the affected area. Afterwards use dandruff taken off the comb of a healthy male. Pinch it into a small cake about one *fen* thick. Place it on the hemorrhoid. Then cut a slice of single-clove garlic as thick as a coin and place it on the dandruff. Use mugwort to apply two times seven cones or three times seven cones of moxibustion. There is no one whose hemorrhoids are not dispersed and dissipated.[59]

凡痔疾腫大勢甚者，先以槐柳枝煎湯，成熱薰洗過後用壯盛男子箆下頭垢捻成小餅約厚一分，置痔上

---

[57] For triangle moxibustion, see also **ZJDC: 9-6-8**, above.

[58] According to Sun's *Prescriptions*, the five types of hemorrhoids are: male hemorrhoids, female hemorrhoids, vessel hemorrhoids, intestinal hemorrhoids, and bleeding hemorrhoids (牡痔，牝痔，脈痔，腸痔，血痔) (Sun 1994, a332). Zhang probably meant "all types of hemorrhoids" when he wrote the "five types of hemorrhoids."

[59] For Sophora & Willow Branch Decoction, see **BCGM: 15-05-25** p. 103. This formula is not taken orally, but is used to steam wash the area before the application of moxibustion.

This method of applying moxibustion over garlic and dandruff cakes was also mentioned by Zhu Danxi in Chapter 67 of the *Heart and Essence of Danxi's Methods of Treatment* (Zhu 2000, 637).

In Chinese, dandruff is literally "head dirt." The properties of dandruff are discussed in **BCGM: 52-03**. According to this passage, Tao Hongjing said: "You should use dandruff from a person with a bright complexion, as their dandruff can be made into pills." Unfortunately, Li Shizhen gives no clues as to why dandruff is useful in treating hemorrhoids. Could it somehow be using the upper to treat the lower?

Single-clove garlic is the type native to China. The kind with many cloves came from the West (Harper 1998, 370n.1). Therefore, single-clove garlic is *xiao suan*, and the many-cloved garlic is *da suan*. For more about garlic see **BCGM: 26-09**, p. 108-12.

，又切獨蒜片厚如錢者置垢上，用艾灸二七壯或三七壯，無不消散。

- **Another treatment:** Simply use fresh ginger.[60] Cut a thin slice and place it on the site of the painful hemorrhoid. Use three mugwort cones on the ginger. Yellow water will promptly come out and the hemorrhoid will spontaneously disperse and dissipate. If there are two or three hemorrhoids, pattern treatment after the previous method and apply moxibustion to them one by one after three to five days have passed. It has magical effects.

又法：單用生薑切薄片，放痔痛處，用艾炷於薑上灸三壯，黃水即出，自消散矣。若有兩三個者，過三五日照依前法逐一灸之，神效。

Prolapse of the rectum:

- Bai Hui [Du 20] (three cones). This point belongs to the governing vessel and is located at the vertex. It is like the drawstring of the yang vessels, uniting the body's yang qi. Whenever there is prolapse of the rectum, it is always because of the downward fall of yang qi. The *Classic* says: "Raise what descends."[61] That is why you should borrow the power of fire in order to lift the downward fall of qi; then spleen qi can upbear and secure the door. It is also this way for children.

脫肛：百會三壯。此穴屬督脈，居巔頂，為陽脈之都綱，統一身之陽氣。凡脫肛者，皆因陽氣下陷。《經》曰：下者舉之。故當藉火力以提下陷之氣則脾氣可升而門戶固矣。小兒亦然。

- Wei Shu [UB 21], Chang Qiang [Du 1]. 胃俞、長強

- There is also prolapse of the rectum from throughflux diarrhea[62] or cold stroke. You must apply 100 cones of moxibustion to Shui Fen [Ren 9]. The patient should take medicinals for warm supplementation internally and he will spontaneously recover.

又有洞泄寒中脫肛者，須灸水分穴百壯，內服溫補藥自愈。

LJTY: 11-3-20 Evil Spirits [邪祟 *Xie Sui*] (Zhang 1991, 948)

Whenever someone is assailed by a corpse ghost, there is fulminant reversal and loss of consciousness. Even though the four limbs are cold and without qi, you can still needle to resuscitate him if you perceive that the expression in his eyes is unchanged, his heart region and abdomen are still warm, there is no drool in his mouth, his tongue is not curled up, his scrotum is not retracted, and if one double-hour has not yet passed. The five evils all are like this. The following treatment methods are from the *Lost Chapters of Elementary Questions*.[63]

---

[60] For more on ginger, see **BCGM: 26-17**, p. 122.

[61] Chapter 69 of *Elementary Questions*.

[62] Throughflux diarrhea is diarrhea with untransformed food in the stool that comes after eating (Wiseman 1998, 612).

[63] This whole section was heavily censored in a modern edition (Zhang, J.Y. 1996, 335-6).
  A corpse ghost is literally the ghost of a dead person. The word 鬼 *gui*, which is often translated as ghost can also mean other types of disembodied spirits, demons, or goblins (Mathews 1943, 536).
  The *Lost Chapters of Elementary Questions* are supposedly the two chapters still missing (72 and 73) after Wang Bing added the seven great treatises during the Tang dynasty. During the Northern Song dynasty, Liu Wenshu came up with the two "lost chapters." The content includes additional information on the five transports and the six qi, but also discussion of ghosts and spirits, something which is noticeably absent from the rest of *Elementary Questions* (Li 1995, 1203).
  Most editions of *Elementary Questions* include Wang's seven chapters but not the two "lost chapters." Some later authors, including Ma Shi (馬蒔《黃帝內經素問注証發微》) and Zhang (in the *Categorized Classic*) included these lost chapters but placed them at the end of *Elementary Questions*, not in numerical sequence. This indicates doubt as to their authenticity.
  This next passage on ghosts comes from Chapter 72 of the "lost chapters" 《素問遺篇・刺法論篇第七十二》. Note that the ghost is the color of the element that controls the weakened organ. In these five sections, acupuncture, not moxibustion is recommended.

凡犯屍鬼暴厥不省人事，若四肢雖冷無氣，但覺
日中神采不變，心腹尚溫，口中無涎，舌不捲，
囊不縮，及未出一時者，尚可刺之復甦也。五邪
皆然。此下治法，出《素問遺篇》。

A patient with lung vacuity sees red corpse ghosts:

- **Fei Shu [UB 13]:** Prick, entering 1.5 *fen*. When qi
  is obtained, supplement. Retain the needle for
  three exhalations. Next, enter one *fen* deeper.
  Retain the needle for one exhalation. Slowly,
  slowly remove the needle.

- **He Gu [LI 4]:** Prick three *fen*. When qi is
  obtained, supplement. Retain the needle for
  three exhalations. Withdraw it one *fen*. Retain
  the needle for one exhalation. Slowly, slowly
  remove the needle.

肺虛者見赤屍鬼：肺俞：刺入一分半，得氣則補，
留三呼，次進一分，留一呼，徐徐出鍼。合谷：刺
三分，得氣則補，留三呼，退一分，留一呼，徐徐
出鍼。

A patient with heart vacuity sees black corpse ghosts:

- **Xin Shu [UB 15]:** Use a fine needle to prick it.
  Obtain qi, retain the needle, and supplement.
  The patient will promptly revive.

- **Yang Chi [SJ 4]:** Prick with the same method.

心虛者見黑屍鬼：心俞：以毫鍼刺之，得氣留補，
即甦。陽池：刺同。

A patient with liver vacuity sees white corpse ghosts:

- **Gan Shu [UB 18]:** Use a fine needle to prick three
  fen. Obtain qi, retain the needle, and supplement.

- **Qiu Xu [GB 40]:** Use a fine needle to prick three

fen. When qi is obtained, supplement. Retain the
needle for three exhalations. You can treat a patient
with sounds in their abdomen using this method.

肝虛者見白屍鬼：肝虛：以毫鍼刺三分，得氣留補
。坵墟：以毫鍼刺三分，得氣則補，留三呼，腹中
鳴者可治也。

A patient with spleen vacuity sees green corpse ghosts:

- **Pi Shu [UB 20]:** Prick three *fen*, retain the needle
  for two exhalations, advance the needle two *fen*
  deeper. When qi arrives, slowly, slowly withdraw
  the needle. The patient will promptly revive.

- **Chong Yang [ST 42]:** Use a fine needle to prick
  three *fen* deep. When qi is obtained, supplement.
  Retain the needle for three exhalations. Next,
  advance the needle one *fen* deeper, and retain it
  for one exhalation. Slowly, slowly withdraw the
  needle, using the hand to feel it.

脾虛者見青屍鬼：脾俞：刺三分，留二呼，進二分
，氣至徐徐退鍼即甦。衝陽：以毫鍼刺三分，得氣
則補，留三呼，次進一分，留一呼，徐徐退鍼，以
手摸之。

A patient with kidney vacuity sees yellow corpse ghosts:

- **Shen Shu [UB 23]:** Prick three *fen* deep [and]
  when qi is obtained, supplement. Retain the
  needle for three exhalations. Again, enter the
  needle two *fen* deeper and retain it for three
  exhalations. Slowly, slowly remove the needle.

- **Someone said:** Located on the two sides below
  15th vertebrae [L3]. I suspected that this is Qi Hai
  Shu [Sea of Qi Transport], in the category of
  non-channel points.[64]

---

[64] Qi Hai Shu is UB 24. Zhang listed it under non-channel points in **LJTY: 10-1-18**. This point was first mentioned in Wang Huaiyin's *Sage-like Prescriptions of the Taiping Era* (Song, 992) (Li 1995, 278). In Wang Zhizhong's *Classic of Nourishing Life with Acupuncture and Moxibustion* (Song, 1220), it was listed as if it were a point on the urinary bladder channel, yet Zhang still included it as a non-channel point.

腎虛者見黃屍鬼：腎俞：刺三分，得氣則補，留三呼，
又進二分，留三呼，徐徐出鍼。○一云在十五椎下兩旁
，疑是奇俞類氣海俞也。

- To use the above pricking method, you must
  first hold the needle in your mouth to make it
  warm and then prick the patient. Then the qi of
  the channels and vessels will not refuse and
  counterflow.[65]

以上刺法，必先以口含鍼，令溫煖而刺之。則經脈
之氣無拒逆也。

Ghosts and demons: Shang Xing [Du 23], Shui Gou
[Du 26] (ghost strike sudden death). For Qin
Chengzu's ghost moxibustion, see the earlier category on non-channel points in the section on the
four limbs.[66]

鬼魅：上星、水溝鬼擊卒死。秦承祖灸鬼法：見前氣
俞類四肢部中。

Oppressive ghost dreams, ghost strike: Ren Zhong
[Du 26] (seven cones), foot Gui Yan [Ghost Eye, non-
channel] (see the category on non-channel points).[67]

夢魘鬼擊：人中七壯、足鬼眼穴在奇俞類

LJTY: 11-3-21 Women's Diseases [婦人病 *Fu Ren Bing*] (Zhang 1991, 949)

Blood bind, menstrual irregularities: Qi Hai [Ren 6],
Zhong Ji [Ren 3], Zhao Hai [KI 6] (absence of men-
struation).

血結月事不調：氣海、中極、照海月事不行

Unceasing flooding: Ge Shu [UB 17], Gan Shu [UB
18], Shen Shu [UB 23], Ming Men [Du 4], Qi Hai
[Ren 6], Zhong Ji [Ren 3] (lower origin vacuity cold,
flooding, white turbidity), Jian Shi [PC 5], Xue Hai
[SP 10], Fu Liu [KI 7], Xing Jian [LV 2].

血崩不止：膈俞、肝俞、腎俞、命門、氣海、中極下
元虛冷，血崩白濁、間使、血海、復溜、行間

Red and white strangury and vaginal discharge:
Ming Men [Du 4], Shen Que [Ren 8], Zhong Ji [Ren
3] (seven cones; extremely effective at treating white
vaginal discharge). Beyond this, use the previous
points for the five stranguries, p. 160.

淋帶赤白：命門、神闕、中極七壯，治白帶極效。餘
用前五淋穴。

Concretions and conglomerations:

- San Jiao Shu [UB 22], Shen Shu [UB 23], Zhong
  Ji [Ren 3], Hui Yin [Ren 1].

癥瘕：三焦俞、腎俞、中極、會陰

- **Zi Gong [Child Palace, non-channel] and Zi Hu
  [Child Door, non-channel]:** Zi Gong is on the left;
  Zi Hu is on the right. They are located three *cun*
  lateral to Guan Yuan [Ren 4]. The supplement to
  Thousand Pieces of Gold calls the point three *cun*
  lateral Qi Men [Qi Gate, non-channel]. For
  details, see the category on non-channel
  points.[68]

---

[65] Obviously we cannot warm the needle in our mouth today. However, it must be possible to warm the needle with other methods
   and still maintain its sterility.
[66] Qin Chengzu was a famous doctor in the Southern and Northern period (Li 1995, 1201). For his ghost moxibustion points, see
   LJTY: 10-1-4-32, above.
   Ghost strike indicates sudden gripping pain of the chest and abdomen or bleeding (vomiting blood, nosebleed, bleeding from
   the lower orifices) (Li 1995, 1110). It feels like an injury from being attacked, yet there was no visible attack.
[67] For oppressive ghost dreams, see the glossary. For the Ghost Eye points, see **LJTY: 10-1-4-32**, above.
[68] Zhang did not discuss Zi Gong (Child Palace, non-channel) in the section on non-channel points. For Zi Hu and Qi Men [non-
   channel], see **LJTY: 10-1-2-13**, above.

子宮子戶：左子宮，右子戶，在關元旁各開三寸，
《千金翼》以三寸為氣門穴，詳奇俞類。

• Fu Liu [KI 7].　復溜

Infertility:

• Ming Men [Du 4], Shen Shu [UB 23], Qi Hai [Ren
6], Zhong Ji [Ren 3], Guan Yuan [Ren 4] (seven
cones up to 100 or 300 cones), Bao Men and Zi
Hu [non-channel] (two points, see the category
on non-channel points for details), Yin Lian [LV
11], Ran Gu [KI 2], Zhao Hai [KI 6] (cold uterus).

不孕：命門、腎俞、氣海、中極、關元七壯至百壯
，或三百壯、胞門子戶二穴詳奇俞類、陰廉、然谷
、照海子宮冷

• **A treatment:** Apply moxibustion to Shen Que
[Ren 8]. First, use clean dry salt to fill the
umbilicus. Apply seven cones of moxibustion.
Then, remove the salt. Change it to 21 pieces of
Chuan Jiao [Pericarpium Zanthoxyli]. Above it,
use a slice of ginger as a cover. Again, apply 14
cones of moxibustion. When the moxibustion is
completed, immediately apply an ointment to it.
Mugwort cones must be the size of a finger,
about five or six *fen* long.[69]

一法：灸神闕穴，先以淨乾鹽填臍中，灸七壯，後
去鹽，換川椒二十一粒，上以薑片蓋定，又灸十四
壯，灸畢即用膏貼之，艾炷須如指大，長五六分許
。

Habitual miscarriage: Ming Men [Du 4], Shen Shu [UB
23], Zhong Ji [Ren 3], Jiao Xin [KI 8], Ran Gu [KI 2].

胎屢雖墮：命門、腎俞、中極、交信、然谷

Difficult delivery, transverse birth: He Gu [LI 4], San
Yin Jiao [SP 6].

產難橫生：合谷、三陰交

• **A treatment for horizontally adverse difficult
childbirth:** This can be critical in an instant.
Talismans and medicinals are ineffective.
Quickly apply three cones of moxibustion the
size of a small grain of wheat on this woman's
right leg, on the tip of the little toe. When you
light the fire, there will be immediate delivery,
like a miracle. This must refer to Zhi Yin [UB 67].

一治橫逆難產，危在頃刻，符藥不靈者，急於本婦
右腳小指尖，灸三壯，炷如小麥，下火立產如神，
蓋此即至陰穴也。

Child high up and unable to descend:

• Ju Que [Ren 14], He Gu [LI 4], San Yin Jiao [SP
6].

子鞠不能下：巨闕、合谷、三陰交

• **Zhi Yin [UB 67]:** Bleed with a three-edged needle.
If horizontal, the fetus will promptly turn
vertical.

至陰：三棱鍼出血，橫者即轉直。

Retention of placenta: San Yin Jiao [SP 6], Kun Lun
[UB 60].

胎衣不下：三陰交、崑崙

Aborting a dead fetus: He Gu [LI 4] (prick to supplement it [and] the fetus will promptly descend).

下死胎：合谷刺補之即下

Inducing childbirth: Jian Jing [GB 21], He Gu [LI 4],
San Yin Jiao [SP 6].

欲取胎：肩井、合谷、三陰交

Postpartum unceasing flow of lochia: Zhong Ji [Ren
3].　產後惡露不止：中極

---

[69] For salt moxibustion, see also **BCGM: 11-01**, p. 121.

Desire to terminate childbearing: 2.3 *cun* below the umbilicus, apply three cones of moxibustion, or up to seven times seven cones. It will immediately cut off pregnancy for the person's whole life.[70]

LJTY: 11-3-22 Children's Diseases [小兒病 xiao er bing] (Zhang 1991, 950)

Avoid moxibustion on San Li [ST 36]. If beyond 30 years of age, you can apply moxibustion to it.

忌灸三里，年三十外，方可灸此。

Marked emaciation, standing bones:[71] Bai Lao [Hundred Taxations, non-channel], Wei Shu [UB 21], Yao Shu [Du 2], Chang Qiang [Du 1].

羸瘦骨立：百勞、胃俞、腰腧、長強

Acute or chronic fright wind: Bai Hui [Du 20] (five times seven cones), Xin Hui [Du 22], Shang Xing [Du 23], Shuai Gu [GB 8] (three cones), Shui Gou [Du 26], Chi Ze [LU 5] (chronic fright), Jian Shi [PC 6], He Gu [LI 4], Tai Chong [LV 3] (five cones).

急慢驚風：百會五七壯、顖會、上星、率谷三壯、水溝、尺澤慢驚、間使、合谷、太衝五壯

Umbilical wind, pursed mouth: This results from qi counterflow while in the mother's abdomen, or they were not careful during childbirth and the baby contracted cold. So it is like this.[72]

臍風撮口：在母腹中氣逆所致或產時不慎受寒而然。

- Cheng Jiang [Ren 24], Ran Gu [KI 2].
  承漿、然谷

- **A treatment:** Apply moxibustion to the umbilicus with small mugwort cones on garlic. Wait to perceive mugwort qi in the child's mouth and he will regain life.[73]

一法：以小艾炷腦蒜灸臍中，俟口中覺有艾氣，亦得生者。

- **Another treatment:** Whenever umbilical wind is fully developed, the path of a vein will be visible, moving across from the lower to the upper abdomen producing two branches. Promptly apply three cones of moxibustion to the head of the vein to stop it. If you see two branches, promptly apply three cones of moxibustion to the heads of both veins. Out of 10 cases, five or six will live. If the patient does not recover, it moves upward to attack the heart and he will die.[74]

又法：凡臍風若成，必有青筋一道，自下上行至腹而生兩岔，即灸青筋之頭三壯截住，若見兩岔，即灸兩處筋頭各三壯，十活五六，不則上行攻心而死矣。

Food accumulation, big belly: Pi Shu [UB 20], Wei Shu [UB 21], Shen Shu [UB 23].

食積杜大：脾俞、胃俞、腎俞

Diarrhea: Wei Shu [UB 21], Shui Fen [Ren 9], Tian Shu [ST 25], Shen Que [Ren 8] (quite wonderful for abdominal pain and milk dysentery).

泄瀉：胃俞、水分、天樞、神闕腹痛乳痢甚妙

Cholera [sudden turmoil]: Shui Fen [Ren 9] (abdomi-

---

[70] There is no channel point located 2.3 *cun* below the umbilicus. This would be between Shi Men (Ren 5) and Guan Yuan (Ren 4). Many books state that nearby Shi Men can induce infertility (Deadman 1998, 504). This point must be related. See also **JYQS: 61-66.**
[71] This is someone so thin, they seem like just bones when you see them standing.
[72] These sentences were missing from the modern edition (Zhang, J.Y. 1996, 337). It is not clear if it was an accidental omission or if it was censored. Umbilical wind is lockjaw in newborns (Wiseman 1998, 637).
[73] To "perceive mugwort qi in the child's mouth" means to smell mugwort and feel warmth in the child's breath.
[74] This treatment is similar to that for red thread boils.

nal cramping), on the tip of the external malleolus (three cones).[75]

霍亂：水分轉筋入腹、外踝上尖三壯

Night crying, heart insufficiency: Zhong Chong [PC 9] (three cones).

夜啼心氣不足：中衝三壯

Eye gan:[76] He Gu [LI 4] (five cones).　疳眼：合谷五壯

Double tongue: Xing Jian [LV 2].[77]　重舌：行間

Weak qi in children, not talking at several years of age: Xin Shu [UB 15].

小兒氣弱數歲不語：心俞

Stool transferred into the mouth: The mother ate cold and cool foods which resulted in this condition. Zhong Wan [Ren 12], nine cones, 14 cones for an adult.[78]

口中轉屎：因母食寒涼所致。中脘：九壯，大人十四壯。

Genital swelling: Kun Lun [UB 60].　陰腫：崑崙

Mounting [or shan] qi: Hui Yin [Ren 1], Da Dun [LV 1].　疝氣：會陰、大敦

The five epilepsies:[79]　五癇：

- **Shen Ting [Du 24]:** Treats wind epilepsy with

protrusion of the tongue and arched-back rigidity. Apply three cones of moxibustion.

神庭：治風癇吐舌，角弓反張，灸三壯。

- **Qian Ding [Du 21]:** Treats all pediatric fright wind patterns. Apply three cones of moxibustion.

前頂：治小兒一切驚癇證，灸三壯。

- **Chang Jiang [Du 1]:** Treats all fright epilepsy. Apply seven cones of moxibustion.

長強：治諸驚癇，灸七壯。

- **Xin Hui [Du 22], Ju Que [Ren 14], Zhang Men [LV 13], Tian Jing [SJ 10], Shao Hai [HT 3], Nei Guan [PC 6], Shao Chong [HT 9].**

顖會、巨闕、章門、天井、少海、內關、少衝

- **A treatment says:** Epilepsy is a pediatric malignity pattern. The ancients said, "Once fright wind occurs three times it becomes epilepsy." There are five epilepsy patterns, namely the categories of ox, goat, pig, horse, and rooster.

The treatment method is to wait for the time when the disease erupts. Place the patient's two thumbs beside each other. Use cotton cord to bind them securely. The point right at the corner of the nails of the two thumbs is named Ghost Eye of the hands.[80] Use seven cones of

---

[75] See **LJTY: 10-1-4-22** for this point.

[76] Child eye gan is "dryness, aversion to light, screens on the dark of the eyes... in severe cases, withering of the eyeball and blindness" (Wiseman 1998, 60).

[77] Double tongue was discussed in *Magic Pivot*, Chapter 9. There is swelling under the tongue that makes it look like there are two tongues. This condition is seen in infants (Li 1995, 1094-5). Moxibustion on Xing Jian (LV 2) for double tongue is found in Sun's *Prescriptions*, Volume 5 (Sun 1994, a80).

[78] The exact nature of this condition is unclear, but it seems to be that the nursing mother ate cold food. The cold food affected her milk, and this affected the baby. The 14 cones for the adult are intended for the mother. It must be the odor of stool in the mouth, as stool itself cannot come back up into the mouth.

[79] The "five epilepsies" is a term used in different books to mean different things. Here Zhang describes epilepsies corresponding to five types of animals (see, p. 168).

[80] For more on the Ghost Eye points, see **LJTY: 10-1-4-32** and **ZJDC: 9-6-2**, above.

mugwort moxibustion. You must apply fire to the four places of nail and flesh. It is effective right then.

You can also apply treatment to these two points on the big toes, using the same method as for the hand points. This point is named Ghost Eye of the feet. Like the previous point, applying moxibustion to it is greatly effective.

In adults, this disease is called withdrawal. It is also best to apply moxibustion like this for such cases.

一法云：癇為小兒惡證，古云驚風三發便爲癇，癇證有五，即牛、羊、豬、馬、雞之類也。治法俟其病發之時，將患者兩手大拇指相並，以綿繩縛定，當兩指爪甲角，是名鬼眼穴，用艾灸七壯，須甲肉四處著火方效。又二穴在足大拇指，亦如取手穴法，是名足鬼眼穴，如前灸之大效，大人病此則名為癲，灸亦如之最良。

Ox epilepsy:[81] Da Zhu [UB 11], Jiu Wei [Ren 15] (apply three cones of moxibustion five *fen* below the tip [of the xiphoid process]. You cannot use a lot of moxibustion).

牛癇：大杼、鳩尾尖下五分，灸三壯，不可多

Goat epilepsy: Staring straight ahead, making goat sounds. Bai Hui [Du 20], Shen Ting [Du 24], Xin Shu [UB 15], Gan Shu [UB 18], Tian Jing [SJ 10], Shen Men [HT 7], Tai Chong [LV 3].

羊癇：目直，作羊聲。百會、神庭、心俞、肝俞、天井、神門、大衝

Pig epilepsy: Phlegm drool like threads, making pig sounds. Bai Hui [Du 20], Ju Que [Ren 14], Xin Shu [UB 15], Shen Men [HT 7].

豬癇：痰涎如綿，作豬聲。百會、巨闕、心俞、神門

Horse epilepsy: Gaping mouth, shaking head, arched-back rigidity. Bai Hui [Du 20], Xin Shu [HT 7], Ming Men [Du 4], Shen Men [HT 7], Pu Can [UB 61], Tai Chong [LV 3], Zhao Hai [KI 6].

馬癇：張口搖頭，角弓反張。百會、心俞、命門、神門、僕參、太衝、照海

Rooster epilepsy: Falling forward with outstretched arms. If you grab them and stop them, they will promptly regain consciousness. Shen Mai [UB 62].

雞癇：張手前仆，提住即醒。申脈

LJTY: 11-3-23 External Medicine [外科 *Wai Ke*] (Zhang 1991, 952)

Eruptions on the back: Xin Shu [UB 15], Wei Yang [UB 39] (someone said it is located 1.6 *cun* below the buttocks, on the thigh where there is a seam), Ride the Bamboo Horse points. For a reachable sore on either side, add Hui Yang [UB 35].[82]

發背：心俞、委陽一曰在尻臀下一寸六分，大腿上有縫、騎竹馬穴、左右搭手，加會陽

Moxibustion on garlic method for abscesses: Whenever someone suffers flat-abscesses and malign toxins on the back, the color of the flesh does not change. It is like carrying stones on the back. It is a diffuse swelling, without a head. This situation is definately serious.

The method to search for the head of the abscess: Rub damp paper on the site of the swelling. See where the paper dries first. This is the head of the welling-abscess, the site where it binds and gathers.

Use a big head of single-clove garlic. Cut it into slices that are three *fen* thick and apply it to the peak of the flat-abscess. Apply mugwort moxibustion on the garlic, replacing the garlic every three cones. Sometimes the eruptions on the back are initially red

---

[81] The other four types of epilepsy all have a little description. This one does not in any edition.
[82] For the Bamboo Horse points, see **ZJDC: 9-9** and **LJTY: 10-1-7** above. For unfamiliar terms, please see the glossary.

and swollen. The center may be like a small yellow grain of rice. Sometimes there are more than 10 of them in an area. It is especially appropriate to use garlic moxibustion on these.[83]

癰疽隔蒜灸法：凡患背疽惡毒，肉色不變，背如負石，漫腫無頭者，勢必重大。尋頭之法：用濕紙搨在腫處，看有一點先乾者，即是癰頭結聚之處。用大獨頭蒜，切作三分厚片，貼疽頂，以艾於蒜上灸之，每三壯一換其蒜。又有背上初發赤腫，中間有如黃小米一粒者，有十數粒一片者，尤宜隔蒜灸之。

The *Green Sack Book* says: The outer form can be the size of a grain of millet and internally it can be the size of a piece of grain. Outside, some are shaped like a coin and internally they can be the size of a fist. Be careful not to see them as unimportant; there is no greater suffering than what they bring about.

In a case where the head of the sore is wide open, take more than 10 heads of purple-skinned garlic, half a *ge* of Dan Dou Chi [Semen Praeparatum Sojae], two *qian* of Ru Xiang [Olibanum], and pound them together to make a paste. Pat it into thin cakes based on the size of the toxins. Place it on the toxins and apply mugwort moxibustion to it.[84]

《青囊書》云：外形如粟，內可容穀；外狀如錢，裏可著拳。慎勿視爲微小，致成莫大之患。設或瘡頭開大，則以紫皮大蒜十餘頭，淡豆豉半合，乳香二錢，同搗成膏，照毒大小拍成薄餅，置毒上鋪艾灸之。

On a person suffering pain, you must apply moxi-

bustion until there is no pain. If there is no pain, apply moxibustion until the patient feels pain. The pain must be [because the fire touches] the good flesh. No pain means it is in the region of the toxic qi. If first there is no pain, and then the patient perceives pain, the toxins are mild and shallow. On the other hand, if first there is pain, and then there is no pain, the toxins are deep and serious. That is why the person performing moxibustion must make the fire qi extend straight into the site of the toxins. You cannot limit or restrict the number of cones; the ancients have applied up to 800 cones of moxibustion to achieve recovery.[85]

務要痛者，灸至不痛，不痛者灸至知痛。蓋痛者爲良肉，不痛者爲毒氣。先不痛而後覺痛者，其毒輕淺；先痛而後反不痛者，其毒深重。故灸者必令火氣直達毒處，不可拘定壯數，昔人有灸至八百壯而愈者。

After the moxibustion, you must give medicinals to supplement the center, internally expel [pus and toxins], reinforce the stomach, or invigorate qi, according to the person's condition of vacuity or repletion. In 10,000 patients, not one will be lost.

When not yet ulcerated, it must be that moxibustion is able to draw out and scatter the depressed toxins; it does not let the opening get bigger. When already ulcerated, moxibustion is able to supplement and receive yang qi, [and] it easily promotes contraction. That is why the best plan is only early detection and early moxibustion together.

灸後須隨人虛實，服補中托裏助胃壯氣等藥，萬無一

---

[83] Zhang switches between welling-abscess (*yong*) and flat-abscess (*ju*) in this discussion. I suspect that he is using the two terms interchangeably, not applying their specific meaning. In any case, before a head has formed, you can find the abscess: it will be hotter than the surrounding skin, so it will dry damp paper first. The method of searching for the head of an abscess with damp paper is also discussed in **BCGM: 15-05-47**, p. 105.

Single-clove garlic is the type native to China. The kind with many cloves came from the West (Harper 1998, 370n.1). For more about garlic see **BCGM: 26-09** p. 98-112.

[84] I am unable to identify the *Green Sack Book*.

This passage points out that while the head may be small, the abscess can be very big inside and can become quite serious. The same formula is found in **BCGM: 26-29-01**, p. 111 and a similar formula is also in **BCGM: 25-01-35**, p. 118.

Age is one-tenth of a *sheng*. These units of measurement are especially used for grains (Zhang 1992, 164).

[85] This idea of differentiating the treatment by the presence or absence of pain is also discussed in **JYQS: 46-11, JYQS: 63-117, BCGM: 15-05-47** p. 105 and **BCGM: 26-09** p. 98-112. In other words, this seems to be a common idea.

As for the ancients applying a lot of cones to sores such as these, Sun's *Prescriptions*, Volume 22 suggests 700-800 cones on top of the sores (Sun 1994, a317).

失。蓋未潰而灸，則能拔散鬱毒，不令開大，已潰而
灸，則能補接陽氣，易於收斂。然惟蚤覺蚤灸，方為
上策。

True Person Liu Yuanran said: If moxibustion is applied to patients with toxins that have erupted for
one or two days, 100 percent will recover. If it has
been three or four days, 60 or 70 percent will recover. If it has been five or six days, 30 or 40 percent
will recover. When past seven days, even if moxibustion is applied, the toxins cannot be dispersed and
scattered. Because the inner pus has already developed, you must needle to remove and loosen it.

Even though it is like this, there are five benign and
seven malign signs within the disease of flat-abscesses.
When facing these patterns, you must first recognize
this. Earlier wise people have said: If you see three of
the five benign signs, it is auspicious. If you see four of
the seven malign signs, it is inauspicious. If perchance,
you see the seven malign signs, be careful not to apply
moxibustion; you will only invite slander.[86]

淵然劉真人曰：毒發一二日者，十灸十愈，三四日者
，六七愈，五六日者，三四愈，過七日，則雖灸不能
消散矣。緣其內膿已成，必須鍼去方得寬鬆也。雖然
疽之為病，有五善七惡，臨證之時，先須識此。前哲
云：五善見三則吉，七惡見四則凶，倘見七惡，慎勿
為灸，徒召謗耳。

There is also the pattern of clove sores. They do not
all have an identical form. They do not all have the
same color. There are some like small scrofula, some
like water blisters, some with pain that cannot be
withstood, some that itch and are difficult to endure, some with numbness of the skin and flesh,
some with heat and cold and headaches, some with
nausea and vomiting, some with hypertonicity of
the limbs. The symptoms have so many causes that
it is difficult to thoroughly describe them. But all
must have early application of moxibustion. When
severe, apply garlic paste all around.

Moxibustion using mugwort to touch the flesh is
only applied to the peak of the dew toxins. Take blistering as the measure of successful treatment. If
there is no blistering, it is difficult to recover. In addition, it is appropriate to apply a lot of moxibustion: 100 cones and above. There is no one who
does not recover.[87]

又有疔瘡一證，其形不一，其色不同，或如小瘰，或
如水泡，或痛不可當，或癢而難忍，或皮肉麻木，或
寒熱頭疼，或噁心嘔吐，或肢體拘急，其候多端，難
以盡狀。皆須用前灸法，甚則以蒜膏徧塗四圍，只露
毒頂，用艾著肉灸之，以爆為度，如不爆者難愈。更
宜多灸，百壯以上，無弗愈者。

Mammary welling-abscess: mammary flat-abscess,
mammary rock, mammary qi, mammary toxins, in-
vading sacs (near Dan Zhong [Ren 17]):[88] Jian Yu [LI
15], Ling Dao [HT 4] (two times seven cones), Wen

---

[86] True Person Liu Yuanran (14th century, Ming) wrote *Immortal's Prescriptions for Emergency* 《濟急仙方》 (Li 1995, 606).
Ji Dezhi (Yuan) described the five benign and seven malign signs in the *Profound Significance of External Medicine*.
齊德之《外科精義·辨瘡疽善惡法》.
A summary of the five benign signs of flat-abscesses: food has taste and breathing and pulse are peaceful; elimination is normal; the
sore ulcerates, the swelling disperses and the fluids from the sore do not smell bad; the spirit is bright and speech is clear; etc.
A summary of the seven malign signs of flat-abscesses: the patient has a concurrent internal syndrome; the pus looks withered
and smells bad; dilated pupils, red whites of the eyes and the eyes are looking upward; wheezing and shortness of breath; unable
to eat and food is tasteless; superficial edema and poor color in face; etc. (Ji 1990, 24-5).
You only invite slander by treating a patient with the seven malign signs because the patient will have a bad outcome regardless
of what you do, yet people will blame you.
[87] "If there is no blistering, it is difficult to recover." 爆 *bao* is to explode, to burst, to crack, to pop. 爆發 means to break out or
erupt. Therefore, I have translated this as blistering, meaning that the moxibustion causes the eruption of blisters. These blisters
may even spontaneously pop open with some force.
Zhang said that dew toxins are the only type of sore in this category that does not use an isolating substance for moxibustion.
This may refer to dew cinnabar 露丹, a pediatric disease with red blistering papules (Li 1995 1743).

Liu [LI 7] (children, seven cones; adults, two times seven cones), Zu San Li [ST 36], Tiao Kou [ST 38] (mammary welling-abscess), Xia Ju Xu [ST 39] (each two times seven cones).

乳癰、乳疽、乳岩、乳氣、乳毒、侵囊：近膻中者是。肩髃、靈道二七壯、溫溜小人七壯，大人二七壯、足三里、條口乳癰、下巨虛各二七壯

Heat toxins: Da Ling [PC 7].　熱毒：大陵

Lung welling-abscess, spitting pus: Shen Shu [UB 23] (three times seven cones), He Gu [LI 4] (two times seven cones), Tai Yuan [LU 9] (two times seven cones).

肺癰吐膿：腎俞三七壯、合谷二七壯、太淵二七壯

Hemilateral pillow on the nape:[89] Feng Men [UB 12] (two times seven cones).

項上偏枕：風門二七壯

Welling-abscess of the stomach:[90] Those growing on the left are flat-abscesses of the stomach opening. Those growing on the right are welling-abscesses of the stomach opening. Qu Chi [LI 11] (bilateral, each three times seven cones), Nei Guan [PC 6] (seven cones).

胃癰：生於左者胃口疽，生於右者胃口癰。曲池二穴各三七壯、內關七壯

Welling-abscess of the kidney:[91] Arises from Shen Shu [UB 23]. Hui Yang [UB 35] (two times seven cones).

腎癰：自腎俞穴起。會陽二七壯

Bone-clinging flat-abscess:[92] When there is pain at Huan Tiao [GB 30], it is probably the growth of a welling-abscess attached to the bone. Da Ling [PC 7], Xuan Zhong [GB 39] (three times seven cones).

附骨疽：環跳穴痛，恐生附骨疽也。大陵、懸鍾三七壯

Bone rotation:[93] Zhou Jian [Tip of the Elbow, non-channel] (seven times seven cones. If the patient does not recover, 100 cones).

骨旋：肘尖七七壯，不愈百壯

Scrofula:[94]　瘰癧：

Bee's nest large scrofula: arising from the left side. The seven times seven holes all exude pus.[95]
蜂窠癧自左邊起，七七竅皆出膿。

• Jian Yu [LI 15] (seven cones or nine cones), Qu

---

[88] These are various kinds of breast abscesses, sores, and lumps.
[89] This seems to mean a stiff neck on one side from sleeping in the wrong position or a wind invasion during the night. If so, it is misplaced here among different types of abscesses; perhaps Zhang is referring to something else.
[90] Wiseman (1998, 670-1) says that this term can refer to a welling-abscess internally on the stomach duct or to an external welling-abscess located in the region of Zhong Wan (Ren 12). Since the next item describes a welling-abscess of the kidneys as arising at Shen Shu (UB 23), it is likely this passage also means an external abscess. It is also possible that the external abscess was viewed as concurrent pathology with one inside the associated internal organ. An axiom of Chinese medicine is that whatever is on the inside will manifest on the outside.
[91] Li says a welling-abscess of the kidney is located in the region of Jing Men (GB 25), the *mu* alarm point of the kidneys (Li 1995, 905). Wiseman does not discuss it.
[92] A bone-clinging flat-abscess is "a headless flat-abscess located on a bony and sinewy part of the body" (Wiseman 1998, 44).
[93] This is likely some kind of problem near the elbow or forearm as that is the area with the most rotation of bones, and the treatment at the tip of the elbow is also in this region. I am unable to locate this condition in any reference book. This entry is placed between abscesses and scrofula, so it is likely related to one or the other. Zhou Jian is commonly used for scrofula. In a later entry, Zhang says that Zhou Jian refers to Qu Chi (LI 11); so perhaps this is not the non-channel point.
[94] Zhang differentiates the scrofula by the appearance, comparing the swellings to a familiar object, as was the custom. *Luo* 瘰 is small scrofula. *Li* 癧 is large scrofula (Wiseman 1995, 543 and 554).
[95] In late stages, scrofula can rupture and exude thin pus (Wiseman 1998, 515). In bee's nest scrofula, many lumps in one area have ruptured, giving the appearance of a honeycomb.

Chi [LI 11]. These two points are a secret method for treating large scrofula.

肩髃七壯，九壯、曲尺，此二穴乃治瘰秘法也。

- Tian Chi [PC 1], Tian Jing [SJ 10] (two times seven cones), San Jian [LI 3] (three times seven cones).

天池、天井二七壯、三間三七壯

Sharp awl large scrofula: A growth arising on the right side. Jian Yu [LI 15], Qu Chi [LI 11], Tian Jing [SJ 10].

錐銳瘰：右邊生起。肩髃、曲池、天井

Coiled serpent large scrofula: A prolonged growth on the neck. Jian Jian [Shoulder Tip] (meaning Jian Yu [LI 15]), Zhou Jian [Elbow Tip] (meaning Qu Chi [LI 11]), Ren Ying [ST 9] (seven cones), Jian Wai Shu [SI 14] (two times seven cones), Tian Jing [SJ 10] (two times seven cones), Ride the Bamboo Horse points (three times seven cones).[96]

盤蛇瘰：延頸生者。肩尖即肩髃、肘尖即曲池、人迎七壯、肩外俞二七壯、天井二七壯、騎竹馬穴三七壯

Melon vine large scrofula: A growth on the front of the chest. Zhou Jian [LI 11], Shao Hai [HT 3], Ride the Bamboo Horse points.
瓜藤瘰：胸前生者。肘尖、少海、騎竹馬穴

Saber lumps:[97] Below the armpits. 馬刀：腋下者。

- Yuan Ye [GB 22], Zhi Gou [SJ 6], Wai Guan [SJ 5], Zu Lin Qi [GB 41] (treats both the neck and armpits).
  淵腋、支溝、外關、足臨泣頸腋俱治

- When large scrofula sores erupt below the

cheeks and near Jia Che [ST 6], you should apply treatment to points of the hand and foot yang brightness channels. Thus, both Jian Yu [LI 15] and Qu Chi [LI 11] are also wonderful.

瘰瘡出於頰下，及頰車邊者，當於手足陽明經取穴治之，然肩髃、曲池二穴亦妙。

- He Gu [LI 4], Zu San Li [ST 36] (each seven cones).

The above points affect deep toxins overall. After the moxibustion, repeat this treatment for two or three more sessions. There is no one who does not recover.

合谷、足三里各七壯。已上凡感毒深者，灸後再二三次報之，無有不愈。

Moxibustion on garlic for scrofula:

- Use a slice of single-clove garlic. First, begin moxibustion on the most recently erupted nucleus. When you reach the mother nucleus from the initial eruption, stop. A lot of moxibustion is spontaneously effective.

瘰瘰隔蒜灸法：用獨蒜片，先從後發核上灸起，至初發母核而止，多灸自效。

- Another effective treatment that was handed down: Use one dried toad [Bufo Siccus]. Break it open and remove the intestines. Cover the large scrofula with it. Outside the toad skin, right on the large scrofula, apply moxibustion with seven or 14 cones of true mugwort from Qizhou, the cones the size of the large scrofula. Use the hot qi [from the moxibustion] to thrust out from the interior, and then stop. Also, apply moxibustion first to the most recent eruption. When you reach the initial eruption, stop. If the toad skin gets

---

[96] Here, Zhang states that Zhou Jian is not the non-channel point; it is Qu Chi (LI 11). This makes it a little difficult to identify which point is meant in the some entries, because the non-channel point called Zhou Jian also treats scrofula.
  For Ride the Bamboo Horse points, see **LJTY: 10-1-7** and **ZJDC: 9-9**, above.
[97] Saber lumps are scrofula that gives the appearance of a saber (Wiseman 1998, 509).

scorched, it must be changed before applying moxibustion to it. When the moxibustion is finished, the patient should take a prescription of decocted medicinals. This prescription uses seven small Ya Zao [Fructus Gleditsiae]; seven Jiang Can [Bombyx Batryticatus]; one Gua Lou [Fructus Trichosanthis] including the skin, cut or broken open; and one berry of Wu Wei Zi [Fructus Schisandrae] for each year of age. Use two cups of water to decoct the above four flavors. Besides this, add lightly brewed Da Huang [Radix Et Rhizoma Rhei] (3-5 *qian*). Measure the person's vacuity or repletion when using these formulas. After taking the formula, the scrofula will immediately disperse. If 100 people try it, it is effective for 100. Do not bother asking if the scrofula has already ulcerated or has not yet ulcerated; as a result of moxibustion, the patient will recover.[98]

又傳驗方：用癩蝦蟆一箇，破去腸，覆瘰上，外以真蘄艾照瘰大小爲炷，於蝦蟆皮上當瘰灸七壯或十四壯，以熱氣透內方住，亦從後發者先灸，至初發者而止。若蝦蟆皮焦，須移易灸之。灸畢服煎藥一劑，其方用牙皂七箇，殭蠶七條、瓜蔞一箇，連皮子切碎、五味子一歲一粒、上四味一水二鍾煎熱，外加生煎大黃三五錢，量人虛實用之，一服即消，百試百效。不問已潰未潰，經灸必愈。

Goiter:[99]

• **Jian Yu [LI 15]:** On males, apply18 cones of moxibustion on the left and 17 cones on the right. On females, apply 18 cones of moxibustion on the right and 17 cones on the left.[100]

肩髃：男左灸十八壯，右十七壯，女右灸十八壯，左十七壯。

• **Tian Tu [Ren 22]:** Treats all goiters when they initially arise. It is wonderful to apply moxibustion on them.

天突：治一切瘻瘤初起者灸之妙。

• Tong Tian [UB 7] (goiter), Feng Chi [GB 20] (100 cones), Da Zhui [Du 14] (neck goiter), Qi She [ST 11] (five cones of moxibustion), Yun Men [LU 2] (goiter), Bi Nao [LI 14] (goiter), Nao Hui [SJ 13] (five cones), Tian Fu [LU 3] (five times seven cones), Qu Chi [LI 11] (goiter), Zhong Feng [LV 4] (goiter), Chong Yang [ST 42] (three cones).

通天瘻、風池百壯、大椎頸瘻、氣舍灸五壯、雲門瘻、臂〔月+需〕瘻、〔月+需〕會五壯、天府五七壯、曲池瘻、中封瘻、衝陽三壯

Warts on the body and face: Apply three cones of moxibustion right on the wart. It will promptly disperse. Also, some only apply one cone of moxibustion and drip water on it. It will spontaneously be eliminated.

身面〔疒+贅〕疣：當疣上灸三壯即消。亦有止灸一壯，以水滴之自去者。

Dormant papules:[101] Qu Chi [LI 11].   癮疹：曲池

Scabby sores:[102] Feng Men [UB 12], Jian Shi [PC 5], He Gu [LI 4], Da Ling [PC 7] (sores and scabs on the front of the chest).

---

[98] Li Shizhen discussed this type of toad in **BCGM: 42-2**. He recommended it for scrofula that has ulcerated, but using a different method: remove the intestines. Bake and grind it. Mix it with oil and apply it to the scrofula. No moxibustion is used.
  "Measure the person's vacuity or repletion when using these formulas" means to modify the formula based on the patient's condition.
  "Do not bother asking if the scrofula has already ulcerated or hasn't yet ulcerated" means that this treatment is effective in either case.

[99] This term can indicate both goiters and tumors, or just goiter (Li 1995, 1714). Here it seems to simply mean goiter.

[100] Males, being yang, are associated with the left side. Females, being yin, are associated with the right side. Odd numbers are yang and even numbers are yin. Here, 18 cones (the yin number) are applied to the main side based on gender, and 17 cones (the yang number) are applied to the secondary side. Hyperthyroidism often accompanies goiter. Perhaps using the yin number of cones on the main side helps counteract some of the yang symptoms of hyperthyroidism.

瘄疥：風門、間使、合谷、大陵胸前瘄疥

Toxic sores that do not close for a long time:

- Whenever someone has suffered a welling-abscess with toxins that has ulcerated but has not closed for a long time, with watery pus that does not smell, and also no bad flesh, it is because it was excessively dispersed and scattered. The result is vacuity cold of the blood and qi so the flesh does not flourish. The treatment has lost its suitability and the condition can become a lifelong affliction. The patient must take medicinals internally, such as Shi Quan Da Bu [Ten {Ingredients} Completely Supplementing {Pill or Decoction}]. Externally, use Da Fu Zi [Aconite] soaked thoroughly in warm water. Cut it into slices two or three *fen* thick. Place them on the hole of the fistula and apply mugwort moxibustion to it. You can also apply moxibustion on cakes made from powdered Aconite mixed with spittle. Every two or three days, you can apply moxibustion to it again. In less than three or five applications, the flesh will grow and fill in naturally and the long-term suffering is quelled.[103]

凡患癰毒潰後，久不收口，膿水不臭，亦無歹肉者，此因消散太過，以致血氣虛寒，不榮肌肉，治失其宜，便為終身之患。須內服十全大補等藥，外用大附子以溫水泡透，切作二三分厚片，治漏孔上，以艾灸之。或以附子為末，用唾和作餅，灸之亦可

。隔二三日再灸之，不三五次，自然肌肉長滿而宿患平矣。

- **Another formula:** Use wheat flour, Liu Huang [Sulfur], and Da Suan [Garlic]. Pound these three flavors to a pulp. Pinch them into cakes that are three *fen* thick, the size of the affected area. Set one on the affected area and apply three times seven cones of moxibustion. Change the cake every three cones. After four or five days, apply moxibustion once again. It is never without effect.

又方：用麥麵、硫磺、大蒜三味搗爛，如患大小捻作三分厚餅，安患上，灸三七壯，每三壯易餅子，四五日後再灸一次，無弗效者。

Eliminating the root of armpit qi: Whenever there is armpit qi, first use a sharp knife to cleanly shave off the armpit hair. Then mix good starch powder and water and apply it to the affected site. Six or seven days later, you will see that there is a black spot below the armpits. It will have a hole the size of a needle or the tip of a hairpin. This is the qi [smell] orifice. Apply moxibustion to it with mugwort cones the size of a grain of rice. Three times four cones will bring recovery. It will never emerge again.[104]

腋氣除根：凡腋氣先用快刀剃去腋毛淨、水調搽患處。六七日後，看腋下有一點黑者，必有孔如鍼大，或如簪尖，即氣竅也。用艾炷如米大者灸之，三四壯愈，永不再發。

---

[101] Dormant papules are "wheals that come and go, so named by their ability to remain latent between eruptions." This is mostly equivalent to urticaria in Western medicine (Wiseman 1998, 145).

[102] This is "a disease characterized by small papules the size of a pinhead that are associated with insufferable penetrating itching and that, when scratched, may suppurate or crust." It is parallel to scabies in Western medicine (Wiseman 1998, 512-3).

[103] Excessively cooling medicinals taken internally can damage qi, blood, and yang. Because of this malpractice, the sores are unable to heal. Sores that do not close up lack yang qi. Just as yang qi holds the interstices shut to prevent sweating or holds the lower orifices shut to prevent incontinence, it also promotes the closing up of sores. The ability of moxibustion to warm yang is increased with Fu Zi (Aconite) in this entry or with Liu Huang (Sulfur), and Da Suan (Garlic) in the next entry.
   In a number of recipes from Zhang and Li Shizhen, aconite powder is made into a cake with spittle. Spittle is the humor of the kidneys, and as such, it theoretically would have a greater medicinal effect than water. See also **BCGM 17-17-1**, above.

[104] Armpit qi means body odor.
   Jingyue's *Complete Works*, Volume 60, says to use seven cones and adds, "If too much moxibustion was applied or if there is turbid qi attacking the heart making pain, you should use medicinals afterwards to precipitate it: Ding Xiang [Flos Caryophylli], Qing Mu Xiang [Radix Aristolochiae], Bin Lang [Semen Arecae], Tan Xiang [Lignum Santali Albi], She Xiang [Secretio Moschi], and Da Huang [Radix Et Rhizoma Rhei]. Brew the above medicinals and take them. Take precipitation as the degree of success."
灸過或有濁氣攻心作痛者，當用後藥下之：丁香、青木香、檳榔、檀香、麝香、大黃。右煎服，以下為度。《景岳全書‧狐腋氣方二九三‧卷之六十》(Zhang, J.Y. 1995, 1630)

LJTY: 11-3-24 All Damage from Toxins [諸毒傷 *Zhu Du Shang*] (Zhang 1991, 956)

Infixation of the five gu toxins:[105] Malign stroke, unable to eat. Zhong Wan [Ren 12], Zhao Hai [KI 6] (gu toxins stroke).

五蠱毒注：中惡不能食。中脘、照海中蠱毒

Rabid dog bite:

Quickly make the person completely suck out the malign blood. Apply 100 cones of moxibustion to the site of the bite. Afterwards, apply moxibustion to it every day, stopping after 100 days. He should avoid pork and wine, being careful about them throughout his life.[106]

瘋犬咬傷：急令人吮盡惡血於咬處灸百壯，已後日日灸之，百日乃止，忌豬肉與酒，一生慎之。

True Person Sun said, "At the end of spring and beginning of summer, many dogs go mad. No one with this type of bite can get through without moxibustion." The method is to apply moxibustion on the teeth marks, only near the site of the bite. Apply three cones of moxibustion per day, stopping after 120 days. It is appropriate to constantly eat fried Chinese leeks [Jiu Cai]. It will never emerge again. This is also a good method.[107]

孫真人曰：春末夏初，犬多發狂，被其咬者，無出於灸。其法只就咬處牙迹上灸之，一日灸三壯，灸至一百二十日乃止。宜常食灸韭菜，永不再發，亦良發也。

Another treatment for all dog bites: If the toxin qi does not come out, you must apply moxibustion to Wai Qiu [GB 36]. Someone said: Quickly use three people with different surnames to apply moxibustion to the site of the bite for immediate recovery.[108]

又治一切犬傷：毒氣不出者，須灸外邱。一曰速用三姓人，灸所嚙處立愈。

Snake venom: Whenever there is a venomous snake bite, apply three times seven cones of moxibustion on the venom. If at so me time you do not have mugwort, burn the bite with the end of a flaming piece of charcoal, matched to the size of the sore's opening.[109]

蛇毒：凡蛇傷中毒者，灸毒上三七壯。若一時無艾以火炭頭稱瘡孔大小〔艸+熱〕之。

All insect and reptile toxins: Whenever there are snake, scorpion, or centipede bites, the pain is extreme and the situation is dangerous. Quickly apply moxibustion to the site of the bite using mugwort fire. This draws out and scatters the venom qi, promptly quieting the situation.

Or use slices of single-clove garlic and apply garlic-isolated moxibustion. Replace the slice every two or three cones. If the toxins are severe, apply 50 cones of moxibustion.

Or it is also wonderful to take Zi Jin Dan [Purple & Gold Elixir] internally.

Or, for horse sweat that has entered a sore as well as

---

[105] For gu toxins and infixation, see the glossary. See also Fruehauf (1998) for further discussion of gu toxins.

[106] This passage is based on Sun's *Prescriptions*, Volume 25 (Sun 1994, a359). Sun took it from *Short Sketches* (Chen 1993, 177). *Elementary Questions*, Chapter 60 says to apply three cones of moxibustion to the site of a dog bite. Only local moxibustion is used; no distal points. The techniques here seem to be a more detailed prescription from these earlier books.

[107] The quote is also from Sun's *Prescriptions*, Volume 25 (Sun 1994, a358). Only local moxibustion is used; no distal points.
  Li Shizhen also includes an internal formula using Chinese leeks (Jiu Cai) to treat rabid dog bites. This medicinal is included in formulas for many other types of toxins, too. See **BCGM: 26-1** (Li 1996, 698).

[108] "Quickly use three people with different surnames," these words were censored in one modern version (Zhang, J.Y. 1996, 343). It must be that the toxins are so potent, it is better to make sure no one person or family has too much exposure to them. A treatment for cold impediment in the legs and knees in Sun's *Supplement*, Volume 28 also contains this phrase (Sun 1994, b262).

[109] Once again, the treatment only consists of local moxibustion to destroy or draw out the venom. It came from Sun's *Prescriptions*, Volume 25 (Sun 1994, a355).

the venom from the likes of silkworms or spiders, moxibustion is effective for all this.[110]

處灸之，拔散毒氣即安。或用獨蒜片膈蒜灸之，二三
壯換一片，毒甚者灸五十壯，或內服紫金丹亦妙。或
馬汗入瘡及蠱毒、蜘蛛等毒，灸之皆效。

CONCLUSION

Zhang's moxibustion treatment formulary is almost a whole volume of the *Illustrated Supplement*. Zhang must have felt that moxibustion was a powerful tool in the treatment and prevention of disease. Perhaps we can judge Zhang's confidence in moxibustion to treat a specific condition by the length of the section on that condition. If so, cold damage, vacuity taxation, bleeding patterns, accumulations, pain in the heart region and abdomen, cough and other kinds of counterflow qi, diseases of the head, face, hands, feet, and the two yin, gynecology, pediatrics, and external medicine all received a significant amout of space. Malaria, jaundice, wasting-thirst, mania-with-drawal, diarrhea, dysphagia-occlusion, drum distention, and reverse flow received fewer words.

One thing to note is that Zhang rarely used an isolating substance for moxibustion except on hemorrhoids, sores, bites, and other kinds of treatment for external conditions. He favored direct moxibustion for diseases of the organs and other internal ailments. Apparently, isolating substances have a direct effect on the tissue they touch and are generally used as part of a topical treatment. If the points and channel system are used, whether for a channel problem or to treat the organs on the inside, direct moxibustion has the best effect. The biggest exception to this statement would be the use of salt or other medicinals with Shen Que (Ren 8).

The next section of the book contains other treatments prescribed by Zhang, Li, and Yang.

---

[110] In **BCGM: 50-6**, Li Shizhen said that horse sweat is very toxic. If it enters a sore, its toxins attack the heart (Li 1996, 1167). See Volume 60 of Jingyue's *Complete Works* (**JYQS: 60-202**), for Zi Jin Dan (Purple & Gold Elixir).

CHAPTER 11
OTHER TREATMENTS WITH MOXIBUSTION

Chapter Contents

In this chapter we will examine additional treatments prescribed by Zhang Jiebin in his *Complete Works* and those described by Li Shizhen and Yang Jizhou in their books.

MOXIBUSTION IN [ZHANG] JINGYUE'S *COMPLETE WORKS*

Besides the extensive section on treatment in the *Illustrated Supplement*, Zhang wote more about moxibustion in his *Complete Works*, which was published 12 years later in 1636. Volumes 7-47 described the treatment of condition after condition. Most often the recommended treatment was in the form of medicinal formulas but Zhang frequently suggested moxibustion and occasionally acupuncture.

Some of the information on moxibustion in the *Complete Works* is repeated from the *Illustrated Supplement*, but most is new. Below, passages are abridged when they repeat those already translated from the *Illustrated Supplement*.

JYQS: 46-11 External Medicine, Discussion on Moxibustion (Zhang 1995, 1069) [abridged]
《景岳全書 • 外科 • 論灸法 • 卷之四十六》

Wang Haicang said: It is not appropriate to apply moxibustion for sores that enter from the exterior. It is appropriate to apply moxibustion for those that come out from the interior. Those entering from the exterior should be drawn out and not internalized. Those coming out from the interior should be caught and made to externalize. That is why the *Classic* says, "Apply moxibustion to what is sunken."[1]

When moxibustion is applied but is not painful, stop when the moxibustion becomes painful. When moxibustion is applied and is not painful, it means the effects first reach the flesh that has ulcerated, so there is no pain. Later, the effects reach good flesh, so there is pain.

---

[1] *Elementary Questions*, Chapter 60 《素問 • 骨空論篇第六十》

When moxibustion is applied and is painful, stop when the moxibustion is no longer painful. When moxibustion is applied and is painful, it means it first reaches flesh that has not ulcerated, so there is pain. Next it reaches the flesh that is about to ulcerate, so there is no pain.

王海藏曰：瘡瘍自外而入者，不宜灸；自內而出者，宜灸。外入者托之而不內，內出者接之而令外。故經曰：陷者灸之。灸而不痛，痛而後止其灸。灸而不痛者，先及其潰，所以不痛，而後及良肉，所以痛也。灸而痛，不痛而後止其灸。灸而痛者，先及其未潰，所以痛，而次及將潰，所以不痛也。

Master Li said: As for methods to treat abscesses, the merits of burning mugwort are superior to using medicinals. Now, moxibustion makes toxic qi discharge through the exterior. This is like a thief entering a household. You must open the gate to expel him. If not, he can enter the house and do harm. Overall, in the initial one or two days when sores erupt, you must use a big head of garlic. Cut it into slices three *fen* thick. Apply them to the peak of the abscess, and apply moxibustion with mugwort on the garlic. Change the garlic every three cones. When the sores ulcerate, apply Shen Yi Gao [Miraculous Paste]. When this is done, sores will not become big ulcers, the flesh will not spoil, and the openings of the sores easily close. With one action, three goals are obtained. People seldom know the wonder of this method. If abscesses appear on the head, this method cannot be used (Recorded in the *Stele of the Ultimate Observation of the Five Palaces* [*Wu Fu Ji Guan Bei*]).[2]

李氏云：治瘡之法，灼艾之功，勝於用藥，蓋使毒氣外泄；譬諸盜入人家，當開門逐之，不然則入室為害矣。凡瘡初發一二日，須用大顆獨蒜，切片三分厚，貼瘡頂，以艾隔蒜灸之，每三壯易蒜，瘡潰則貼神異膏，如此則瘡不開大，肉不壞，瘡口易斂，一舉三得，此法之妙，人所罕知。 若頭頂兒疽，則不可用此法。《五府極觀碑》載。

Master Chen said: The brain is the meeting of all yang. The neck is near the throat. Shen Shu [UB 23] is the place of mortality. Mugwort cannot be burned on any of these places.

Master Wu said: As for using garlic cake moxibustion, the flavor of garlic is acrid, warm, and toxic. It governs scattering abscesses. You must rely on the influence of fire in order to move the power of the medicine [garlic]. Some only use mugwort cone moxibustion for treating abscesses; it can be applied for such things as stubborn abscesses and intractable eruptions. Generally, when red swellings and purple or black toxins are severe, moxibustion with both garlic and mugwort is wonderful.

He also said: Whenever treating abscesses, eruptions on the back, and clove sores, if there is pain when moxibustion is initially applied, it is from toxic qi that is mild and shallow. If there is no pain when moxibustion is applied, it is deep and serious toxic qi. It is completely appropriate to take medicinals internally to expel the toxins and pus. Externally, apply medicinals to disperse toxins. Generally, abscesses should not be painless but they also should not have great pain, oppression, and derangement. Those that are painless are difficult to treat.

He also said: Whenever applying moxibustion on garlic, the number of cones is not discussed. In this way, the evil will not be permitted and true qi will not be harmed.[3] However, it is appropriate to use the Ride the Bamboo Horse method as well as to apply moxibustion to Zu San Li [ST 36] for sores appearing on the head and nape.

陳氏曰：腦為諸陽之會，頸項近咽喉，腎俞乃致命之所，皆不可灼艾。
伍氏曰：凡用蒜餅灸者，蓋蒜味辛溫有毒，主散癰疽，假火勢以行藥力也。有只用艾炷灸者，此可施於頑疽瘤發之類，凡赤腫紫黑毒甚者，

---

2   Next Zhang repeats the "moxibustion on garlic method for abscesses" that was in the *Illustrated Supplement to the Categorized Classic*, **LJTY: 11-3-23**, translated p. 168.

3   In other words, use as many cones as it takes to remove the evil. The evil will not get amnesty if it is able to survive a specific prescribed number of cones.

須以蒜艾同灸為妙。又曰：凡治疽，癰，發背，疔瘡，
若初灸即痛者，由毒氣輕淺，灸而不痛者，乃毒氣深重，
悉宜內服追毒排膿，外傳消毒之藥。
大抵癰疽不可不痛，又不可大痛悶亂。不知痛者難治。
又曰：凡隔蒜灸者，不論壯數，
則邪無所容而真氣不損。但頭項見瘡，宜用騎竹馬法，
及足三里灸之。

Thousand Pieces of Gold says: When abscesses start to develop, some are quite painful. Some have little pain. Some erupt like a grain of rice, meaning they exude pus. It is appropriate to quickly abstain from flavorful food and disinhibit and remove the toxins. Use Ride the Bamboo Horse moxibustion or burn mugwort near the affected site. If it is severe, apply a total of 100 or 200 cones of moxibustion in the center of each of the four sides. Further, use the external application of medicinals. The effect is very fast.[4]

《千金》云：癰疽始作，或大痛，或小痛，
或發如米粒，即便出膿，宜急斷口味，利去其毒，
用騎竹馬灸法，或就患處灼艾，
重者四面中央總灸一二百壯，更用敷藥，其效甚速。

Xue Lizhai said:[5] Now, in patterns of sores "what is in the center must appear on the outside." Lead and draw out sores that are located on the exterior. Course and descend those located in the interior. The merits of burning mugwort are very great. If toxic qi is depressed and bound up and static blood congeals and stagnates, when it is mild, it can perhaps be scattered with medicinals. If it is severe, medicinals do not have perfect results.

Li Dongyuan said: If acupuncture and cautery is not used, the toxic qi lacks something to follow in order to be resolved. That is why someone who is good at treating toxins must use moxibustion on garlic. Perhaps you can reject this and use the likes of bitter cold prescriptions that vanquish toxins on those with vigorous repletion and internal heat. Those who are timid and weak with qi vacuity are always defeated with this type of prescription. There is also toxic qi that is deep and hidden. Some people are advanced in years and their qi is weak. Some have taken a prescription that restrains and attacks [implying an improper prescription]. In these cases, the qi becomes more vacuous. Because the pus has not ulcerated, you must rely on the power of fire in order to achieve results. Generally speaking, if the sore has not ulcerated, steaming or moxibustion draws and leads out depressed toxins. When it has already ulcerated, steaming or moxibustion joins and supplements yang qi, and dispels and scatters cold evils. The opening of the sore will spontaneously close. The results are very great.

I have treated sores on the four limbs when qi and blood was insufficient and only used the previous method of applying moxibustion to it. All have recovered. Only moxibustion is appropriate for severe clove sore toxins. Heat toxins seem to make a partition in the middle so the interior and exterior do not communicate. If you do not effuse and discharge them, they will not resolve and scatter. If the place where the patient lives is impoverished or the residence is out of the way [not near herb stores], sometimes there may be no medicinals. In that case, using moxibustion on garlic is especially convenient. Change the slice of garlic every three cones. The general guideline is to use 100 cones. Use garlic for its acrid flavor and ability to scatter. Use the mugwort cones for the power of fire which is able to thrust outward. If you apply this method of moxibustion to them, the sores will exude pus and open up. Then apply Shen Yi Gao [Miraculous Paste] to them. They will spontaneously recover in less than a day. One, it is able to prevent the sore from opening big. Two, the interior flesh does not spoil. Three, the sore is easy to close. Its effectiveness is very miraculous.

---

[4] This is paraphrased quite a bit from *Prescriptions Worth a Thousand Pieces of Gold*, Volume 22, Chapter 2 on abscesses (Sun 1994, a310). Of course Sun did not mention the Ride the Bamboo Horse technique, as that was developed after his time.

[5] In this whole long section, Zhang is quoting Xue Lizhai.

Zhu Danxi said: The head is the only place where all yang gathers, so it is appropriate to apply just a few small cones.

Official Cao already had eruptions on his back for 18 days. The head of the sores was the size of a grain of millet. The inside of the sore was like an awl. The pain was extreme. Sometimes there was chest oppression and visual distortion. He had no thought of food or drink, so his qi became more vacuous. More than 10 big cones of mugwort moxibustion were applied on garlic. He still did not feel it and the pain was not eliminated. Following that, more than 20 cones of direct moxibustion were applied. The inside of the sore was completely removed. Lots of toxic qi came out. He gradually began eating and drinking. Further, he used strong medicinals to supplement and also burned mulberry wood moxibustion. The stasis in the flesh gradually ulcerated.

Liu Guanqing had already suffered clove sores on his feet for 11 days. His qi was weak. More than 50 cones of moxibustion were applied. Further, he used internal expulsion medicinals and recovered.

Huang Jun had leg abscesses. The pus was green and his pulse was weak. A woman's arm had a bound up lump, already ulcerated. In both cases, the sore did not close. Moxibustion on Dou Chi [Semen Praeparatum Sojae] cakes was applied to both of them. They also drank internal expulsion medicinals and recovered.

A male had a swelling on his chest. It did not disperse for half a year. One hundred cones of direct moxibustion were applied and then it ulcerated. He also took strong medicinals for supplementation, but it did not close. Moxibustion was applied again using Fu Zi [Radix Lateralis Praeparatae Aconiti] cakes and he recovered.

A male suffered eruptions on his back. There were quite a lot of sores with heads. The swellings were hard and purple. It was not extremely painful. Nor was it putrid or ulcerating. Mugwort was spread on the af-

fected sites and moxibustion was applied. Further, he used strong medicinals to supplement. After a few days, the dead flesh sloughed off and he recovered.

Official Chen had already suffered eruptions on his back for four or five days. Although the head of the sore was small, the root was recalcitrant and quite large. More than 30 cones of moxibustion on garlic were applied. The root dispersed internally. Only the head of the sore made pus. After a few days, he recovered.

In a bing zi year, I was suddenly nauseated. The Da Zhui [Du 14] bone [C 7] itched a lot. In a short while, I was unable to lift my arm. My spirit was very fatigued. This was a perished flat abscess, a critical disease. I quickly applied moxibustion on garlic to it. The itching was more severe. Again, I applied more than 50 cones of direct moxibustion. The itching then stopped. I recovered in ten days. *Essentials [Jing Yao]* says: Moxibustion has the merit of being able to return life. This is true. (Xue's Notes)

立齋云: 夫瘡瘍之證, 有諸中必形諸外,
在外者引而拔之, 在內者疏而下之。灼艾之功甚大,
若毒氣鬱結, 瘀血凝滯, 輕者或可藥散,
重者藥無全功矣。東垣曰: 若不鍼烙, 則毒氣無從而解,
是故善治毒者, 必用隔蒜灸, 舍是而用苦寒敗毒等劑,
其壯實內熱者或可, 彼怯弱氣虛者,
未有不敗者也。又有毒氣沉伏, 或年高氣弱,
或服剋伐之劑, 氣益?以虛, 膿因不潰者,
必假火力以成功。大凡蒸灸, 若未潰則拔引鬱毒,
已潰則接補陽氣, 祛散寒邪, 瘡口自合,
其功甚大。嘗治四肢瘡瘍, 氣血不足者,
祇以前法灸之皆愈。疔毒甚者尤宜灸, 蓋熱毒中隔,
內外不通, 不發泄則不解散。若處貧居僻, 一時無藥,
則用隔蒜灸法尤便。每三壯一易蒜片,
大概以百壯為度。用大蒜取其辛而能散,
用艾炷取其火力能透, 如法灸之, 必瘡發膿潰,
繼以神異膏貼之, 不日自愈。一能使瘡不開大,
二內肉不壞, 三瘡口易合, 見效甚神。丹溪云:
惟頭為諸陽所聚, 艾炷宜小而少。曹工部發背已十八日,
瘡頭如粟, 瘡內如錐, 痛極, 時有悶瞀, 飲食不思,
氣則愈虛。以大艾隔蒜灸十餘壯, 尚不知而痛不減,
遂明灸二十餘壯, 內瘡悉去, 毒氣大發,
飲食漸進。更以大補藥, 及桑木燃灸,

瘀肉漸潰。劉貫卿足患疔瘡已十一日，氣弱，
亦灸五十餘壯，更以托裏藥而愈。黃君腿癰，膿清脈弱；
一婦臂一塊，已潰，俱不收斂，各灸以豆豉餅，
更飲托裏藥而愈。一男子胸腫一塊，半載不消，
令明灸百壯方潰，與大補藥不斂，
復灸以附子餅而愈。一男子患發背，瘡頭甚多，
腫硬色紫，不甚痛，不腐潰，以艾鋪患處灸之，
更以大補藥，數日，
死肉脫去而愈。陳工部患發背已四五日，瘡頭雖小，
根畔頗大，以隔蒜灸三十餘壯，其根內消，惟瘡頭作膿，
數日而愈。余丙子年，忽惡心，大椎骨甚癢，
須臾臂不能舉，神思甚倦，此夭疽，
危病也。急隔蒜灸之，癢愈甚，又明灸五十餘壯，
癢遂止，旬日而愈。《精要》云：灸法有回生之功，
信矣。薛按

Master Shi's Supporting Evidence says: Specialists in sores and wounds often use instruments to operate on them. In a jia xu year, I examined the mother of Master Shi, and said: Inside there is an amassment of heat. Guard against it becoming an abscess. In the sixth month of the xin si [year, seven years later], as anticipated, her back and shoulder blade itched slightly and a sore developed the size of a grain of millet. Moxibustion was burned and it promptly dispersed. After a night, she relapsed and used a plaster to cover it. A halo opened around it for about six *cun* and the pain was unbearable. The woman blamed it on mugwort.

By chance, I met a monk who said, "The disease of sores is very critical. Once, I applied more than 800 cones of moxibustion before recovery." In the end, I used big mugwort cones the size of ginkgo nuts to apply moxibustion to the head of the sore as well as the four sides, a few cones in each place. The pain stopped. When more than 30 cones were reached, the red halo had completely retreated. I also used mugwort to make 40 cones shaped like balls, the size of plums or apricots, and then the patient ate por-

ridge and rested quietly. The sores protruded four *cun*, with about 100 small openings. The affected flesh all spoiled and then the patient recovered.[6]

史氏引證曰：瘍醫常器之，於甲戌年診太學史氏之母，
云：內有蓄熱，防其作疽。至辛巳六月，果背胛微癢，
瘡粒如黍，灼艾即消。隔宿復作，用膏藥覆之，
暈開六寸許，痛不可勝，歸咎於艾。適遇一僧自云：
病瘡甚危，嘗灸八百餘壯方甦。 遂用大艾壯如銀杏者，
灸瘡頭及四傍各數壯，痛止，至三十餘壯，赤暈悉退，
又以艾作團如梅杏大者四十壯，乃食粥安寢，瘡突四寸，
小竅百許，患肉俱壞而愈。

Li Zhai said: In the method of burning mugwort, moxibustion must be applied on a patient with painful sores until there is no pain. When there is no pain, apply moxibustion until there is pain so that the toxins follow the fire and scatter. Otherwise, not only is there no advantage, but on the contrary, it harms the patient.

My [Zhang's] humble idea is that all abscesses, when they cause suffering, are due to congested blood and stagnant qi. This is because the qi and blood lingers, bound up, unmoving. Overall, great bindings and great stagnation are the most difficult to scatter. You must desire to scatter them. If you do not borrow the power of fire, you are unable to scatter them quickly, so it is quite appropriate to use moxibustion. Thus, there is also *Daoist Immortal Sun's Fumigation Formula*.[7] This method is particularly essential, particularly wonderful. When toxic evils are somewhat chronic, the evil is deep, or the channel is distant, [right] qi cannot extend to it, so applying moxibustion to it is good. When toxic evils blaze exuberantly, the condition is a fierce disease and the patient falls into danger. It is appropriate to use the fumigation formula, which is superior to moxibustion in cases like this.[8]

---

[8] It is obvious that Zhang thought moxibustion on garlic was the best treatment for abscesses and sores. He writes extensively on it here, and also in **LJTY: 11-3-23**, p. 168, **JYQS: 49-229**, p. 112, **JYQS: 63-117**, p. 113, and **JYQS: 64-115**, p. 113.
   This section also has some interesting insights into the mechanism of moxibustion, which will be discussed in the Conclusion of this book.

立齋曰：灼艾之法，必使痛者灸至不痛，
不痛者灸至痛，則毒必隨火而散，
否則非徒無益而反害之。愚意癰疽為患，
無非血氣壅滯，留結不行之所致。凡人結大滯者，
最不易散，必欲散之，非藉火力不能速也，
所極宜用灸。然又有孫道人神仙熏照方，其法尤精尤
妙。若毒邪稍緩，邪深經遠而氣有不達，灸之為良；
若毒邪熾盛，其勢猛疾而亟危者，則宜用熏照方，
更勝於灸也。

JYQS: 11-1-15 Wind Stroke, Moxibustion (Zhang 1995, 233) [abridged]
《景岳全書・非風・灸法・卷之十一》

Overall, you must use moxibustion for fulminant de-sertion of original yang as well as for unregulated construction and defense of blood and qi. If you want to receive quick efficacy, only mugwort fire is good. But, using the method of fire is only appropri-ate for yang vacuity, lots of cold, or congealed and stagnant channels and vessels. When there are symptoms such as exuberant fire, debilitated metal, depleted water, lots of dryness, rapid pulse, fever, dry throat, red face, thirst, and hot defecation or urina-tion, you cannot rashly add mugwort fire. If you mistakenly use it, it will result in the blood becom-ing dryer and the heat becoming more severe. This, on the contrary, quickens the peril.

Moxibustion for critical patterns such as windstroke or fulminant reversal: ... Dan Tian [Cinnabar Field] and Qi Hai [Ren 6]: Both these points connect to life gate. They really are the sea of living qi and the root of the channels and vessels. Applying moxibustion to both of these points is very efficacious.[9]

凡用灸法，必其元陽暴脫，及營衛血氣不調，
欲收速效，惟艾火為良。然用火之法，惟陽虛多寒，
經絡凝滯者為宜。若火盛金衰，水虧多燥，
脈數發熱，咽乾面赤，口渴便熱等證，
則不可妄加艾火。若誤用之，必致血愈燥而熱愈甚，
是反速其危矣… …灸非風卒厥危急等證： …

…丹田，氣海：二穴俱連命門，實為生氣之海，
經脈之本，灸之皆有大效。… …

JYQS: 19-3-7 Hiccough, Moxibustion (Zhang 1995, 436)
《景岳全書・呃逆・灸法・卷之十九》

The two breast points treat hiccoughs which will im-mediately stop.

Method to find the point: On a female, the point is where the nipple reaches as it hangs down. Since males cannot hang down, use one finger below the nipple as the guideline. The point is directly below the nipple, in the depression between the bones [in-tercostal space]. Apply moxibustion unilaterally to the left on males, and to the right on females, using mugwort cones the size of a small grain of wheat. When the fire touches, the hiccoughs will promptly stop. Apply three cones of moxibustion. If they do not stop, they cannot be treated.

Dan Zhong [Ren 17], Zhong Wan [Ren 12], Qi Hai [Ren 6], San Li [ST 36].

兩乳穴，治呃逆立止。取穴法：
婦人以乳頭垂下到處是穴。男子不可垂者，
以乳頭下一指為率，與乳頭相直，骨間陷中是穴。男左，
女右，灸一處。艾炷如小麥大，著火即止，灸三壯，
不止者不可治。膻中，中脘，氣海，三里。

JYQS: 22-1-8 Swelling & Distention, Acupuncture & Moxibustion (Zhang 1995, 500)
《景岳全書・腫脹・針灸法・卷之二十二》

Pi Shu [UB 20] (treats distention. Apply moxibustion to it. The number of cones is based on the years of age), Gan Shu [UB 18] (treats distention. Apply 100 cones of moxibustion), San Jiao Shu [UB 22] (treats distention and swelling of the heart region and ab-domen with reduced food intake, inhibited urina-

---

[9] For Zhang's treatment of wind stroke, see also **LJTY: 11-3-1**, p. 141.

tion, marked emaciation, shortage of qi), Shui Fen [Ren 9] (treats abdominal distention winding around the umbilicus with binding pain and inability to eat. If it is water disease [edema], only moxibustion is appropriate), Shen Que [Ren 8] (governs water swelling, drum distention, rumbling intestines like the sound of water. It is extremely effective), Shi Men [Ren 5] (governs water swelling and water moving in the skin, yellow urination), Zu San Li [ST 36] (governs water swelling and abdominal distention), Shui Gou [Du 26] (governs all water swelling).

Note that water swelling patterns should only be needled at Shui Gou [Du 26]. If the rest of the points are needled, the water will become severe and the patient will promptly die. This warning came from the *Bright Hall* and the *Bronze Man*. A vulgar healer often needles Shui Fen [Ren 9]. Many people make this mistake. If by chance someone obtains a cure by needling other points, he is unusually fortunate and that is all. Generally, acupuncture is contraindicated for water swelling; you cannot perform this method.[10]

脾俞治脹，隨年壯灸之。　肝俞治脹，灸百壯。
三焦俞治心腹脹滿，飲食減少，小便不利，羸瘦少氣。
分水治腹脹繞臍結痛，不能食。　若是水病，尤宜灸之。
神闕主水腫臌脹，腸鳴如水之聲，極效。
石門主水腫水行皮中，小便黃。　足三里主水腫腹脹。
水溝主一切水腫。按水腫證惟針水溝，若針餘穴，
水盡即死，此《明堂》《銅人》所戒也。
庸醫多為人針分水，
誤人多矣。若其他穴，或有因針得瘥者，特幸焉耳。大
抵水腫禁針，不可為法。

JYQS: 23-1-5 Accumulations & Gatherings, Acupuncture & Moxibustion (Zhang 1995, 510) [abridged]
《景岳全書・積聚・針灸法・卷之二十三》

If an accumulation glomus is located in the upper body, it is appropriate to apply moxibustion to points such as Shang Wan [Ren 13], Zhong Wan [Ren 12], Qi Men [LV 14], and Zhang Men [LV 13]. If an accumulation lump is located in the lower body, it is appropriate to apply moxibustion to points such as Tian Shu [ST 25], Zhang Men [LV 13], Shen Shu [UB 23], Qi Hai [Ren 6], Guan Yuan [Ren 4], Zhong Ji [Ren 3], and Shui Dao [ST 28].

The general method for moxibustion: It is appropriate to first apply moxibustion above and then below. It is appropriate that cones used in the umbilical region are a little larger. For all, first apply 7 or 14 cones of moxibustion. Afterwards, gradually increase it each time. The more moxibustion, the more wonderful it is.

All the above points are able to treat glomus. Select the appropriate ones and use them. However, sometimes you cannot treat this based on points; for example [sometimes you must use] the hardest place of the glomus, or the head, or the tail, or the protrusion, or the moving place. In any case, look for the source of the vessels and network vessels. You should apply moxibustion based on all these sites. When the power of fire arrives, the qi of the hard gathering will gradually resolve and scatter naturally. It has the wonder of miraculous transformation.

However, in the method of applying moxibustion to the glomus, one treatment will not be effective in a short time. You must select what is essential, either this or that, and repeatedly apply moxibustion to it in succession. There is no one who does not recover.[11]

積痞在上者，宜灸：上脘，中脘，期門，
章門之類。積塊在下者，宜灸：天樞，章門，腎俞，
氣海，關元，中極，水道之類。凡灸之法，
宜先上而後下，臍腹之壯用宜稍大，皆先灸七壯，
或十四壯，以後漸次增加，
愈多愈妙。以上諸穴皆能治痞，
宜擇而用之。然猶有不可按穴者，如痞之最堅處，
或頭，或尾，或突，或動處，但察其脈絡所由者，
皆當按其處而通灸之，火力所到，

---

[10] For Zhang's treatment of swelling and drum distention, see also **LJTY: 11-3-6**, p. 147.
[11] For Zhang's treatment of accumulations and gatherings, see also **LJTY: 11-3-7**, p.148.

則其堅聚之氣自然以漸解散，
有神化之妙也。第灸痞之法，非一次便能必效，
務須或彼或此，擇其要者，至再至三，
連次陸續灸之，無有不愈者。

JYQS: 25-2-4 Pain of the Rib-sides, Moxibustion (Zhang 1995, 563)
《景岳全書・脅痛・灸法・卷之二十五》

To treat sudden unendurable pain of the rib-sides, use a waxed string horizontally to measure the distance between the two nipples. Bend the string in half. From the breast run it obliquely down the painful rib-side. Apply 30 cones of moxibustion to the site at the end of the string. Furthermore, apply moxibustion to Zhang Men [LV 13] (seven cones) and Qiu Xiu [GB 40] (three cones. You can needle, entering five *fen*).

治卒脅痛不可忍者，用蠟繩橫度兩乳中，半屈繩，
從乳斜趨處痛脅下，繩盡處灸三十壯，更灸章門七壯，
丘墟三壯，可鍼入五分。

JYQS: 27-1-5 Eyes, Acupuncture & Moxibustion (Zhang 1995, 600)
《景岳全書・眼目・針灸法・卷之二十七》

Qing Ming [UB 1], Feng Chi [GB 20], Tai Yang [Supreme Yang, non-channel], Shen Ting [Du 24], Shang Xing [Du 23], Xin Hui [Du 22], Bai Hui [Du 20], Qian Ding [Du 21], Zan Zhu [UB 2], Si Zhu Cong [SJ 23], Cheng Qi [ST 1], Mu Chuang [GB 16], Ke Zhu Ren [GB 3], and Cheng Guang [UB 6]. Use all the above points. All can be needled, or use a three-edged needle to bleed. Generally, all points near the eyes are contraindicated for moxibustion.

Da Gu Kong [Thumb Bone Hollow, non-channel]: The point is located on the tip of the second joint of the thumb. Apply nine cones of moxibustion. Use the mouth to blow the fire out.

Xiao Gu Kong [Little Finger Bone Hollow, non-channel]: The point is located on the tip of the second joint of the little finger. Apply seven cones of moxibustion. Use the mouth to blow the fire out.

The above two points are able to treat patterns such as tearing when exposed to wind cold and wind eye with ulceration on the rim of the eyelid.

He Gu [LI 4]: Treats yang brightness heat depression and red swollen eye screens or tearing on exposure to wind. Apply seven cones of moxibustion. It is often appropriate to apply moxibustion to this point for eye disease. It will never relapse. It can also be needled.

Yi Feng [SJ 17]: Apply seven cones of moxibustion. It treats red and white screen membranes and eyes that are not bright.

Gan Shu [UB 18]: Apply seven cones of moxibustion. It treats liver wind visiting heat, tearing on exposure to wind, and sparrow vision [night-blindness].

Zu San Li [ST 36]: Applying moxibustion to it can make fire qi descend to brighten the eyes.[12]

Er Jian [LI 2]: Moxibustion.

Ming Men [Du 4]: Moxibustion.

Shui Gou [Du 26]: Can be needled, moxibustion can be applied to it. It treats forward-staring eyes.

Shou San Li [LI 10]: If the right is affected, apply moxibustion to the left. If the left is affected, apply moxibustion to the right.

Great Pricking of the Eight Passes: Treats unendurable eye pain with desire to take them out. To

---

[12] Moxibustion on ST 36 for the eyes was recommended by Wang Tao and Sun Simiao. This is also discussed in **LJTY: 4-27-4** and **LJTY: 6-3-36**, above.

recover, you must prick to cause bleeding at the 10 finger seams.

睛明，風池，太陽，神庭，上星，囟會，百會，前頂，
攢竹，絲竹空，承泣，目窗，客主人，承光。以上諸穴，
皆可用鍼，或以三稜鍼出血。凡近目之穴，
皆禁灸。大骨空穴在手大指第二節尖。灸九壯，
以口吹火滅。小骨空穴在手小指第二節尖。灸七壯，
以口吹火滅。上二穴能治迎風冷淚，
風眼爛弦等證。合谷治陽明熱鬱，赤腫翳障，
或迎風流淚。灸七壯。大抵目疾多宜灸此，水不再發也，
亦可鍼。 翳風灸壯。治赤白翳膜，
目不明。肝俞灸七壯。 治肝風客熱，迎風流淚，
雀目。足三里灸之可令火氣下降明目。二間灸。命門灸
。水溝可鍼可灸。治目睛直視。手三里灸，右取左，
左取右。八關大刺治眼痛欲出，
不可忍者。須刺十指縫中出血愈。

JYQS: 28-3-6 Teeth, Acupuncture & Moxibustion (Zhang 1995, 630) [abridged]
《景岳全書・齒牙・針灸法・卷之二十八》

A method to treat all toothaches: Use a piece of straw to measure from the tip of the middle finger to the horizontal line proximal to the palm [the wrist crease]. Take the straw and break it into quarters. Remove three and keep one. Use it to measure the center of the arm proximal to the horizontal line [wrist crease]. Apply three cones of moxibustion to the left or right according to the pain. The patient will promptly recover.

Item: A treatment from experience: In front of the ear inside the tip of the hair on the temples,[13] there is the site of a moving pulse. Apply five times seven small mugwort cones of moxibustion to the left or right according to the pain. It is miraculously effective. In addition, you must not apply a plaster. If the toothache occurs again, apply moxibustion again. You can promptly sever the root of the pain.

一法治一切牙痛：以草量手中指，至掌後橫紋止，
將草折作四分，去三留一，於橫紋後量臂中，
隨痛左右灸三壯，即愈。一，經驗法：
於耳前鬢髮尖內有動脈處，隨痛左右用小艾炷灸五七壯，
神效。亦不必貼膏藥。如再發，再灸，即可斷根。

JYQS: 32-1-8 Leg Qi, Acupuncture & Moxibustion (Zhang 1995, 705)
《景岳全書・腳氣・針灸・卷之三十二》

Whenever leg qi is initially perceived, promptly apply 20 or 30 cones of moxibustion to the affected site, or use the thunder fire needle [translated above, p. 130-1] in order to conduct damp qi out through the exterior. In addition, drink unstrained sweet wine [*laoli*] in order to free the channels and scatter the evils. This is an important method.

If congestion has already developed and the evil is exuberant, there will be extreme swelling, pain, and heat. If medicinals cannot scatter it in a short time, it is appropriate to use a healing stone to remove malign blood in order to disperse the heat and swelling. After pricking with the healing stone, follow it with medicinals.[14]

凡腳氣初覺，即灸患處二三十壯，
或用雷火鍼以導引濕氣外出，及飲醪醴以通經散邪，
其要法也。若壅既成而邪盛者，必腫痛熱甚，
一時藥餌難散，宜砭去惡血，以消熱腫，砭刺之後，
以藥繼之。

JYQS: 35-2-15 Moxibustion for Gu Toxins (Zhang 1995, 773)
《景岳全書・諸毒・灸蠱毒法・卷之三十五》

Overall, to apply moxibustion to treat all gu toxins: Apply three cones of moxibustion to the tips of both little toes. Something will promptly come out. For wine stroke, it will come out along with wine. If it

---

[13] "The tip of the hair on the temples" is the inferior end of the sideburns. This may be harder to find on Caucasian males, as their sideburns blend into their beard.
[14] Leg qi is also discussed in **LJTY: 11-3-18**, p. 159.

was in drink and food, it will come out with drink and food. It is proven repeatedly.[15]

凡灸一切蠱毒，於兩足小指盡處，各灸三壯，
即有物出。酒中者，隨酒出，飲食中者，隨飲食出，
屢驗。

JYQS: 60-239 Rabid Dog Bite (239) (Zhang 1995, 1620) [abridged]
《景岳全書 • 瘋犬傷人二三九 • 卷之六十》

A formula: Pull out red hair from the vertex. Quickly make the person suck out the malign blood. Use five times seven cones of mugwort moxibustion at the site of the bite. If severe, apply 100 cones of moxibustion. It is miraculously effective.[16]

一方：拔去頂上紅髮，急令人吮去惡血，
以艾灸傷處五七壯，甚者灸百壯，神效。

JYQS: 60-243 Moxibustion for all Dog & Insect Bites[17] (243) (Zhang 1995, 1621)
《景岳全書 • 諸犬咬蟲傷灸法二四三 • 卷之六十》

Generally, the pain is extreme and the condition is critical from all wolf, dog, snake, scorpion, or centipede bites. Some contract wind from the bite and suffer clenched jaw, arched rigidity of the lumbar and back, and loss of consciousness. Quickly cut garlic slices or pound garlic into a pulp and cover the site of the bite. Apply moxibustion on garlic, maybe 20 or 30 cones, maybe 40 or 50 cones. Everyone recovers smoothly. Applying treatment like this is very effective.

Thus, the *Materia Medica* says garlic cures sore toxins and has the effect of returning life. Now, even though accumulations in the intestines and stomach

are difficult to cure, compare it to when the four limbs are affected; since the severed channels and network vessels are far away, medicinals do not easily reach them. That is why the ancients had methods such as soaks, washes, moxibustion, and pricking — precisely because they free the channels, expel evils, and conduct qi and blood.

凡狼犬蛇蝎蜈蚣諸傷痛極危急，
或因傷受風而牙關緊急，腰背反脹，不省人事者，
速切蒜片或搗爛罨傷處，隔蒜灸之，或二三十壯，
或四五十壯，無不應手而愈，取效多矣，
故《本草》謂蒜療瘡毒，有回生之功。夫積在腸胃，
尚為難療，況四肢受患，則經絡遠絕，藥不易及，
故古人有淋洗灸刺等法，正為通經逐邪，
導引氣血而設也。

JYQS: 60-278 Formula for Cold Stroke Abdominal Pain after Sexual Activity (278) (Zhang 1995, 1627)
《景岳全書 • 事後中寒腹痛方二七八 • 卷之六十》

Overall, a person with cold stroke and reversal cold after sexual activity who has nausea, vomiting, and abdominal pain can take scallion and ginger pounded to a pulp and drenched in hot wine. Then, they should sleep for a little while. They will sweat and then promptly recover. If abdominal pain is severe, use scallion whites pounded to a pulp. Spread them on the umbilicus. Apply mugwort moxibustion on them, or they can also be ironed. When the tip of the nose sweats, all the pain will promptly stop.

凡房事後中寒厥冷，嘔噁腹痛者，用蔥，
薑搗爛衝熱酒服之，睡少頃。
出汗即愈。如腹痛甚者，以蔥白頭搗爛攤臍上，
以艾灸之或熨之亦可解。得鼻尖有汗，其痛痛即止。

---

[15] In other words, there will be vomiting of wine, food, or drink, depending on the situation and something, probably resembling worms, will come out with the vomitus. For gu toxins, see also **LJTY: 11-3-24**, p. 175.

[16] I am unable to find an earlier source for this. It is unclear if the red hair is growing out of the dog's or the victim's head. However, if the dog is rabid, it is not safe to approach it, and in any case, it may have run off. Therefore, I surmise it is on the victim's head. Since head hair is the surplus of the blood, perhaps the hair was thought to manifest a red color when such potent toxins entered the blood. Of course, red hair is unusual on a Chinese person. For dog bites, see also **LJTY: 11-3-24**, p. 175.

[17] For dog and insect bites, see also **LJTY: 11-3-24**, p. 175.

JYQS: 61-66 Moxibustion to Terminate Childbirth (66) (Zhang 1995, 1646)
《景岳全書・斷產灸法六六・卷之六十一》

A formula that has been passed on: If you desire to sever childbirth forever, apply three cones of moxibustion 2.3 *cun* below the umbilicus on the yin pulsating vessel. Regard the area from the center of the umbilicus to the border of the pubic bone as broken into five equal *cun*.[18]

一傳方欲絕產者，
灸臍下二寸三分陰動脈中三壯。此當自臍中至骨際折作五寸約之。

JYQS: 64-265 Moxibustion for Lockjaw (265) (Zhang 1995, 1778)
《景岳全書・破傷風灸法二六五・卷之六十四》

Treats knocks and falls or insect and animal wounds breaking the skin resulting in wind evils entering inside, clenched jaw, arched back rigidity, or hemilateral numbness. There is unconsciousness if it is severe. Quickly pound garlic into a pulp and apply it to the site of the damage. Place mugwort cones on the garlic and apply moxibustion to it. A lot of moxibustion is good. Further, apply a plaster to protect it and take Yu Zhen San [Jade True Powder] internally. If it is a venomous snake or a rabid dog bite, first prick the affected site to let out the toxic blood. Then treat it using the previous method.

治跌打損傷，或蟲獸傷破皮膚，以致風邪入內，
牙關緊急，要背反張，或遍體麻木，
甚者不知人事。急用蒜搗爛塗傷處，
將艾壯於蒜上灸之，多灸為善，仍用膏藥護貼，
內服玉真散。如毒蛇瘋犬咬傷，先刺患處去毒血，
如前法治之。

JYQS: 60-237 Snake Venom (237) (Zhang 1995, 1619) [abridged]
《景岳全書・蛇毒二三七・卷之六十》

Item: Whenever snakes enter the seven orifices, quickly use mugwort moxibustion on the snake's tail.[19]

Another treatment: Use a knife to break the snake's tail open a little bit. Insert a number of grains of Chuan Jiao [Pericarpium Zanthoxyli] and use paper to seal it. The snake will spontaneously exit. Promptly use Xiong Huang [Realgar] and Zhu Sha [Cinnabar] powder and brew Ren Shen Tang [Ginseng Decoction]. Mix them and pour them on, or eat garlic and drink wine. The inner toxins will promptly resolve.

Item: For snake bite, people who reside in the mountains quickly use urine to wash the site of the bite. They wipe it dry and apply mugwort moxibustion to it. It is immediately effective.

Another formula: Cut a head of garlic into slices and place them on the affected site. Apply mugwort moxibustion on the garlic. Change the garlic every three cones. A lot of moxibustion is wonderful. Overall, it is effective for all venomous snake bites.

一，凡蛇入七竅，
急以艾灸蛇尾。又法以刀破蛇尾少許，入川椒數粒，
以紙封之，蛇自出。即用雄黃，
朱砂末煎人參湯調灌之，或食蒜飲酒，
內毒即解。一，山居人被蛇傷，急用溺洗咬處，
拭乾，以艾灸之立效。又方：
用獨頭大蒜切片置患處，以艾於蒜上灸之，
每三壯換蒜，多灸為妙，凡被毒蛇所傷皆效。

---

[18] This point is 0.3 *cun* below Shi Men Ren 5, which is said to cause infertility in many old books, going as far back as the *Systematic Classic*. See also **LJTY: 11-3-21**, p. 164.

[19] Moxibustion on the snake's tail was recommended for the distressing problem of "snakes entering into a person's mouth and not exiting" by Chen Yangzhi in *Short Sketches* (Chen 1993, 160). While that book has been lost, this passage was quoted in *Emergency Prescriptions to Keep Up Your Sleeve*, Volume 7, by Ge Hong (Ge 1996, 220). For snake bites, see also **LJTY: 11-3-24**, p. 175.

JYQS: 60-279 Damp Mounting Testicular Pain (279) (Zhang 1995, 1627)
《景岳全書・濕疝陰丸作痛二七九・卷之六十》

Qi mugwort, Zi Su Ye [Folium Perillae] (bake with dry heat), Chuan Jiao [Pericarpium Zanthoxyli] (stir-fried hot, each three *liang*). Mix the above three medicinals evenly. When they are hot, use a pouch to hold them and wedge it around the scrotum. Do not let the qi run away. When it gets cold, promptly change it.[20]

蘄艾、紫蘇葉烘乾熱、川椒炒熱，各三兩。右三味，拌勻，乘熱用絹袋盛夾襄下，勿令走氣，冷即易之。

YANG JIZHOU ON TREATMENT OF SOME SPECIFIC CONDITIONS

ZJDC: 9-12 through 9-17, plus 9-21 and 9-30 discuss the treatment of a few conditions: heart qi, hemorrhoids, mounting, diarrhea, and chills and fever. ZJDC: 9-21 is a discussion of preventive moxibustion.

ZJDC: 9-12 Method to Apply Moxibustion for Heart Qi (what follows is all gathered by Master Yang)[21] (Huang 1996, 989)
《針灸大成・取灸心氣法（以下俱楊氏集）・卷之九・卷之九》

First, take a long straw. Compare it to the left hand on males and the right on females. Begin measuring at the horizontal crease at the root of the thumb on the palmar side. Stop at the inside of the nail. Use ink to mark the spot on the straw. Next, compare the index finger, middle finger, ring finger, and lit-

tle finger: compare all five fingers using the previous method. [Each time, adding the length of the finger on the same piece of straw.] Also, mark one additional body-*cun*.[22] Use another stalk of straw and make it the same length as the straw that was measured before, up to the added one *cun* ink mark. Tie them together in a knot. Then make the patient sit straight and remove his clothing. Open and separate the straws and put them on the patient's neck. Use a finger to firmly press the knot onto the bone at Tian Tu [Ren 22]. Let them hang down behind on both sides of the back. Make the two straws even. The site where the ends hang down on the spine is the point. Apply seven cones of moxibustion. It is effective.

先將長草一條，比男左女右手，掌內大拇指根，橫紋量起，至甲內止，以墨點記。次比鹽指，中指，四指，小指，五指皆比如前法。再加同身寸一寸點定，別用稈草一條，與前所量草般齊，至再加一寸墨上，共結一磊。卻令病人正坐，脫去衣，以草分開，加於頸上，以指按定，磊於天突骨上，兩邊垂向背後，以兩條草取般齊，垂下脊中盡處是穴，灸七壯效。

ZJDC: 9-13 Method to Apply Moxibustion for Hemorrhoids & Fistulas (Huang 1996, 989)
《針灸大成・取灸痔漏法・卷之九》

For hemorrhoids and fistulas that have not been there for long, only applying moxibustion to Chang Qiang [Du 1] is very effective. If it has lasted for years, you can use a handful of Huai Zhi [Ramulus Sophorae Japonicae] and Ma Lan Cai Gen [Radix Kalimeris]. Decoct them in three cups of water. Use 1.5 cups in a small-mouth bottle to steam-wash [the affected area] in order to take advantage of its heat. Make the swelling abate. Apply moxibustion to the base of the "mouse breast." Applying moxibustion

---

[20] "Do not let the qi run away" probably means to hold the legs shut around the pouch so the hot acrid qi of the medicinals does not escape.

[21] This note that says the sections that follow were gathered by Master Yang or his family. Huang (2000, 989) tells us that the original does not have this annotation. Some later editor must have added it. However, this section is almost identical to the corresponding one in Xu Feng's *Great Completion* (Huang 1996, 541).

[22] Perhaps the extra body-*cun* added to the straw at the end of the measuring process is to compensate for the length used to make the knot.

to the tip is not effective. Some use a basin of medicinal water to wash it. The swelling will abate slightly. Then they apply moxibustion to it. When the patient perceives a ball of fire qi pass through, entering into the intestines and radiating to the chest, it will be effective. Apply more than 20 cones of moxibustion. In addition, the patient should avoid toxic things in order to permanently recover. At the same time, use slices of bamboo to protect the good flesh on the two sides from the fire qi. Do not damage it.[23]

痔疾未深，止灸長強甚效。如年深者，可用槐枝，馬藍菜根一握，煎湯取水三碗，用一碗半，乘熱以小口瓶薰洗，令腫退，於原生鼠奶根上灸之，尖頭灸不效。或用藥水盆洗腫微退，然後灸，覺一團火氣通入腸至胸，乃效。灸至二十餘壯。更忌毒物，永愈。隨以竹片護火氣，勿傷兩邊好肉。

ZJDC: 9-14 Method to Apply Moxibustion to Points for Small Intestine Mounting Qi (Huang 1996, 989)
《針灸大成 • 灸小腸疝氣穴法 • 卷之九》

If someone suddenly suffers small intestine mounting qi, all cold qi, bound pain radiating to the umbilical region, and dribbling and weak urination, apply treatment to Da Dun [LV 1] bilaterally. This point is located at the end of the big toe, about the width of a Chinese leek leaf from the nail, in the clump of three hairs. Apply three cones of moxibustion.

If someone suffers sudden mounting of the small intestine, pain in the umbilical region, inability to lift the limbs, difficult urination, heavy body, and wilt-

ing of the legs, apply treatment to San Yin Jiao [SP 6] bilaterally. This point is located three *cun* above the medial malleolus. It is appropriate to needle to a depth of three *fen* and apply three cones of moxibustion. It is extremely wonderful.[24]

若卒患小腸疝氣，一切冷氣，連臍腹結痛，小便遺溺，大敦二穴，在足大指之端，去爪甲韭菜許，及三毛叢中是穴，灸三壯。
若小腸卒疝，臍腹疼痛，四肢不舉，小便澀滯，身重足痿。三陰交二穴，在足內踝骨上三寸是穴，宜針三分，灸三壯，極妙。

ZJDC: 9-15 Method to Apply Moxibustion for Intestinal Wind & Bloody Diarrhea (Huang 1996, 989)
《針灸大成 • 灸腸風下血法 • 卷之九》

Take the left middle finger on males and the right on females as the standard. [Holding it] upside down, compare it from the end of the tip of the coccyx up the midline to the site on the lumbar vertebra that is at the end of the one finger-length.[25] This is the first point.

Then take the index finger. In the center point, use the "center" character to divide and open the ends of the finger.

Apply seven cones of moxibustion to each point. Increase the number of cones until it is effective. If the patient has suffered this for a long time, apply more moxibustion the next year. However, only use the middle finger as the standard. At the time of

---

[23] This passage seems to have originated in the *Classic of Nourishing Life*, Volume 3 (Huang 1996, 282), although it has been edited quite a bit. I suspect there was another version between *Nourishing Life* and the *Great Compendium*, as the variation in wording is much greater than in anything else Master Yang copied. Parts of this passage are reminiscent of **BCGM: 26-21** and **15-05-25**.
  Radix Kalimeris is discussed in **BCGM: 14-46**. It is used to treat hemorrhoids. *Nourishing Life* says to boil three cups of water down to 1.5 cups.
  "Mouse breast" is a description of the appearance of the hemorrhoid. Sun's *Prescriptions* also uses this term (Sun 1994, a332). It is even found in the *Formulas for Fifty-Two Illnesses* (MSI.E.143) from the Mawangdui medical manuscripts (Harper 1998, 270).

[24] Zhang Jiebin writes in **LJTY: 8-2** that *Qian Kun Shengyi* by Zhu Quan 朱權《乾坤生意》 (Ming, 1391) says Da Dun (LV 1) is used with San Yin Jiao (SP 6) "to treat small intestine qi pain. It also treats all cold qi, bound pain radiating to the umbilical region, and dribbling and weak urination" (Zhang 1996, 268) This sentence is virtually identical to Yang's indications for Da Dun (LV 1).

[25] Note that 腰 *yao* does not mean only lumbar but the whole low back region, including the sacral area.

treatment, estimate [the number of cones based on the patient's condition].[26]

取男左女右手，中指為準，於尾閭骨尖頭，從中倒比，上至腰背骨一指盡處，是第一穴也。
又以第二指，於中穴取中一字分開指頭各一穴，灸七壯。已上加至壯數多為效。患深，次年更灸，但以中指一指為準，臨時更揣摸之。

ZJDC: 9-16 Moxibustion for Bound Chest & Cold Damage (Huang 1996, 989)
《針灸大成 • 灸結胸傷寒法 • 卷之九》

Huang Lian [Radix Coptidis] from Xuancheng [in Anhui province] (seven *cun* [long], pounded into powder); Ba Dou [Semen Crotonis] (seven pieces, remove the shell, do not remove the oil). Grind them together finely to make a paste. If it is dry, drip two drops of water into it. Put it in the umbilicus. Use mugwort moxibustion on top until the patient is unblocked. Diarrhea and cramping are the measure of success.[27]

宣黃連七寸，搗末，巴豆七個，去殼不去油，一處研細成膏，如乾，滴水兩點，納於臍中，用艾灸腹中通快痛為度。

ZJDC: 9-17 Moxibustion for Yin Toxins Binding the Chest (Huang 1996, 989)
《針灸大成 • 灸陰毒結胸 • 卷之九》

Put 10 pieces of Ba Dou [Semen Crotonis] (ground to a pulp) into one *qian* of flour. Pound it into a cake. Put it in the heart of the umbilicus. Use mugwort cones about the size of a bean on top. Apply seven cones of moxibustion. The patient will feel rumbling and roaring within his abdomen. It is good if this lasts a while: it will free itself.[28]

Next use a bunch of Cong Bai [Bulbus Allii Fistulosi] tightly bound up. Slice it to make cakes. Apply moxibustion and iron the region below the umbilicus to make it hot.[29]

Further, iron the cakes with a hot ash iron to make the patient engender true qi. He will gradually feel warmth and heat in his body. Then use two *qian* of Wu Ji San [Five Accumulations Powder], mixing in one *qian* of Fu Zi [Radix Lateralis Praeparata Aconiti] powder, 1.5 cups of water, ginger, Zao [Fructus Jujubae], and add a pinch of salt. Decoct them together until [the volume of water is down to] 70 percent. Take it warm. Altogether take take two or three doses per day. When the patient spontaneously sweats, the condition will be secure.[30]

---

[26] The source of this passage is unknown. The first point should be in the vicinity of Yao Shu Du 2. The location of the second point is unclear. Possibly, the 中 character is made on the finger with the middle phalange as the 口. The vertical line bisects the finger. The moxa is placed where the vertical line intersects the 口, in two places.
"However, only use the middle finger as the standard." This means you don't need the point on the low back if you do it again on the second year.

[27] **BCGM: 35-47-1-14** has a similar recipe. Li attributes it to *Collection of Formulas from the Yang Family* 《楊氏家藏方》 [*Yang Shi Jia Cang Fang*], a Song dynasty book by Yang Tan 楊〔人+炎, published in 1178, 20 Volumes (Li 1995, 716). Even though the family name is Yang, this book was written more than 400 years before Yang Jizhou's, so they may not be related.

[28] This is also in **BCGM: 35-47-1-17**. Li Shizhen attributes it to 《仁齋直指方》 [*Ren Zhai Zhi Zhi Fang*] by Yang Shiying 楊士瀛, published in 1264 (Song), 26 Volumes (Li 1995, 289). Even though the family name is Yang, this book was written more than 300 years before Yang Jizhou's, so they may not be related.

[29] **BCGM 03-59-3**, p. 194 has a similar remedy for bound up stool or blockage of urine and stool.
A hot ash iron is literally an iron filled with hot ashes.

[30] *Five Accumulations Powder* [*Wu Ji San*] was originally from *Professional and Popular Prescriptions from the Taiping Era* 《太平惠民和劑局方》 [*Tai Ping Hui Min He Ji Ju Fang*] (p 16), published in 1208 (Song) (Bensky 1990, 62).

巴豆十粒研爛，入麵一錢，搗作餅子，實搭臍中心，上
用艾炷如豆許，灸七壯，覺腹中鳴吼，良久自通利；次
用蔥白一束緊札，切作餅餤，灸令熱，與熨臍下；更用
灰火熨斗烙其餅餤，令生真氣，漸覺體溫熱，即用五積
散二錢，入附子末一錢，水盞半，薑棗加鹽一捻，同煎
至七分，溫服，日併三兩服，即汗自行而安。

ZJDC: 9-21 Moxibustion from *A Thousand Pieces of Gold* (Huang 1996, 990)
《針灸大成 • 〈千金〉灸法 • 卷之九》

Prescriptions Worth a Thousand Pieces of Gold says, "Officials traveling to Wu and Shu must constantly apply moxibustion to two or three sites on their body. When the moxa sores are not allowed to heal even for a short while, miasmic pestilence and warm malaria toxins are unable to touch the person. That is why people traveling to Wu and Shu frequently apply moxibustion."

Thus it is said, "If you desire to be secure, San Li [ST 36] must not be dry." For someone who has wind, it is especially suitable to keep that in mind.[31]

《千金方》云：宦遊吳蜀，體上常須三兩處灸之，切令
瘡暫瘥，則瘴癘，溫瘧毒不能著人，故吳蜀多行灸法。
故云：若要安，三里常不乾。有風者，尤宜留意。

ZJDC: 9-30 Moxibustion for Chills and Fever (Huang 1996, 991)
《針灸大成 • 灸寒熱 • 卷之九》

Method to apply moxibustion for chills and fever: First apply moxibustion to Da Zhui [Du 14]. Use the years of age for the number of cones. Next, apply moxibustion to Jue Gu [Du 1].[32] Use the years of age for the number of cones. If you observe a sunken back transport point, apply moxibustion to it. Apply moxibustion to sunken places on the arms and shoulders.[33] Apply moxibustion to the region of the two free ribs.[34] Apply moxibustion to Jue Gu [GB 39], near the end of the external malleolus. Apply moxibustion between the little toe and the fourth toe.[35] Apply moxibustion to sunken vessels below the calf.[36] Apply moxibustion behind the external malleolus.[37] Apply moxibustion to the site on the clavicle that feels hard like a sinew when pressed, and pulsates.[38] Apply moxibustion to the sunken space between the bones on the breast.[39] Apply moxibustion to Guan Yuan [Ren 4], which is three *cun* below the umbilicus. Apply moxibustion to the pulsating vessel in the pubic hair region.[40] Apply moxibustion to the divided space three *cun* below the knees.[41] Apply moxibustion to the pulsating vessel of the foot yang brightness channel on the dorsum of the foot.[42] Apply moxibustion to the point on the vertex.[43]

灸寒熱之法：先灸大椎，以年為壯數，次灸撅骨，以

---

[31] The first quotation is from Sun's *Prescriptions*, Volume 29 《千金要方 • 卷三十九 • 灸例》. Sun discussed *ashi* points there (Sun 1994, a415). This paragraph was repeated in *Nourishing Life*, Volume 2 (Huang 1996, 268) and Gao Wu's *Gatherings*, Part 2, Volume 3 (Huang 1996, 732), both under the heading of *ashi* points. Apparently Sun, Gao, and Wang Zhizhong did not associate this statement with Zu San Li ST 36.
   The second paragraph is from Southern Song medical doctor Zhang Gao from Volume 2 of *Medical Explanations* 張杲 《醫說 • 卷二》, published in 1224 (Gu and Zhao 1994, 3). It seems likely that Yang first connected these two paragraphs, giving momentum to the use of Zu San Li (ST 36) for prevention of contagious diseases.
[32] Note this is not Jue Gu (GB 39). It has different characters in Chinese although the pinyin is similar.
[33] This may refer to Jian Yu (LI 15) which makes a depression when the arm is raised. In *Elementary Questions*, Chapter 60, it says to raise the arm. The character for "raise" 舉 is omitted here.
[34] Perhaps Zhang Men (LV 13) or Jing Men (GB 25).
[35] Probably Xia Xi (GB 43) or Di Wu Hui (GB 42).
[36] Maybe Cheng Shan (UB 57) or Fei Yang (UB 58).
[37] Likely Kun Lun (UB 60).
[38] Maybe Que Pen (ST 12).
[39] This one is harder to guess. It could be Zhong Fu (LU 1).
[40] This could be Qi Jie (ST 30).
[41] Zu San Li (ST 36).
[42] Chong Yang (ST 42).
[43] Bai Hui (Du 20). This whole section is from *Elementary Questions*, Chapter 60. It is also included in Gao Wu's *Gatherings*, Part 1, Volume 2 (Huang 1996, 641).

年為壯數。視背俞陷者灸之，臂肩上陷者灸之，兩季
脅之間灸之，外踝上絕骨之端灸之，足小指次指間灸
之，〔月+尚〕下陷脈灸之，外踝後灸之，缺盆骨上
切之堅動如筋者灸之，膺中陷骨間灸之，臍下關元三
寸灸之，毛際動脈灸之，膝下三寸分間灸之，足陽明
跗上動脈灸之，顛上一穴灸之。

SELECTIONS FROM VOLUMES 3 & 4 OF THE *GREAT PHARMACOPEIA* ON VARIOUS INDICATIONS

Most of the *Great Pharmacopeia* was organized by medicinal, but Li Shizhen arranged two volumes (Volumes 3 and 4) by indication or chief complaint. These short entries could be used to quickly pick the most effective medicinals for a condition. If the reader then wanted more information, he could refer to the larger section on that medicinal.

Many of these entries involved various types of external heat treatments, including moxibustion. A selection of them is translated below. However, in order to show the variety of external heat treatments, they are arranged here by treatment method, not by symptom or disease.

Direct Moxibustion

BCGM: 03-04-2 Epilepsy – wind, heat, fright, and phlegm: Mugwort leaf: for epilepsy and all wind, apply moxibustion to the main gate of the grain path [the anus], right in the center. The number of cones is based on the years of age.

《本草綱目・主治第三卷・百病主治藥・癲癇・風熱驚痰
》艾葉：癲癇諸風，灸穀道正門當中，隨年壯。

BCGM: 03-61-4 Hemorrhoids & fistulas – fuming & moxibustion: Mugwort leaf: apply moxibustion on the swollen node.

《本草綱目・主治第三卷・百病主治藥・痔漏・熏灸》艾
葉：灸腫核上。

Moxibustion on Isolating Substances

BCGM: 03-20-2 Sudden turmoil [cholera] – cold damp: Boil Chinese garlic and drink the juice. At the same time, apply it to the umbilicus, burning seven cones of moxibustion on it.

《本草綱目・主治第三卷・百病主治藥・霍亂・寒濕》小
蒜：煮汁飲，并貼臍，灸七壯。

BCGM: 04-19-2 Scrofula – external treatment: Cut Shang Lu [Radix Phytolaccae] into slices. Apply mugwort moxibustion.

《本草綱目・主治第四卷・百病主治藥・瘰癧・外治》商
陸：切片，艾灸。

BCGM: 04-19-2 Scrofula – external treatment: If the scrofula has already ulcerated, make cakes of Ting Li [Semen Lepidii/Descuraniae] and apply moxibustion on it.

《本草綱目・主治第四卷・百病主治藥・瘰癧・外治》葶
藶：已潰，作餅灸。

BCGM: 04-22-1 Various sores, part 1 – clove sores: Liu Pi [Pericarpium Punica-granati]: apply moxibustion to the clove sore.

《本草綱目・主治第四卷・百病主治藥・諸瘡上・疔瘡》
榴皮：灸疔。

BCGM: 04-28-1 Various types of worm or insect bites – snake & serpent bites: Isolate mugwort leaf with garlic and apply moxibustion to it.

《本草綱目・主治第四卷・百病主治藥・諸蟲傷・蛇、虺
傷》艾葉：隔蒜灸之。

BCGM: 04-29-3 Various types of animal bites – dog & rabid dog bite: Mugwort leaf: for rabid dog bite, apply seven cones of moxibustion, or isolate it with earth taken from under a bed and apply moxibustion to it.

《本草綱目・主治第四卷・百病主治藥・諸獸傷・犬、〔犬+折〕傷》艾葉：〔犬+折〕犬傷，灸七壯，或隔床下土灸之。

BCGM: 04-41-2 Fright epilepsy – yin patterns: Apply moxibustion on single-clove garlic to the umbilicus and sniff the juice.

《本草綱目・主治第四卷・百病主治藥・驚癇・陰證》獨頭蒜：灸臍及汁嗅鼻。

BCGM: 04-40-21 Various pediatric and newborn diseases – umbilical wind:

- Place single-clove garlic on the umbilicus. Apply moxibustion until garlic qi [smell] comes out of the mouth. In addition, sniff the juice up the nose.

- Put salted fermented soybeans in the umbilicus and apply moxibustion to it.

- **Zao Mao [Jujube Cat]:**[44] Apply it with various medicinals, and apply moxibustion.

- First apply moxibustion with mugwort on Ren Zhong [Du 26] and Cheng Jiang [Ren 24]. Burn silver carp and grind it. Take it with wine.

《本草綱目・主治第四卷・百病主治藥・小兒初生諸病・臍風》獨蒜：安臍上，灸至口出蒜氣，仍以汁〔口+畜〕鼻。
　　鹽豉：貼臍灸之。
　　棗貓：同諸藥貼，灸。
　　鯽魚：先以艾灸人中、承漿，燒研酒服

BCGM: 03-30-2 Cramping – external treatment:
Pound garlic with salt and apply it in the umbilicus. Apply seven cones of moxibustion. Rub it into the heart of the foot and eat a clove.

《本草綱目・主治第三卷・百病主治藥・轉筋・外治》蒜：鹽搗敷臍，灸七壯。擦足心，并食一瓣。

Application of Medicinals to the Umbilicus

BCGM: 03-06-4 Cold damage febrile disease – warming the channels: For yin toxins, apply Jie Zi [Semen Sinapis] to the umbilicus. It will induce sweating.

《本草綱目・主治第三卷・百病主治藥・傷寒熱病・溫經》芥子：陰毒，貼臍，發汗。

BCGM: 03-20-2 Sudden turmoil [cholera] – cold damp: For abdominal pain from sudden turmoil [cholera], iron it with stir-fried salt. For cramping and feeling as if about to die, fill up the umbilicus with salt and apply moxibustion to it.

《本草綱目・主治第三卷・百病主治藥・霍亂・寒濕》炒鹽：霍亂腹痛，熨之。轉筋欲死者，填臍灸之。

BCGM: 03-21-4 Diarrhea – external treatment: Apply garlic to the hearts of the two feet. It can also be applied to the umbilicus.

《本草綱目・主治第三卷・百病主治藥・泄瀉・外治》大蒜：貼兩足心，亦可貼臍。

BCGM: 03-22-5 Dysentery – external treatment:

- **Mu Bei Zi [Semen Momordicae]:** Grind six, dig an opening into a hot flour cake, place half in the opening, heat, and apply on the umbilicus. Change it in a short while. It will promptly stop.

- **Jie Zi [Semen Sinapis] with fresh ginger:** Pound it into a paste and seal the umbilicus with it.

- **Huang Dan [Minium]:** Pound it with garlic and seal the umbilicus with it. Also apply it to the heart of the foot.

- **Shui Wa [water frog]:** Add She [Xiang, Secretio Moschi] and pound it. Apply it in the umbilicus.

- **Tian Luo [freshwater snail]:** Add She [Xiang,

---

[44] For Jujube Cat, see **BCGM: 40-5** p. 127.

Secretio Moschi] and pound it. Apply it in the umbilicus.

• **Bi Ma [Semen Ricini Communis]:** Pound it with Liu Huang [Sulfur] and fill the umbilicus with it.

• **Needle filings:** Mix them with Guan Gui [quilled Cortex Cinnamomi], calcined Ku Fan [Alum] and water. Apply it in the umbilicus.

《本草綱目•主治第三卷•百病主治藥•痢•外治》
木鱉子：六個研，以熱麵餅挖孔，安一半，熱貼臍上，少頃再換即止。
芥子：同生姜，搗膏封臍。
黃丹：同蒜搗，封螺，仍貼足心。
水蛭：入麝搗，貼臍。
田螺：入麝搗，貼臍。
蓖麻：同硫黃搗，填臍。
針砂：同官桂、枯礬，水調貼臍。

BCGM: 03-59-3 Dry, bound stool – guiding the qi: For blockage of stool, pound Zao Jiao [Fructus Gleditsiae] with garlic and apply it inside the umbilicus.

《本草綱目•主治第三卷•百病主治藥•大便燥結•導氣》皂莢：……便閉，同蒜搗，敷臍內。

BCGM: 04-43-3 Pox sores – external treatment: Burn ox hoof to a powder and apply it to the umbilicus.

《本草綱目•主治第四卷•百病主治藥•痘瘡•外治》牛蹄甲：燒末貼臍。

BCGM: 03-53-8 Dribbling block and stranguary – external treatment: Iron the umbilicus with garlic and salt. Apply garlic, salt, and Zhi Zi [Fructus Gardeniae] to the umbilicus. Apply garlic with Gan Sui [Radix Euphrobiae Kansui] to the umbilicus and apply two times seven cones of mugwort moxibustion. When hundreds of medicinals are ineffective, using this is very effective.

《本草綱目•主治第三卷•百病主治藥•癃淋•外治》大蒜：同鹽熨臍。蒜、鹽、栀子貼臍。同甘遂貼臍，以艾灸二七壯。百藥無效，用此極效。

BCGM: 03-59-3 Dry, bound stool – guiding the qi: For blockage due to large intestine vacuity, pound Cong Bai [Bulbus Allii Fistulosi] with salt and apply them to the umbilicus. For blockage of urine and stool, mix them with vinegar, apply them to the small abdomen, and apply seven cones of moxibustion.

《本草綱目•主治第三卷•百病主治藥•大便燥結•導氣》葱白：大腸虛閉，同鹽搗貼臍；二便閉，和醋敷小腹，仍灸七壯。

Heavenly Moxibustion & Medicinal Application Moxibustion

Heavenly moxibustion causes blisters; medicinal application moxibustion does not. I have included the application of medicinals to acu-moxa points in this section, but usually not topical application of medicinals to an affected site.

BCGM: 03-01-5 All wind – external application for deviation of the eyes & mouth: Apply garlic paste to He Gu [LI 4].

《本草綱目•主治第三卷•百病主治藥•諸風•貼歪》大蒜膏：貼合谷穴。

BCGM: 03-01-5 All wind – external application for deviation of the eyes & mouth: Apply Ba Dou [Semen Crotonis] to the heart of the palms of the hands.

《本草綱目•主治第三卷•百病主治藥•諸風•貼歪》巴豆：貼手掌心。

BCGM: 03-70-5 Mounting with prominence [*i.e.*, swelling of the testes] – yin prominence [or swelling of the testes]: Pound Bai Tou Weng [Radix Pulsatillae] and apply it. It will make a sore in one night. The patient will recover in 20 days.

《本草綱目•主治第三卷•百病主治藥•疝〔疒+貴〕•陰〔疒+貴〕》白頭翁：搗塗，一夜成瘡，二十日愈。

BCGM: 04-02-5 Headache – external treatment: Apply these to the Tai Yang [Supreme Yang, non-channel] point: Quan Xie [Scorpio] with Di Long [Pheretima], Tu Gou [mole cricket], and Wu Bei Zi [Galla Rhois] powdered; You Ye [Folium Citris Grandis] with Cong Bai [Bulbus Allii Fistulosi]; Shan Dou Gen [Radix Sophorae Subprostratae] and Nan Xing [Rhizoma Arisaematis] with Chuan Wu [Radix Praeparata Aconiti]; Wu Tou [Radix Aconiti] and Cao Wu Tou [Radix Aconiti Kusnezoffi] with Zhi Zi [Fructus Gardeniae] and scallion juice; Ru Xiang [Olibanum] with Bi Ma Ren [Semen Ricini Communis]; or Jue Ming Zi [Semen Cassiae].[45]

《本草綱目・主治第四卷・百病主治藥・頭痛・外治》全蠍：同地龍、土狗、五倍子末。柚葉：同蔥白。山豆根、南星：同川烏。烏頭、草烏頭：同梔子、蔥汁。乳香：同蓖麻仁。決明子：并貼太陽穴。

BCGM: 04-02-5 Headache – external treatment: Collect dew water on the first day of the eighth lunar month at dawn.[46] Grind ink with it and dab it on Tai Yang [Supreme Yang, non-channel]. It will stop the headache.

《本草綱目・主治第四卷・百病主治藥・頭痛・外治》露水：八月朔旦取，磨墨點太陽，止頭疼。

Ironing

BCGM: 03-06-4 Cold damage febrile disease – warming the channels: For yin toxins, stir-fry Cong Bai [Bulbus Allii Fistulosi] until hot and iron the umbilicus with it.

《本草綱目・主治第三卷・百病主治藥・傷寒熱病・溫經》蔥白：陰毒，炒熱熨臍。

BCGM: 03-06-4 Cold damage febrile disease – warming the channels: For yin toxins, mix Wu Zhu Yu [Fructus Evodiae] with wine and steam or iron the heart of the foot.

《本草綱目・主治第三卷・百病主治藥・傷寒熱病・溫經》吳茱萸：陰毒，酒拌蒸熨足心。

Fuming, Steaming, or Washes

BCGM: 03-28-5 Leg qi – ironing and fuming: Jing Ye [Folium Schizonepetae]: Make the patient lie down and use steam heat to make him sweat. Burn it and fume Yong Quan [KI 1] with the smoke.

《本草綱目・主治第三卷・百病主治藥・腳氣・熨熏》荊葉：蒸熱臥之，取汗。燒煙熏涌泉穴。

BCGM: 04-22-5 Various sores, part 1 – scabs & lichens: Burn mugwort leaf to make smoke for fuming. Boil mugwort in vinegar and apply it. Burn mugwort and apply the ash.

《本草綱目・主治第四卷・百病主治藥・諸瘡上・疥、癬》艾葉：燒煙熏，煎醋塗，燒灰搽。

BCGM: 04-22-8 Various sores, part 1 – hand sores: Fume mugwort leaf and ox dung together for goose foot wind [see the glossary].

《本草綱目・主治第四卷・百病主治藥・諸瘡上・手瘡》艾葉、牛屎：并熏鵝掌風。

BCGM: 04-22-10 Various sores, part 1 – shank sores: Burn mugwort leaf to make smoke to fume the sores. Malign water will come out. Or burn it with Xiong Huang [Realgar] and cloth. Or burn it with Jing Ye [Folium Schizonepetae] and chicken droppings. Burn them in a pit to fume the sores. It will conduct the worms out.

《本草綱目・主治第四卷・百病主治藥・諸瘡上・臁瘡》艾葉：燒煙，熏出惡水，或同雄黃、布燒；或同荊葉、雞屎，坑中燒熏，引蟲出。

---

[45] This is not one formula. It is a listing of a few small formulas or individual medicinals.
[46] The first day of the lunar month is the new moon day.

BCGM: 04-23-7 Various sores, part 2 – invisible-worm sores [see the glossary]: Burn mugwort leaf to make smoke and fume the sores.

《本草綱目・主治第四卷・百病主治藥・諸瘡下・〔匿+虫〕瘡》艾葉：燒煙熏。

BCGM: 03-61-2 Hemorrhoids & fistulas – washes & soaks: Wash a hemorrhoid that is swollen like a cucumber with a decoction of Liu Zhi [willow twig]. After, apply mugwort moxibustion.[47]

《本草綱目・主治第三卷・百病主治藥・痔漏・洗漬》柳枝：洗痔如瓜，後以艾灸。

BCGM: 04-21-3 Abscesses – ulcerated sores: Fu Zi [Radix Lateralis Praeparata Aconiti]: For abscesses with outcroppings [see glossary], boil it with concentrated vinegar and use it as a wash. For sore openings that do not close due to enduring cold, make cakes and apply moxibustion to them. In a few days it will promptly engender flesh. You can also apply garlic-isolated moxibustion to them.

《本草綱目・主治第四卷・百病主治藥・癰・疽・潰瘍》附子：癰疽弩肉，濃醋煎洗；瘡口久冷不合，作餅灸之，數日即生肉。隔蒜灸亦可。

BCGM: 04-21-3 Abscesses – ulcerated sores: For abscesses and sores erupting on the back, decoct Yin Zhu [Vermillion] with Fan [Alum] and use it as a wash. Apply moxibustion to it with fire from mulberry.

《本草綱目・主治第四卷・百病主治藥・癰・疽・潰瘍》銀朱：疽瘡發背，同礬湯洗，以桑柴火灸之。

Moxibustion with Substances other than Mugwort

BCGM: 04-22-1 Various sores, part 1 – clove sores: Make cones of arrow shaft shavings and apply moxibustion to the clove sore.

《本草綱目・主治第四卷・百病主治藥・諸瘡上・疔瘡》箭〔竹+可〕茹：作炷，灸疔。

BCGM: 04-22-1 Various sores, part 1 – clove sores: Human lice, 10 of them. Put them in the sore. Apply moxibustion to it with a rope of Bo Sheng [silvergrass].

《本草綱目・主治第四卷・百病主治藥・諸瘡上・疔瘡》人虱：十枚，著瘡中，箔繩灸之。

Unclassified

BCGM: 04-05-3 Ears – external treatment: Stop up the ears with Tu Gua Gen [Radix Curcubitae] and apply moxibustion for deafness.

《本草綱目・主治第四卷・百病主治藥・耳・外治》土瓜根：塞耳，灸聾。

BCGM: 04-18-2 Goiter, tumors, warts & moles – warts & moles: Filter the juice of a mugwort leaf with mulberry ash and dab it on warts, moles, tumors, and spots on the face. Apply three cones of moxibustion to a mole and it will promptly be removed.

《本草綱目・主治第四卷・百病主治藥・瘦瘤疣痣・疣痣》艾葉：同桑灰淋汁，點疣、痣、瘤、臁；灸痣，三壯即去。

BCGM: 04-23-4 Various sores, part 2 – condensed eyebrow sores:[48] Grind Huang Lian [Radix Coptidis] into a fine powder, mix it with oil, and apply it. Inside a bowl, make mugwort smoke to fume it. Add one grain of Zao Fan [Melanterite] and a little Qing Fen [Calomel] and apply it.

《本草綱目・主治第四卷・百病主治藥・諸瘡下・煉眉》黃連：研末，油調塗。碗內艾煙熏過，入皂礬一粒、輕粉少許塗之。

---

[47] There are related entries in **BCGM: 15-05-25**, p. 103, **35-16** and **35-29**.

[48] Condensed eyebrow sores [*lian mei*] are damp open sores on or between an infant's eyebrows (Li 1995, 1281).

Treating Moxa Sores

BCGM: 03-40-2 Bleeding & sweating – external treatment: Apply Han Lian [Camptotheca] to moxibustion sores for incessant bleeding.

《本草綱目•主治第三卷•百病主治藥•血汗•外治》旱
蓮：敷灸瘡，血出不止。

BCGM: 4-24-3 Various sores due to external damage – moxa sores:

- For moxa sores that bleed incessantly, take two *qian* of Huang Qin [Radix Scutellariae] in wine. It will promptly stop.

- **White fish:** When moxa sores do not erupt, make rich food and eat it.

- Apply the ash of dark blue cloth and Li Chang [Herba Ecliptae] to moxa sores.

- **Xie Bai [Bulbus Allii Macrostemmi]:** Decoct it with pig fat and apply it.

- Tian Cai [beet], Mao Hua [Flos Imperatae], Wa Song [roof pine], Mu Fu Rong [cotton rose], Qiu Gen Pi Ye [root bark of Manchurian catalpa and its leaf], axle grease, Hai Piao Xiao [Os Sepiae], ash of ox dung, rabbit skin or hair: Apply them for moxibustion sores that do not recover.

- For moxa sores that are swollen and painful, mix the white part of goshawk feces with human semen and apply it.

- Boil Zao Zhong Huang Tu [Terra Flava Usta], filter the 'juice,' and wash the sore.

《本草綱目•主治第四卷•百病主治藥•外傷諸瘡•灸
　瘡》
　黃芩：灸瘡血出不止，酒服二錢即止。
　白魚：灸瘡不發，作膾食。
　青布：灰；鱧腸：并貼灸瘡。
　薤白：煎豬脂塗。
　菾菜、茅花、瓦松、木芙蓉、楸根皮、葉、
　　車脂、海螵蛸、牛屎：灰、兔皮及毛：并塗
　　灸瘡不瘥。
　鷹屎白：灸瘡腫痛，和人精塗。
　灶中黃土：煮汁淋洗。

CHAPTER 12
CASE STUDIES USING MOXIBUSTION

A SMALL SAMPLING OF YANG'S CASE STUDIES

Yang Jizhou included over 30 case studies at the end of Volume 9 of the *Great Compendium*. They are all cases that he himself treated. Yang combined acupuncture, medicinals, and moxibustion in his treatment of patients. I have selected four that are representative of his use of moxibustion.

ZJDC: 9-36 Appended Case Studies of Master Yang (Huang 1996, 992-7)
《針灸大成 • 附楊氏醫案 • 卷之九》

ZJDC: 9-36-5 In the summer of a *jia xu* year [1598], Official Xiong Keshan suffered unceasing dysentery and vomiting blood at the same time. His body was hot, he was coughing, and he had a painful lump around his umbilicus. He was approaching death. His pulse qi was critical and about to expire. The crowd of doctors said, "He cannot be treated."[1]

The Ministers of Public Works, Wei Yuetan and Gong Sushan, invited me to see him. Although his pulse was critical and expiring, his chest was still warm. In the middle of the umbilicus, a high lump had grown up the size of a fist.

This day was not suitable for acupuncture; so he had not received it. I quickly needled Qi Hai [Ren 6]. In addition, I applied moxibustion. He revived after reaching 50 cones. The lump promptly scattered and the pain promptly stopped. Afterwards, I treated the dysentery and he recovered. Next, I treated the coughing blood[2] in order to regulate him so he could recover. The next year, he was promoted to a higher position.

He asked the reason [why I treated him on a day that was inappropriate for acupuncture, but there was a good outcome]. I said, "In disease, there is branch and root; in treatment there is moderate and acute. If I had been constrained by the daily

---

[1] This statement means that the other doctors thought the patient could not be saved. In addition, it says later that this was a day when acupuncture (and possibly moxibustion) was contraindicated. See Chapter 13: Timing of Treatment for details.

[2] Above Yang said the patient is vomiting blood, but here he said he is coughing blood.

prohibitions and had not needled Qi Hai [Ren 6], then how could the lump scatter? Once the lump was dispersed and scattered, qi could be freed up so the pain stopped and your pulse returned. The idea that is called "when acute, treat the tip [or branch]" is correct. Although your body is secure now, in order to preserve the harmony of the root you cannot let yourself get very angry after drinking and eating. Otherwise, right qi will become perverted and liver qi will become exuberant. This will result in spleen earth receiving control. You can calculate day for revenge."[3]

甲戌夏，員外熊可山公，患痢兼吐血不止，身熱咳嗽，繞臍一塊痛至死，脈氣將危絕。眾醫云：不可治矣。工部正郎隗月潭公素善，迎予視其脈雖危絕，而胸尚暖，臍中一塊高起如拳大，是日不宜針刺，不得已，急針氣海，更灸至五十壯而蘇，其塊即散，痛即止。後治痢，痢愈。治嗽血，以次調理得痊。次年升職方，公問其故，予曰：病有標本，治有緩急，若拘於日忌，而不針氣海，則塊何由而散？塊既消散，則氣得以疏通，而痛止脈復矣。正所謂急則治標之意也。公體雖安，
飲食後不可多怒氣，以保和其本；否則正氣乖而肝氣盛，致脾土受剋，可計日而復矣！

> **Notes:** In this case, only one point was mentioned in the initial treatment. Both acupuncture and moxibustion were applied to Qi Hai [Ren 6] which is able to move and regulate qi in the abdomen. It dispersed the lump and rescued the patient.

In many of Yang's case studies, the patient not only recovers, he also gets a promotion. It seems Yang took this as a sign of the patient's new vigor for life.

ZJDC: 9-36-18 In the summer of a *ren shen* year [1600], Ministry of Finance Secretary[4] Wang Shu suffered intensely exuberant phlegm fire and it was difficult for him to stretch out his arms. I saw that his physique was strong. This condition is often damp phlegm flowing inside the channels and network vessels. I needled Jian Yu [LI 15] to free the hand greater yin and hand yang brightness channels of damp phlegm. I repeatedly applied moxibustion to Fei Shu [UB 13] in order to rectify the root so that the phlegm qi would clear, and he was able to lift his arms. He was promoted to a higher position and his physique increased in strength.

壬申夏，戶部尚書王疏翁患痰火熾盛，手臂難伸，予見形體強壯，多是濕痰流注經絡之中，針肩髃，疏通手太陰經與手陽明經之濕痰，復灸肺俞穴，以理其本，則痰氣可清，而手臂能舉矣。至吏部尚書，形體益壯。

> **Notes:** Apparently Secretary Wang suffered phlegm fire internally, but phlegm damp also flowed in the channels of his arms. Yang needled Jian Yu [LI 15] to open up the channels of his arms. He applied moxibustion to Fei Shu [UB 13] to treat what he considered the root: phlegm in the lungs. Even though Yang diagnosed it as phlegm fire, he felt that moxibustion was an appropriate treatment. Also note the simplicity of the treatment.

ZJDC: 9-36-26 In a *ji mao* year [1593], Mrs. Zhang Jingchen experienced flooding that would not stop. She had generalized feverishness, bone pain, vexation and agitation. The disease was serious. I was summoned for a consultation. I took the six pulses which were rapid and skipping beats. The disease

---

[3] "You can calculate day for revenge." *Elementary Questions*, Chapter 40 says, "The spleen is earth and it is adverse to wood. If [the wrong] medicinals are taken, it will worsen on *jia* and *yi* days." *Jia* and *yi* days are wood like the liver, so they add to the burden on the spleen. *Jia* and *yi* days would be the days for revenge on the spleen.

[4] Job titles are hard to translate: the exact position at that time may not be obvious today.

must have been externally contracted. It would be a mistake to use cooling medicinals. I gave her *Qiang Huo Tang* [Notopterygium Decoction] and the fever abated. The rest of the disease could gradually resolve. However, her original qi had difficulty returning. I repeatedly applied moxibustion to Gao Huang [UB 43] and San Li [ST 36] and she recovered. Generally, the doctor's use of medicinals must rely on pulse theory. If the disease is externally contracted and you mistakenly cause internal damage by replenishing repletion or evacuating vacuity, decreasing the insufficient or boosting the surplus, how can the patient not come to a premature end, their life extinguished?

己卯歲，行人張靖宸公夫人，崩不止，身熱骨痛，煩燥病篤，召予診，得六脈數而止，必是外感，誤用涼藥。與羌活湯，熱退，餘病漸可。但元氣難復，復灸膏肓，三里而愈。凡醫之用藥，須憑脈理，若外感誤作內傷，實實虛虛，損不足而益有餘，其不夭滅人生也，幾希？

> **Notes:** After recovery from a serious illness, repeated moxibustion to Gao Huang [UB 43] and San Li [ST 36] restored Mrs. Zhang's original qi. Note, that even though Yang is known for acupuncture and moxibustion because of this book, he chose a medicinal formula to treat the original disease. Yang advocated using all modalities, choosing them as appropriate for the specific condition.

ZJDC: 9-36-30 In a *jia xu* year [1598], the father of Inspector Tian Chunye suffered spleen-stomach disease. He was recuperating near the Altar to Heaven.[5] He had to travel many *li* to reach my house. Mr. Chunye accompanied his father every time he came,

doing his utmost to carry out filial piety. I was moved by his sincerity, and that he did not dread the distance. I hurried out to greet them whenever they came.[6]

I told them that the spleen-stomach are the root of the entire body. They establish the foundation of the five phases and are the mother and father of the tens of thousands of things. How can you not try to make them extremely healthy and smooth-functioning? If they are not extremely healthy and smooth-functioning, the calamity of deep illness will arrive. Because it is like this, the father's disease was not caused in one day. However, the spleen likes sweetness and dryness and is averse to bitterness and dampness. When medicinals are hot, they disperse the flesh. When medicinals are cold, they reduce the intake of drink and food [by reducing the appetite]. The doctor who treats the patient after he has had the condition for a long time does not obtain good results. This is not as good as early application of moxibustion to Zhong Wan [Ren 12] and Shi Cang [Food Grainery, non-channel].[7]

They were happy to go along with this. I applied nine cones of moxibustion to each point. In addition, I needled them, moving the needle nine times, the number of yang. Moxa sores erupted and he gradually recovered.

Today, Mr. Chunye has been appointed to be a military quartermaster, and his father and younger brother both passed the civil service exams and are abundantly strong.

甲戌歲，觀政田春野公乃翁，患脾胃之疾，養病天壇，至敝宅數里，春野公每請必親至，竭力盡孝。予感其誠，不憚其遠，出朝必趨視。告曰：脾胃乃一身之根蒂，五行之成基，萬物之父母，安可不由其至健至順哉？苟不至健至順，

---

[5] An important temple in Beijing.
[6] Master Yang was at a much higher social position and therefore should wait in his office for them to arrive, but he was so moved by the situation that he treated them as if they were his superiors.
[7] Shi Cang [Food Grainary, non-channel] is located three *cun* lateral to Zhong Wan [Ren 12] (O'Connor and Bensky 1981, 373).

則沉痾之咎必致矣。然公之疾，非一朝所致，但脾喜甘燥，而惡苦濕，藥熱則消於肌肉，藥寒則減於飲食，醫治久不獲當，莫若早灸中脘食倉穴。忻然從之，每穴各灸九壯，更針行九陽之數，瘠發漸愈。春野公今任兵科給事中，迺翁迺弟俱登科而盛壯。

> **Notes:** Here, Yang feels that the patient would suffer side effects from medicinal formulas due to the weakness of his middle burner. Instead, acupuncture and moxibustion were used to supplement spleen qi and yang. Yang Jizhou relied on the extreme yang nature of the number nine to enhance his treatment. Not only is nine odd and, therefore, yang, it is three times three. The number two only represents yin and yang. Three represents heaven, earth, and humanity; three includes humans, which are in the center and, therefore, also the central nature of the middle burner, the spleen-stomach. Squaring the number three amplifies it. In addition, nine is the number used to represent extreme yang in *Change* theory, while seven represents younger yang. All this would help to fortify spleen yang and qi, thereby benefiting the post-heaven qi of the body as a whole.

ZHANG'S CASE STUDIES

Zhang did not have a section on case studies. A few can be found here and there in his *Complete Works*. The entry below is found in Zhang's volumes on formulas, but it is a case study from an earlier time. In addition to this case study, there are a few cases on treating sores in **JYQS: 46-11**, above.

JYQS: 58-115 Decoction to Support Yang and Reinforce the Stomach (115), Volume 58 (Zhang 1995, 1555)

《景岳全書·扶陽助胃湯百十五·卷之五十八》

Luo Qianfu [Li Dongyuan's disciple] treated Cui Yunshi's eldest son, Yunqing, who was 25 years old. His body was obese and thickly nourished. He often ate cold things and took cold medicinals. As a result, malaria developed in the autumn. He again swallowed medicinals such as *Pi Shi* [Arsenic] with water. Contrarily, it increased his vomiting and diarrhea, and his central qi became more vacuous. This lasted until the fourth month of the next year. Again because of taxation and anger, the earlier pattern worsened. Luo examined his pulse and found it to be bowstring, fine, and faint. His hands and feet were slightly cold. His facial complexion was green and yellow. His food intake was reduced, and he had glomus oppression, sour vomiting, hasty breathing, and he was sweating.

Luo considered that the *Inner Canon* says, "In central qi insufficiency, urination and defecation are changed, and the intestines suffer rumbling. When qi of the lower body is insufficient, there is wilting reversal, and vexation and oppression of the heart."[8] It also says, When cold qi settles in the intestines and stomach, there is sudden pain.[9] This is a case where very hot prescriptions are able to bring about recovery, so Luo prepared this formula:

Fu Zi [Radix Lateralis Praeparata Aconiti] (blast-fried, remove the skin and "umbilicus," two *qian*), Gan Jiang [dry Rhizoma Zingiberis] (blast-fried, 1.5 *qian*), Cao Dou Kou [Fructus Amomi Katsumadai], Yi Zhi Ren [Fructus Alpiniae Oxyphyllae], Jian Shen,[10] mix-fried Gan Cao [Radix Glycyrrhizae], Guan Gui [quilled Cortex Cinnamomi], Bai Shao Yao [Radix

---

[8] *Magic Pivot*, Chapter 28 《靈樞·口問第二十八》
[9] Paraphrased from *Elementary Questions*, Chapter 39 《素問·舉痛論篇第三十九》
[10] I am unable to identify the medicinal *Jian Shen* at this time.

Alba Paeoniae] (each one *qian*), Wu Zhu Yu [Fructus Evodiae], Chen Pi [Pericarpium Citri Reticulatae], Bai Zhu [Rhizoma Atractylodis Macrocephalae] (each five *fen*).

Break the above into pieces, add two cups of water, two *Zao* [Fructus Jujubae], and two slices of ginger. Decoct it to 80 percent of the water and take it warm before eating.

After three doses, the general situation was removed and the pain had decreased by half. When autumn arrived, moxibustion was applied to Zhong Wan [Ren 12] in order to reinforce stomach qi. Next, more than 100 cones of moxibustion were applied to Qi Hai [Ren 6] to engender and effuse original qi. The next year, two times seven cones of moxibustion were again applied to San Li [ST 36], also to reinforce stomach qi, and draw qi to move downward. He carefully nursed his health for a year and he was cured.

羅謙甫治崔運使長男雲卿，年二十五，體肥養厚，
常食涼物寒藥，以致秋間瘧發，復用水吞砒石等藥，
反增吐瀉，中氣愈虛，延至次年四月，復因勞怒，

前證大作。診其脈得弦細而微，手足稍冷，
面色青黃，食少痞悶嘔酸，
氣促汗出。予思《內經》云：中氣不足，
溲便為之變，腸為之苦鳴。下氣不足，
則為痿厥心悗。又曰：寒氣客于腸胃之間，
則卒然而痛。非大熱之劑不能愈，
遂製此方。附子炮去皮臍，二錢。 乾薑炮，
錢半。草豆蔻，益智仁，揀參，甘草炙，官桂，
白芍藥，各一錢。吳茱萸，陳皮，白朮，
各五分。右㕮[口+父]咀。水二盞，棗二枚，薑三片，
煎八分。食前溫服。三服後，大勢去，
痛減半。至秋灸中脘以助胃氣，次灸氣海百餘壯，
生發元氣。明年復灸三里二七壯，亦助胃氣，
引氣下行。仍慎加調攝，一年而平復。

LI'S CASE STUDIES

Like Zhang Jiebin, Li Shizhen never wrote a section on case studies. However, there are some cases spread throughout the *Great Pharmacopeia*. Most are historical cases, not Li's personal patients. The ones translated in this book are located in Chapter 8: The Materials of Moxibustion. Sometimes very few details are given for a case. Please see the following table:

CASE STUDIES IN THE *GREAT PHARMACOPEIA* RELATING TO MOXIBUSTION	
ITEM IDENTIFICATION	**CONDITION**
BCGM: 15:05:25	Hemorrhoids
BCGM: 15:05:52	Toothache
BCGM: 26-09	Sores (there are a few case studies in this section)

CHAPTER 13
TIMING OF TREATMENT

Heaven and earth cycle through day and night. They bring us winter, spring, summer, and autumn. The new moon waxes to full and then wanes in endless cycles.

observable chronicity relates to the cycles mentioned above. Even a layperson can tell if it is day or night, summer or winter. No special knowledge is needed to observe the phase of the moon. Observable

---

人身小天地。張介賓《類經附翼·醫易義》
The human body is a small heaven and earth.
Appended Supplement to the Categorized Classic—Medicine and Yijing,
by Zhang Jiebin

This idea was emphasized from the time of the *Inner Canon* through the Ming dynasty, although it is less evident or almost absent in modern texts on Chinese medicine. Since the human body is a small *tai ji* surrounded by the big universe, it must respond to these natural cycles. It must also have its own cycles of day and night and change to mirror the moon and the four seasons. This concept has many implications for etiology, progression, prevention, and treatment of disease, including the harvesting and processing of medicinals.

We can divide chronicity into two types. What I call

chronicity would include methods such as picking mugwort on the third day of the third lunar month, which is also close to the spring equinox, in order to give the mugwort a surge of yang qi rising up within it. Another example would be the recommendation to practice moxibustion after noon, after the patient has eaten but before yin becomes too strong.

Calculated chronicity requires some special knowledge, or at least a check of the calendar. The simplest kind only involves the stems and branches. If the doctor feels the patient should receive or avoid treatment on a *zi* branch day, he must check the calendar, not the sky, to find when that is. Some types of calculated chronicity become very complicated, for example midnight-noon flowing and pooling (*zi wu liu zhu*), a method of chrono-acupuncture. Here, certain points are "open" during specific time periods during the 10-day cycle of the heavenly stems. The five transports and the six qi (*wu yun liu qi*) theory is another example of complex calculated chronicity.

In some cases, it is hard to determine if an aspect of timing is observable or calculated; there is some overlap. If a treatment needs to take place during the *wu* hour (11AM – 1 PM), is it simply because the sun is at its peak at noon? Or is it because there is a specific qi associated with the *wu* hour, somewhat independent of the fact that it is also noon? Different cases will have different answers.

The use of both types of chronicity in treatment seems to have declined from the Qing dynasty to the present. However, based on the writings of the three authors here, it was still flourishing during the Ming dynasty.

This chapter will present the recommendations of these Ming masters in regards to using or avoiding moxibustion at particular times.

OBSERVABLE CHRONICITY

Observable chronicity is older than calculated chronicity, as it is simpler and and based on perceptible cycles of the universe. First we will examine the recommended time to pick mugwort.

ZJDC: 9-23 says mugwort "is picked on the third day of the third lunar month or the fifth day of the fifth lunar month." Yang also said that burning mugwort is effective to "keep away malignity and kill ghosts" if it is picked on the fifth day of the fifth lunar month.

Li made similar statements. In **BCGM: 15-05**, he quoted previous authors who said that mugwort

should be picked on the third day of the third lunar month or the fifth day of the fifth lunar month. These authors also advised drying it in the sun. Li himself described it as common practice: "On the fifth day of the fifth lunar month, everyone cuts the stalks with the leaves, and dries this harvest in the sun."

The third day of the third lunar month occurs at the end of March or in the first half of April in the Western calendar. This is around the time of the vernal equinox (春分). It is the time when daylight becomes as long as the night and is still growing. Yang is now predominant and is getting stronger by the day.

The fifth day of the fifth lunar month usually occurs in June, often very near the summer solstice (夏至) when yang is at its peak. For example, in 1977, the solstice occurred exactly on the fifth day of the fifth lunar month. (See next page)

Of course, one reason mugwort is picked at these times is because the plant is at an optimum state in its growth cycle for use as moxibustion. The leaves are big enough but not old and tough. However, if that were the only reason, the books would say it could be picked *between* these two dates, not right on them.

Li said, "When processed into floss, mugwort is pure yang." Gathering it on these two dates enhances the yang nature of mugwort by picking it at the most yang times of the year. In addition, the numbers three (third day of the third lunar month) and five (fifth day of the fifth lunar month), being odd, are yang. Up until recently, most Chinese would feel this enhanced the effect.

The sun, called greater yang (*tai yang*) by the ancients, is the most yang object in the known universe. Picking mugwort when the sun is giving out the most yang increases the yang nature of the plant, as does drying it in the sun. In addition, Li told us that the best way to light a moxa cone was with a yang speculum or fire bead (BCGM: 06-06), both methods that use the rays of the sun.

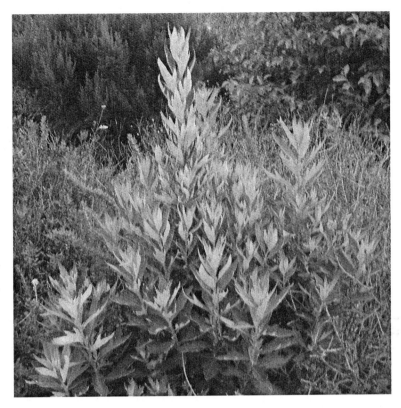

**Mugwort as seen on the fifth day of the fifth lunar month, June 11, 2005
(photo by the author)**

There is another reason for choosing the fifth day of the fifth lunar month. In addition to being the Dragon Boat Festival day and near to the summer solstice, it is also a day for expelling the five toxic creatures (五毒): snakes, toads, lizards, scorpions, and centipedes (Mathews 1943, 1072). In fact, the fifth lunar month is also known as the "toxin month" (毒月). This word toxin or poison (*du*) can also mean malevolent or evil (Mathews 1943, 947) and has connotations of a supernatural evil.

Because this day contains so much yang, the fifth day of the fifth lunar month is a potent day to expel yin evils, including poisonous creatures and ghosts. Mugwort has a long history of being used in this way. Vivienne Lo (2005, 228) stated that "There is good evidence that the development of moxibustion with mugwort was related to an earlier use of mugwort to ward off inauspicious entities and drive away demons."

This type of practice was passed on by Li in his citation of Zong Lin, "On the fifth day of the fifth lunar month, before the rooster crows... pick mugwort that is in the shape of a man, and hang it over the doorway. It can exorcise toxin qi." Being in the shape of man, it has a resonance or affinity with the human body, and is better able to treat or protect it.

Meng Xian gave a recipe for dumplings with young mugwort leaves. Eating these "treats all ghosts and malign qi."

Zhen Quan advised, "Pound mugwort into juice to drink for treating cold qi and ghost qi of the entire heart region and abdomen."

Looking through Li's collection of formulas that use mugwort externally, we see they often treat worms, bugs, parasites, snake bites, and various toxins or wind diseases such as epilepsy. All these would be attributed to ghost qi by some.

While mugwort may or may not be effective for these ailments from a biomedical point of view, it seems clear that this herb retained some of its magical properties from the past. Its extreme yang nature, derived in part from the sun, is used to expel or counteract yin toxins and evils harassing the body.

The timing of moxibustion treatment was discussed by Yang Jizhou. In these two passages, we can see the shift of attitude over time from observable toward calculated chronicity.

ZJDC: 9-20 Reading the Weather & Time,[1] (Huang 1996, 990)

《針灸大成 • 相天時 • 卷之九》

Thousand Pieces of Gold says: You can apply moxibustion after noon, meaning yin qi is not yet extreme. There is nothing moxibustion will not affect. Grain qi is vacuous before noon at daybreak, making a person withdrawn and dizzy; acupuncture-moxibustion cannot be applied then. If the case is sudden and urgent, do not use this rule.

The Lower Canon says:[2] If you meet clouds and fog,

great wind and snow, violent rain, blazing heat, thunder and lightning, or rainbows at the time moxibustion is applied, stop and wait for clear bright weather to apply moxibustion again. If you have an acute and difficult situation, do not be constrained by this.

Note: During the day, qi flows into the heart channel at noon. In the *wei* time [1-3 PM], it pours into the small intestine channel; so you can only apply moxibustion to points like Ji Quan [HT 1], Shao Hai [HT 3], Ling Dao [HT 4], Tong Li [HT 5], Shen Men [HT 7], Shao Fu [HT 8], Shao Chong [HT 9], Shao Ze [SI 1], Qian Gu [SI 2], Hou Xi [SI 3], Wan Gu [SI 4]. The rest of the channels and network vessels each have their own time when qi arrives so the *Precious Mirror* says:[3] If qi has not arrived [in a channel at the time of moxibustion], moxa sores will not erupt. It is *Thousand Pieces of Gold* that says the words "after noon apply moxibustion." I fear this is not True Person Sun's own formula.[4]

《千金》云：正午後乃可，謂陰氣未至，灸無不著，午前平旦穀氣虛，令人癲眩，不可針灸。卒急者，不用此例。《下經》云：灸時若遇陰霧、大風雪、猛雨、炎暑、雷電、虹蜺、停候晴明再灸。急難亦不拘此。按：日正午，氣注心經，未時注小腸經，止可灸極泉，少海，靈道，通里，神門，少府，少衝，少澤，前谷，後谿，腕骨等穴，其餘經絡，各有氣至之時。故《寶鑑》云：氣不至，灸之不發。《千金》所云：午後灸之言，恐非孫真人口訣也。

---

[1] Yang quotes all of this passage, including the note at the end, from Gao Wu's *Gatherings*, Part 2, Volume 3 (Huang 1996, 732-3). Gao took the first part, without the note, from Volume 3 of *Nourishing Life* (Huang 1996, 270). It is likely that Gao is the original author of the note, although it is possible that he copied it from an earlier unknown source.

The idea of the first paragraph came from Sun's *Prescriptions*, Volume 29 《千金要方·卷三十九·灸例》 (Sun 1994, a414). It is interesting that in Sun's *Supplement*, Volume 28, a similar statement is made, except that it is regarding acupuncture, not moxibustion (Sun1994, b262). **LJTY: 4-27-5** makes the same statement in regard to acupuncture.

[2] The *Lower Canon* refers to Volume 100 of 《太平聖惠方》 *Sage-like Prescriptions of the Taiping Era* by 王懷隱 Wang Huaiyin (Huang 1996, 235). This book was published in 992, on the order of the Song Emperor Taizong.

[3] The *Precious Mirror* refers to 《衛生寶鑑》 the *Precious Mirror of Protecting Life* by 羅天益 Luo Tianyi (Yuan, 1220-1290). The statement here from the *Precious Mirror* is given in a more complete form in the next entry.

[4] Meaning these words are apocryphal, in error, and not written by Sun Simiao.

Notes: The first part of this passage, which is from Sun Simiao (or was added falsely to *Prescriptions* according to Gao Wu's note at the end), advises acupuncture-moxibustion after noon, especially after the patient has eaten. This way, the patient is not weak because there is enough grain qi in the body. However, the treatment should still be relatively early in the day, before yin qi is too strong. This is somewhat odd; if the prohibition is based on insufficient grain qi at that time of day, it could be easily remedied by eating. Most patients would probably have had breakfast well before noon. If not, they could be instructed to eat before receiving treatment.

The author of the note disagrees with recommending or prohibiting specific times of the day for all moxibustion. He does not want to use moxibustion unless the channel is open (in its own time period according to the circadian circulation of qi in the twelve channels). It is likely that this controversy arose because of the difference in time when these passages were originally written. Sun's *Prescriptions* was published in 652. Chrono-acupuncture (and chrono-moxibustion) was not highly developed during the Tang dynasty, so Sun based his idea on observation of his patients' physical state at different times of the day (observable chronicity).

By the Song and Yuan dynasties, the calculation arts were much more developed, so the *Precious Mirror* did not emphasize the balance of yin and yang according to the time of day; instead, it emphasized the location of the high tide of qi-blood in the channels. Gao Wu favored this later, more theoretical approach based on calculation of the qi according to the clock (calculated chronicity).

The advice of the *Lower Canon* here is to avoid treatment during unusual weather (observable chronicity).

We are told twice in this section that if the case is urgent, the appropriate treatment must be given right away, without regard for the time.

ZJDC: 9-22 Method to Make Moxa Sores Erupt from the *Precious Mirror* (Huang 1996, 990) 《針灸大成 • 〈寶鑑〉發灸法 • 卷之九》

The *Precious Mirror* says: When qi does not arrive, moxibustion is not effective. In addition, moxa sores do not erupt. It seems that the twelve channels respond to the twelve double-hours. In each of them, the qi arrives based on the time so if you do not know the amount of qi and blood in the channels and network vessels and the corresponding time of arrival [of qi in the channel] when you apply moxibustion, moxa sores will not erupt. For generations of doctors, no one knew this.[5]

《寶鑑》云：氣不至而不效，灸亦不發。
蓋十二經應十二時，其氣各以時而至，故不知經絡氣血多少，應至之候，而灸之者，則瘡不發，世醫莫之知也。

Notes: This passage reveals the consequences of applying moxibustion at a time when the channel is not open: moxa sores will not erupt and the treatment will not be effective. Since the prevailing attitude of the time was that moxibustion was not therapeutic without making sores, the timing of the treatment was used to insure that these sores would develop.

One reason for a lack of moxa sores after treatment is that when the patient's qi and blood are insufficient, the body does not react properly (see **ZJDC: 9-31**

---

[5] This section is quoted by Yang from a note in *Gatherings* (Huang 1996, 732). The contents are related to **ZJDC: 9-20**, above.

above). Therefore, when moxibustion is performed at the time when qi and blood is strongest in the channel, it aids even a weak patient to develop moxa sores.

This passage favors a simple calculated chronicity and acknowledges that this idea is a newer development by saying, "For generations of doctors, no one knew this."

CALCULATED CHRONICITY

Doctors of the Ming dynasty commonly observed prohibitions for treatment on specific days or for treatment of certain body parts at specific times. In addition, some days were considered auspicious for treatment. Finally, a few special treatments were reserved for specific times. These ideas are examined below.

Day Selection for Treatment with Moxibustion

Day selection (擇日 *ze ri*) is the determination of the suitability of a day for a specific activity based on the Chinese calendar and sometimes on the individual's birth information. Day selection is a bit of a misnomer as it can involve larger or smaller periods of time, for example, the double-hour, the month, the season, or the year. Day selection was used by people in general for many things: weddings, grand openings, and ground breaking for construction, as well as for medical treatment. It is still used by many Chinese today.

Day selection was used for medical treatment at least as far back as the *Inner Canon*. For example, *Magic Pivot*, Chapter 41 prohibits piercing of specific channels during each season. *Magic Pivot*, Chapter 61 pro-

hibits certain needling techniques on various body parts on specific days according to the heavenly stems. As centuries passed, the calculations became more complicated and many different calculations evolved. Judging by the contents of the various acupuncture-moxibustion manuals, this practice was quite common during the Yuan and Ming dynasties.[6]

Yang included many types of day selection in Volume 4 of the *Great Compendium*. Most apply to acupuncture, but a few specifically mention moxibustion. There are also days to avoid treatment on different body parts, or days for males or females to avoid treatment. Zhang included a smaller section on this in Volume 4 of the *Illustrated Supplement*. Li Shizhen did not discuss day selection in the *Great Pharmacopeia*.

The passages on day selection are often written into poems to make them easy to memorize. In these poems, there are extra or missing words to make the rhythm and rhyme match.

The sampling below is not comprehensive, but should give the reader the general idea of medical day selection. I am presupposing on the part of the reader a background in the Chinese calendar, including the ten heavenly stems and twelve earthly branches.[7]

ZJDC: 4-31-4 Four Seasons Human Spirit Song (Huang 1996, 872)
《針灸大成 • 九部人神禁忌歌 • 四季人神歌 • 卷之四》

> During spring and autumn: the left and right rib-sides,
> During winter and summer: the lumbar and umbilical regions.

---

[6] A related topic is chrono-acupuncture, picking open points based on the time and date. This includes midnight-noon flowing and pooling (子午流注 *zi wu liu zhu*), the eight methods of the spirit tortoise (靈龜八法 *ling gui ba fa*) and the eight methods of flying and soaring (飛騰八法 *fei teng ba fa*). Chrono-acupuncture was popular during the Ming dynasty. Volume 5 of the *Great Compendium* contained a discussion of these methods. However, this topic is beyond the scope of a book on moxibustion.

[7] The topic of the stems and branches and the Chinese calendar is beyond the scope of this book. The *American Feng Shui Institute* has an on-line class on this topic at www.amfengshui.com

These are the sites of the human spirit in the
  four seasons;
Do not rashly apply acupuncture and moxibustion.[8]

春秋左右脅，冬夏在腰臍，四季人神處，針灸莫妄施。

> **Notes:** The human spirit prohibitions have
> many subcategories. The basic idea is that
> a type of human spirit travels from one
> part of the body to another at regular inter-
> vals based on time, just like the constella-
> tions change position in the sky. It also has
> the image of the emperor surveying his
> lands. According to this, we need to avoid
> applying treatment to the area inhabited
> by the human spirit or else we may cause it
> harm (Li 1995, 34).

Human spirit prohibitions were included in books
like the *Bronze Man*, *Nourishing Life*, the *Compass for
the Acupuncture Classic*, the *Great Completion of
Acupuncture - Moxibustion*, *Gatherings from Eminent
Acupuncturists*, and of course the *Great Compendium*.

In the *Great Compendium*, Yang gave human spirit
prohibitions based on the day stem, the day branch,
the season, the day of the lunar month, and the
double-hour.

In addition, Zhang Jiebin cautioned about violating
the human spirit in **LJTY: 8-3-8** regarding Shen Que
[Ren 8]: "In the summer months, the human spirit is
in the umbilicus, so it is not appropriate to apply
moxibustion at that time."

Zhang addressed the human spirit in Volume 4 of
the *Illustrated Supplement*. He covered five types calculated by: 1) the eight seasonal markers, 2) the day
of the lunar month, 3) the day stem, 4) the day
branch, and 5) the 12 double-hours. It is odd however, that the five types of human spirit discussed by
Zhang do not include avoiding the umbilicus in the
summer months even though he prohibited moxibustion on Shen Que [Ren 8] at that time. However,
we saw above that the *Great Compendium*, Volume 4
covered the human spirit in the four seasons: in
winter and summer it is located in the lumbar and
umbilicus.

Because so many important books repeated these
prohibitions, it is likely that many or most doctors
respected them.

ZJDC: 4-31-8 Song of Selecting the Blood Branch Day by Month[9] (Huang 1996, 872)
《針灸大成 • 九部人神禁忌歌 • 逐月血支歌 • 卷之四》

You must avoid acupuncture and moxibustion on a
blood branch day.
  First month: *chou* days,
  Second month: *yin* days,
  Third month: the *mao* position,
  Fourth month: *chen* days,
  Fifth month: *si* days,
  Sixth month: on *wu* days,
  Seventh month: *wei* days,
  Eighth month: *shen* days,
  Ninth month: in the *you* region,
  Tenth month: month in *xu* days,
  Eleventh month: *hai* days,
  Twelfth month: it appears on *zi* days.

血支針灸仍須忌，正丑二寅三卯位，四辰五巳六午中
，七未八申九酉部，十月在戌十一亥，十二月於子上
議。

---
[8] This whole passage is almost word-for-word from Li Chan's *Entering the Gate of Medicine*. Zhang did not include it in the *Illustrated Supplement*.
[9] "Branch" refers to the twelve earthly branches. This whole section is almost word-for-word the same as in Li Chan's *Entering the Gate of Medicine*. It is also in Gao Wu's *Gatherings from Eminent Acupuncturists*.

LJTY: 4-17 Blood Avoidance Song (Avoid Acupuncture, Moxibustion, and Pricking to Bleed)

《類經圖翼・卷四・血忌歌》（忌針灸刺血）

Blood avoidance: First month the ox [*chou*];
Second month the sheep [*wei*];
Third should avoid the tiger [*yin*];
Fourth is the monkey's [*shen*] homeland.
Fifth is rabbit [*mao*], sixth is rooster [*you*], both to be feared;
Seventh is dragon [*chen*], eighth is dog [*xu*], these are truly staunch.
Ninth is located in the snake [*si*] palace, tenth is located in *hai*;
Eleventh leans toward disliking the horse's [*wu*] ambush.
In the twelfth month, meet the rat [*zi*] position;
These are called blood avoidance and must be guarded against.

血忌正牛二月羊，三當避虎四猴鄉。五兔六雞皆可畏
，七龍八狗正剛強。
九在蛇宮十在亥，十一偏嫌馬伏藏。十二月中逢鼠位
，是名血忌必須防。

Notes: In Volume 4 of the *Illustrated Supplement*, besides the human spirit, Zhang Jiebin only discussed one other type of day for avoiding treatment: blood avoidance days. These days are calculated differently than the blood branch days (see p. 211), but the concept is similar. In both cases, anything that can cause bleeding is deemed harmful on these days. A doctor would look at the calendar, and in a particular month, he would avoid the prohibited treatments on days belonging to the forbidden branch. Of course, he could use medicinals, massage, or other treatments if they would not cause bleeding.

ZJDC: 4-31-12 Auspicious Days for Acupuncture, Moxibustion & Taking Herbs (Huang 1996, 872)

《針灸大成・九部人神禁忌歌・針灸服藥吉日・卷之四》

Ding mao, geng wu, jia xu, bing zi, ren wu, jia shen, ding hai, xin mao, ren chen, bing shen, wu xu, ji hai, ji wei, geng zi, xin chou, jia chen, yi si, bing wu, wu shen, ren zi, gui chou, yi mao, bing chen, ren wu, bing xu, open days, heavenly doctor, invite peace.[10]

丁卯，庚午，甲戌，丙子，壬午，甲申，丁亥，辛卯
，壬辰，丙申，戊戌，己亥，己未，庚子，辛丑，甲
辰，乙巳，丙午，戊申，壬子，癸丑，乙卯，丙辰，
壬戌，丙戌，開日，天醫，要安。

Notes: These are days that are considered beneficial for medical treatment (if no other prohibition taints them). It includes 25 stem-branch combinations (which repeat every 60 days).

Open days are from a series of 12 days called the "12 on-duty positions" [十二值位]. They were discussed as far back as *Huananzi*, Chapter 3 (Major 1993, 119). The 12 on-duty positions are calculated according to the branch of the month and the branch of the day. Once you calculate the first position, the rest simply follow in order as a series, repeating until the new month begins. This series of days is commonly used in non-medical day selection, but some of the days also have medical implications. Yang did not describe their calculation in the *Great Compendium*. He must have felt that giving the calculation was not necessary as these days are listed in every almanac.

For heavenly doctor and invite peace days, see below.

---

[10] This whole section is similar to one in Li Chan's *Entering the Gate of Medicine*. However, Yang added *yi wei*, the heavenly doctor, and invite peace days. He left out *ding chou, ji wei* and hold [執 *zhi*] days. Volume 6 of the *Great Completion* added open [開 *kai*], achieve [成 *cheng*], and hold [執 *zhi*] days. Open, achieve, and hold days are part of the 12 on-duty positions.

ZJDC: 4-31-13 Days to Avoid Acupuncture-Moxibustion (Huang 1996, 872)

《針灸大成・九部人神禁忌歌・針灸忌日・卷之四》

Xin wei (this is the day of Bian Que's death), white tiger, month repression, month slaughter, and month punishment.[11]

Notes: *Xin wei* is a stem-branch combination.

Yang did not describe the calculation for most of these days in the *Great Compendium*, assuming that the reader had access to this information. Below are tables for determining these days, according to a few different sources.

DAY SELECTION FOR ACUPUNCTURE—MOXIBUSTION			
GOOD FOR ACUPUNCTURE—MOXIBUSTION			
MONTH	HEAVENLY DOCTOR	OPEN DAY	INVITE PEACE
1st	MAO / CHOU	ZI	YIN
2nd	YIN / YIN	CHOU	SHEN
3rd	CHOU / MAO	YIN	MAO
4th	ZI / CHEN	MAO	YOU
5th	HAI / SI	CHEN	CHEN
6th	XU / WU	SI	XU
7th	YOU / WEI	WU	SI
8th	SHEN / SHEN	WEI	HAI
9th	WEI / YOU	SHEN	WU
10th	WU / XU	YOU	ZI
11th	SI / HAI	XU	WEI
12th	CHEN / ZI	HAI	CHOU
SOURCE	GREAT COMPENDIUM AND EMINENT ACUPUNCTURISTS / GREAT COMPLETION	SECRET CANON OF DAY SELECTION KNOWLEDGE[12]	GREAT COMPLETION

---

[11] Li Chan's *Entering the Gate* mentions "*Xin wei* (the day of Bian Que's death)" but does not have the rest. Volume 6 of the *Great Completion* has this whole passage.

[12] (Chen 1993, 111) This is a modern book on day selection. I could not find the calculation for the open day in any medical books of the era. This is probably because the twelve on-duty positions were so common in non-medical day selection, that it was assumed everyone knew how to calculate them.

| | DAY SELECTION FOR ACUPUNCTURE - MOXIBUSTION | | | | |
	AVOID ACUPUNCTURE - MOXIBUSTION				
MONTH	**BLOOD BRANCH**	**WHITE TIGER**	**MONTH REPRESSION**	**MONTH SLAUGHTER**	**MONTH PUNISHMENT**
1ST	CHOU	WU	XU	CHOU	SI
2ND	YIN	SHEN	YOU	XU	ZI
3RD	MAO	XU	SHEN	WEI	CHEN
4TH	CHEN	ZI	WEI	CHEN	SHEN
5TH	SI	YIN	WU	CHOU	WU
6TH	WU	CHEN	SI	XU	CHOU
7TH	WEI	WU	CHEN	WEI	YIN
8TH	SHEN	SHEN	MAO	CHEN	YOU
9TH	YOU	XU	YIN	CHOU	WEI
10TH	XU	ZI	CHOU	XU	HAI
11TH	HAI	YIN	ZI	WEI	MAO
12TH	ZI	CHEN	HAI	CHEN	XU
SOURCE	GREAT COMPENDIUM AND EMINENT ACUPUNCTURISTS	GREAT COMPLETION	EMINENT ACUPUNCTURISTS AND GREAT COMPENDIUM	EMINENT ACUPUNCTURISTS AND GREAT COMPENDIUM	EMINENT ACUPUNCTURISTS

Day selection is a vast topic. The medical books from the Tang through the Ming dynasties are full of many other calculations, mostly prohibitions. If the practitioner did not follow an almanac and calculated them all on his own, it would take a considerable amount of time. Treatment would be totally prohibited on many days, and at other times, certain body parts or specific modalities could not be used.

However, not all doctors followed this reasoning without question. One of Yang Jizhou's case studies

(**ZJDC: 9-36-5**, p. 199) illustrates this. The patient had an acute life-threatening condition, but the day was inauspicious for treatment. Yang did not tell us which type of prohibition was in effect, but he chose to treat the patient anyway; otherwise the patient would have died. While it is not clearly stated, Yang gave the impression that he would have preferred not to violate the prohibition. He did not dispute its validity; he only determined that the patient could not wait until the next day for treatment. In fact, in the last sentence of this case study, Yang warned the patient that if he did not take proper care of himself, the day on which he would have a relapse could be predicted based on the heavenly stems.

While day selection is a fascinating topic, following this line of thought takes us out of range for the topic of moxibustion.

OTHER TREATMENTS INVOLVING CALCULATED CHRONICITY

In addition to day selection and the application of moxibustion to a channel during its open time, other references to calculated chronicity for specific treatments appear in these texts. Below are a few.

In **LJTY: 10-1-6**, on the Four Flowers and Six Points of Master Cui, Zhang wrote, "On all the above six points, it is appropriate to select a *li* [*gua*] day, a fire [*bing* or *ding* stem] day, to apply moxibustion to them." Apparently, Zhang wanted to increase the yang or fire element of the moxibustion by applying it at a time when fire qi was prevalent in the universe.

LJTY: 10-1-2-20 and **ZJDC: 9-6-4** discuss the extraordinary point called *Yao Yan* (Lumbar Eyes), also known as *Gui Yan* (Ghost Eye) point. Both texts recommend moxibustion on this point to be applied on a *gui hai* day. The time should be around midnight according to Zhang or the *hai* double-hour (9-11 PM) according to Yang. In addition, Yang specified that it should be done during the sixth lunar month on this day and time.

Gui hai is the last stem-branch combination in the cycle of 60 before it begins again with *jia zi*. *Gui* and *hai* both correspond to yin water. The *hai* hour on a *gui hai* day would be the last hour of the cycle of

sixty, the moment before the *jia zi* day starts the next cycle of sixty. This time of water phase and ending is strongly associated with yin.

Yang recommended that this treatment take place in the sixth lunar month, associated with the *wei* branch. The sixth month generally overlaps quite a bit with July in the Western calendar. It is the time shortly after the summer solstice, a time when yin begins to creep back into heaven and earth. The sixth month is the last month of summer. It is one of the four months associated with the earth phase and the transition between seasons. Note that a *gui hai* day will not occur every year in the sixth month, as *gui hai* comes only once every 60 days.

Zhang said that the end of the *gui hai* day is when the "six spirits all gather."[13] We often talk about the five spirits, one for each of the five viscera, but what are the six spirits? The gallbladder, an extraordinary bowel as well as a normal bowel, also stores a spirit (Hu 1995, 204). This totals six.[14] Since this point is named Gui Yan (Ghost Eye) point, it is used in special cases when the disease seems unusual: perhaps caused by a ghost, evil spirit, or something supernatural. The word "eye" in the name of the point can also mean an opening or aperture. Perhaps moxibustion on this point opens up an exit route for the ghost. Since the patient's spirits all gather at this time, maybe they are strong enough and can team up to expel the ghost evil through the opening of the moxa sore at the Ghost Eye point. Both Zhang and Yang warn us not to let people know what you are doing. This way the ghost evil does not have a warning, so there is no time for it to hide or protect itself.

Yang Jizhou's *Method of Steaming the Umbilicus to Treat Disease* (**ZJDC: 9-19**) uses nine ingredients ground into a fine powder and placed in the umbilicus. A "coin" of Huai Pi [Sophora Bark] is set on top.

---

[13] Actually, this is a direct quote from Wei Yilin's *Effective Formulas Obtained from Generations of Doctors*.

[14] According to http://www.ttcsec.gov.tw/a01/pp01_c104.htm viewed on 5/12/06, these six are the soul [靈 *ling*], nature or temperament [性 *xing*], spirit [神 *shen*], ideation [意 *yi*], ethereal soul [魂 *hun*], and corporeal soul [魄 *po*]. However, other sites list the six spirits differently. In any case, it is clear that when the six spirits gather, the patient will have a greater ability to throw off the disease, especially if it is caused by a supernatural force.

Then mugwort moxibustion is applied to it.

Yang suggested two ways of timing this special treatment. It could be done on an open day (see the section on day selection, p. 211) to "take in the right qi of heaven and earth and bring it into the five viscera so that no evils can invade, the hundreds of diseases cannot enter, long life can withstand aging, and the spleen-stomach are strong."

The umbilicus is the location in the body where the fetus receives pre-heaven nourishment from the mother. Here Yang uses the umbilicus in a similar way to nourish life. The use of an open day is likely intended to help "open" the umbilicus so that the qi of heaven and earth can enter more easily.

The second suggestion for when to apply this treatment is a little more complicated. Yamg prescribes a specific time for each of the eight seasonal markers in the table below.

Because these are the seasonal markers, Yang said, "This combines the right qi of the four seasons."

Besides the obvious benefit of insuring that the treatment will occur eight times evenly spaced throughout the year, there are other factors. Why are these particular times chosen on these days? I believe it is associated with a relationship of the earthly branches called the "six combinations" (六合). Note that when Yang said, "This combines the right qi of the four seasons," the word "combine" is a translation of 合 *he2*, the same as the name of this branch relationship.

Branches that are related by the six combinations tend to be harmonious and beneficial to each other, and when they combine in this way, they are able to mutually produce another element. When the branches are arranged in a circle, the six combinations are found across from each other like this:

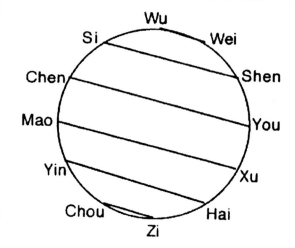

	Date		Time	
Seasonal Marker	**Approximate Date in Western Calender**		**Branch**	**Hour**
Spring begins	February 4 (first month, *yin* branch)		*si*	9-11AM
Spring equinox	March 21 (second month, *mao* branch)		*wei*	1-3AM
Summer begins	May 5 (fourth month, *si* branch)		*chen*	7-9AM
Summer solstice	June 22 (fifth month, *wu* branch)		*you*	5-7AM
Autumn begins	August 8 (seventh month, *shen* branch)		*xu*	7-9AM
Autumnal equinox	September 22 (eighth month, *you* branch)		*wu*	11a-1PM
Winter begins	November 7 (tenth month, *hai* branch)		*hai*	9-11PM
Winter solstice	December 22 (eleventh month, *zi* branch)		*yin*	3-5AM

The pattern of the six combinations can also be seen using a diagram of the 12 palaces:

si	wu	wei	shen
chen			you
mao			xu
yin	chou	zi	hai

When the pairs of branches are able to combine, they produce another phase, as follows:

THE SIX COMBINATIONS		
BRANCHES	COMBINE	TO MAKE
Chou	Zi	Earth
Yin	Hai	Wood
Mao	Xu	Fire
Chen	You	Metal
Si	Shen	Water
Wu	Wei	Fire

With this background,[15] we can now examine Yang's treatment schedule.

Summer begins and the summer solstice are given the *chen* and *you* hours for treatment. These two branches combine to make metal.

Winter begins and the winter solstice use *hai* and *yin* hours. These two combine to make wood.

The elements produced by the combinations of winter and summer have a curious aspect in the graph at the bottom of the page.

Metal gives downbearing to the yang, while wood promotes upbearing of the yin. This helps keep qi circulating as a unified system. If not, yin and yang could separate, allowing yang to float upward and yin to sink down.

The treatment times for the spring and autumn equinoxes are *wei* and *wu* respectively. These two combine to make fire.

The last two are problematic. The treatment times for spring begins and autumn begins are *si* and *xu*. These two do not make up a combination. I wonder if autumn begins should have used the *shen* hour. Then *si* and *shen* would combine to make water. In this way all four of the outer phases would be used in one of the combinations. The only phase missing is earth, the center, which corresponds to the umbilicus, the site of the treatment.

Obviously this explanation is flawed. However, I have not been able to uncover any other way to explain the timing of treatment.

YANG			YIN		
Phase of jing well points of the yang channels			Phase of jing well points of the yin channels		
Phase of the yang channel used in the four gates (He Gu L 14)	metal		Phase of the yin channel used in the four gates (Tai Chong LV 3)	wood	
Phase of the combination for the most yang season (summer)			Phase of the combination for the most yin season (winter)		

---

[15] The background information on the six combinations is standard information in the beginning chapter of any book on Chinese astrology, *Feng Shui*, or *Yi Jing* calculations. For reference, I cite *Essentials of Calculation Skills* (Bai 1996, 14-15).

In any case, during the Ming dynasty, doctors advocated applying the various cycles of time to the treatment of patients. Most modern doctors do not seem to give timing a lot of consideration. This is an area where Western-style research could be useful in determining whether the timing affects the therapeutic effects.

CHAPTER 14
MAGICAL MOXIBUSTION

Chapter Contents

Chinese medicine has always incorporated aspects of magic, the supernatural, divination, and religion. The ancient kings who divined through the oracle bones attributed toothaches and other ailments to the curse of an ancestor. The Mawangdui medical manuscripts are full of magic. The *Inner Canon* has very little, but it can be found; for example, the *tai yi* wind oracle in *Magic Pivot* Chapters 77 and 79 relies on a type of epidemiological divination based on the direction of the wind on certain days. Unschuld (1985 & 2003) has documented all this.

Since ancient times, authors have included, in greater or lesser amounts, writings on magic. This continued through the late Qing dynasty, when the movement to modernize medicine gained impetus. Wang Qingren is one example of a Qing doctor who wanted to modernize. The trend continued until 1949, when the current government of China took control of medical education. At that point, anything with the least scent of magic became completely forbidden (Fruehauf, 1999). This is even evident in Zhang Jiebin's writings. One edition I have was censored in several places containing medical magic (Zhang 1996, pages 331, 335-336, 343, for example).

However, at the end of the Ming dynasty, even the writings of the most literate doctors still acknowledged the influence of the supernatural. We will examine this sort of passage in the writings of Zhang, Li, and Yang.

According to Gordon (1970, 32), there are four kinds of magic:

- **Imitative (or image) magic:** things that are alike influence each other in some way. For example, a shaman dances until sweat falls like rain to make rain fall from the sky.
- **Contagious magic:** things once related or in contact with each other continue to be linked to each other. This is why hair, fingernails, or even a person's name can be used in black magic to harm a person.
- **Sequential magic:** one event causes another. For example, a Western superstition is that breaking a mirror brings seven years of bad luck.
- **Divination:** telling the future by using omens, oracles, etc.

The first three types can be used to cause harm (black magic) or to enact a remedy (white magic). In medicine, only white magic is used. With this background, let's look at the medical magic described by Zhang, Yang, and Li.

EXAMPLES OF MAGICAL MOXIBUSTION

LJTY: 11-3-17 discusses the application of moxibustion for lumbar pain. A bamboo pole is used to measure from the ground to the center of the umbilicus on a standing patient. The pole is marked, and then used to find the same height on the spine. Moxibustion is applied on that spot, but also to the end of the bamboo pole without anyone knowing that the doctor does it. Although this passage originally came from Sun's *Prescriptions* (Sun 1994, a275), Zhang did not need to pass it on unless he felt it had some merit. Perhaps the magic is in the image. Bamboo grows in segments that can resemble the vertebral column. Bamboo grows straight, strong, and flexible, like the back should be. In addition, this could be contagious magic, as it is marked to the height of the patient's umbilicus and has been in contact with his body.

BCGM: 38-42 discusses the scrapings from an arrow, made into cones and used for moxibustion to treat damage from a splinter or thorn. This is imitative magic, as the arrow has a resonance with the sharpness of the splinter or the thorn.

LJTY: 11-3-24 contains a treatment for rabid dog bites. Zhang tells us an unnamed source recommends using three people with different surnames to apply moxibustion to the site of the bite. It must be that the toxins are so potent, it is better to make sure no one person or family has too much exposure to them. This admonition was also used by Sun Simiao in the treatment of cold impediment in the legs and knees in *Supplement*, Volume 28 (Sun 1994, b262). This is contagious magic. The evil is so strong that it is magically contagious to the person who administers treatment. Since the person who applies moxibustion needs to touch the patient, the evil needs to be dispersed into a few different people

or families, rather than be concentrated into one.

In **LJTY: 11-3-4**, Zhang recommended using the *Lotus Sutra* and chanting a Buddhist mantra to aid in the treatment of corpse-transmitted consumption, a serious condition associated at the time with worms or bugs. Worms or bugs are also the etiology in the conditions treated by lumbar eyes (**LJTY: 10-1-2-20**), which also has aspects of medical magic according to Zhang and Yang. (See above for discussion of Yao Yan [Lumbar Eyes].) Worms or bugs were often seen as going beyond what is natural. They need an extra powerful treatment, incorporating the help of a mantra or special timing. Purely natural medicine may not be potent enough to cure this type of patient. Bugs and worms were considered an etiology of illness (sometimes natural, sometimes demonic) since the times of the Mawangdui manuscripts and before (Unschuld 2003, 180; Harper 1998, 74).

GHOST EVILS

LJTY: 11-3-20 discusses evil spirits [邪祟 xiesui]. Some of it is based on the two *Lost Chapters of Elementary Questions* (Chapters 72 and 73, see above for details). Here, vacuity of each of the five viscera causes the person to see ghosts of the color associated with the element that controls the affected organ. For example, a patient with lung vacuity sees red corpse ghosts. Red corresponds to fire, which melts the metal of the lungs. The treatment generally uses acupuncture on the associated back transport point. It often also includes the *yuan* source point of the paired yang channel. In the example of the lungs, Fei Shu (UB 13) and He Gu (LI 4) were recommended for needling. While the disease is supernatural, the treatment is not. We could even debate the supernatural nature of the disease. It is not clear that the ghost exists; the patient may only see the hallucination of a ghost (See Unschuld 1985, 220-221, 332-333).

Other points to treat ghosts include Thumbnail and Big Toenail Points (**LJTY: 10-1-4-32**), which are two of Sun Simiao's Ghost Points. They are related to Qin

Chengzu's "ghost moxibustion," also called the "Ghost Crying Points." Yang discussed the ghost crying points in **ZJDC: 9-6-1**. The patient's two thumbs are bound together side by side. A moxa cone is placed so it touches the nails and skin on both thumbs at the same time. When the cone is lit, the ghost is actually supposed to speak through the person and say that it is going.

This is more clearly an exorcistic treatment. Here the ghost is perceived as real, since it can speak through the patient. These points are in the region of Gui Xin or Shao Shang (LU 11) and Gui Lei or Yin Bai (SP 1), both *jing* well points. *Magic Pivot*, Chapter 1 says that *jing* well points are where qi *exits* or *comes out* (氣出). This is often interpreted as meaning it is where qi begins flowing in the channel, but that is not the only way to understand this phrase. Bleeding the *jing* well points is used to make evil qi exit the body. Moxa sores make an opening that allow the evil to leave as well. Yang said in **ZJDC: 9-33**, "If perchance the moxa sore opening closes easily, the diseased qi is unable to exit." In **9-34**, he added that the medicinal wash "allows the expulsion of wind evils, exiting from the opening of the sore." The binding of the thumbs or big toes immobilizes the ghost. The yang of the mugwort and fire expels the yin ghost evil through the opening of the *jing* well points.[1]

MOXA ROLLS AND PEACH BRANCHES

Both Li and Zhang included the moxa roll under the same heading as the peach branch (**JYQS: 51-54** Thunder Fire Needle and **BCGM: 06-07** Fire from a Miraculous Needle). They were discussed together as both were imbued with special powers of healing.

Daoist incantations are also prescribed by both Zhang and Yang to be used while applying the thunder fire needle in **ZJDC: 9-18** and **JYQS: 51-54**. Zhang's incantation is recited three times and used with an east-growing peach branch picked on the fifth day of the fifth lunar month. Yang's incantation is used with the moxa roll and is chanted nine times. The mantra mentioned earlier for corpse-transmitted consumption is Buddhist, but these are Daoist.

In addition, Yang warned, "While engaged in this, it is important that you are sincere and respectful. Do not let women, chickens, or dogs see. This formula is completely genuine and has often been self-kept as a secret, because people have not followed the principles of the ancients. If your heart is not united with the *dao*, the treatment will not easily bring about a cure." This shows the reverence Yang felt for the healing power of the moxa roll.

Li Shizhen did not use magic in the description of his moxa roll, but he did when discussing peach in **BCGM: 06-07** and **BCGM: 29-06**. He said peach treats "evil ghost malignity stroke… demonic influx and visiting hostility… resolves gu toxins, prevents epidemic pestilence… and kills all worms in sores." In **BCGM: 29-06**, Li discussed various parts of the peach tree. He often specified the east-growing branch for decoctions that are used as a wash. In **29-06-8-6**, Li quoted the recommendation from Sun's *Prescriptions* to carve such a branch into a human figure and attach it to the patient's clothes for amnesia due to a debilitated heart. In **29-06-8-2**, Li repeated a formula for jaundice using peach. In it, he said, "Do not let chickens, women, and dogs see." This same admonition was found in Yang's recipe for making moxa rolls.

Peach was thought to have special properties. It had the ability to protect against ghosts and demons, so talismans were often made of peach wood (a practice which continues to the present). The fruit also symbolizes long life, and therefore may have a protective

---

[1] In bleeding the *jing* well points, the yin blood expels the yang evil of wind or fire. This is the opposite side of the same coin. Ghosts are yin evils and are expelled by the yang of mugwort fire through the moxa sore opening.

effect on health. Peach symbolizes the third month of the year, the time around the vernal equinox, and a time associated with the east, when yang is growing (Eberhard 1986, 227-9).

The gathering of medicinals such as peach branches or mugwort on special days has already been discussed in Chapter 13 on timing. Both are to be picked on the fifth day of the fifth lunar month. Beyond this, the form can also be important. Special powers accumulate in an east-growing peach branch, a branch carved into a human figure, or the mugwort in the shape of a man which is hung over the doorway (**BCGM: 15-05**). Mugwort such as this "can

exorcise toxin qi… mugwort treats all ghosts and malign qi." Once again, the strength of yang coming from the time of gathering or the eastward growth is useful to fight against yin evils such as ghosts and spirits. The shape of a man is image magic, helping to direct the healing powers into the human body.

Through these examples, it is apparent that magic was still a part of the medicine practiced by the literati and intelligentsia of the Ming dynasty. It is also obvious that this was only a small part of their medical practice. The vast majority of the material from these authors deals with natural medicine.

PART 3
CONCLUSION

CONCLUSION

After reviewing the information from these three Ming dynasty masters of moxibustion, there is still much that can be discussed. Two issues will be given priority here. In China, in the past and even in the present, moxibustion has been used in many conditions where most practitioners in the West today would not. The Chinese see a broader scope of functions for moxibustion than most Western practitioners do. Is moxibustion limited to warming, moving, and supplementing? What other functions did the ancients attribute to moxibustion and what are the mechanisms of these neglected functions? I will also discuss the relevancy today of these varied moxibustion techniques. In this age of lawsuits, predominance of Western medicine, and advanced knowledge about transmission of infection, can we expand the scope of moxibustion in our treatments? What aspects of the past are clinically relevant in the West today?

WHAT ARE THE MECHANISMS OF MOXIBUSTION TREATMENT?

The ancient books described types of moxibustion treatment that are not commonly used in the West.

Do we have a better understanding of what works now or have we lost something? Today, it is most commonly said that moxibustion warms coldness, moves qi-blood, and supplements qi-blood and yang. For example, *Chinese Acupuncture and Moxibustion* (Cheng 1987, 340) lists only the most obvious functions of moxibustion:

- warming the channels and expelling cold;
- inducing the smooth flow of qi-blood;
- strengthening yang from collapse; and
- preventing disease and keeping healthy.

The reasoning behind these four functions is as follows:

Moxibustion is warming because the nature of mugwort is warm and because moxibustion involves fire.

Moxibustion moves qi-blood because mugwort, being acrid and warm, also does so when used internally and because the heat of mugwort fire speeds up movement.

Moxibustion can strengthen yang when it is collapsing because of its warm and supplementing nature.

Even though mugwort taken internally does not supplement, it is generally agreed that it can when applied as moxibustion to points like Zu San Li (ST 36), Guan Yuan (Ren 4), or Qi Hai (Ren 6). This is due to the nature of these specific points, plus the vague idea of adding qi to the body through the heat of mugwort fire. In this way, it can keep people strong and healthy.

It is easy to imagine moxibustion supplementing qi and yang, since it is warm. Yet it is generally acknowledged that moxibustion on certain points can also nourish blood. Perhaps, this is because mugwort has an affinity for the blood and because many people with blood vacuity retain some coldness within their body. Or perhaps, because it supplements post-heaven qi when applied to points like Zu San Li (ST 36), the body is also able to generate more blood.

Today, it is rarely said that moxibustion can nourish yin; modern doctors worry that it is too hot and drying for yin vacuity. It is also rarely used for repletion, except repletion cold or stagnation of qi and stasis of blood.

This is a very limited, mechanical, and materialistic point of view. It is based in part on assuming that the fire used in moxibustion will cause heat in the body. But if fire always causes heat, would we decoct medicinals that are used to clear heat? Would the effect of a heat-clearing formula be improved by drinking it cold from the refrigerator? Obviously, the answer is no. Why do we apply this idea to moxibustion but not medicinal formulas?

Another reason for the limited view on moxibustion is based on the idea that mugwort moxibustion has more or less the same functions as mugwort taken internally. As seen in **BCGM: 15-05** and **ZJDC: 9-23** (in the discussion of mugwort in Chapter 8), no less an authority than Zhu Danxi stated that the functions of mugwort differ when applied as moxibustion than when used internally.

Classically, we find that moxibustion was used to:

- prevent disease or prevent progression of disease;
- nourish life (which goes beyond simply preventing disease);
- supplement all aspects of the body (including yin);
- expel evils (including heat);
- descend what has risen;
- raise what has fallen; and
- circulate where there is stagnation, stasis, or depression (even depressed heat).

It is true that some of these extended uses involve specific techniques and the selection of special moxibustion points (whether channel or non-channel points). The number of cones and length of treatment is also important.

First let us differentiate and give an overview of some of the above terms:

- *Nourish life:* When there is no disease, moxibustion is applied to increase longevity or vitality and prevent the effects of aging. This is often done at specific times of the year.
- *Supplement:* Supplementation (unlike nourishing life) implies that there is already a vacuity. Techniques to supplement are related, but not identical to techniques for nourishing life. Supplementation is sometimes used to rescue a patient in emergency conditions of extreme vacuity.
- *Prevent disease:* These techniques are sometimes, but not always, related to supplementation of right qi. They may be done when traveling or when certain diseases are prevalent. They are applied when no disease exists in the body.
- *Prevent progression of disease:* The body already has disease so moxibustion is performed to prevent it from worsening; for example, to prevent wind stroke in a patient who already has internal wind.
- *Expel evils:* Disease already exists but is made to exit the body through the moxa sores, which are exit gates, and through the outward radiating action of heat.

- *Circulate stagnation:* Moxibustion can move qi-blood through the channel system, thereby increasing circulation. Through circulation even heat accumulation in an area can be dissipated.
- *Descend what has risen:* Moxibustion can drain repletion down from the upper body. Often, there is repletion above and vacuity below, so once qi circulates, it will even out in all parts of the body. This is also important when moxibustion has been used on the upper body to prevent side effects such as accumulation of heat above.
- *Raise what has fallen:* This goes beyond the mechanism of heat rising. Otherwise, moxibustion on Bai Hui (Du 20) could not raise prolapsed. If the heat applied to Bai Hui rose up, it would not even enter the body.

In fact, it seems that moxibustion (or specific techniques on certain points) attracts qi toward the site where it is applied. That is why moxibustion on points of the upper body raises qi, and moxibustion on points of the lower body descends qi. It is also how moxibustion expels evils; it can attract the evil qi to it and then radiate the evil out of the body.

Let us examine some of the above ideas through the writings of these three masters. Yang Jizhou, Li Shizhen, and Zhang Jiebin never wrote chapters discussing the mechanisms of moxibustion. However, they left a number of clues throughout their writings. Many of these statements are quoted from earlier sources, but their inclusion suggests agreement.

Moxibustion descends qi & treats heat conditions:

BCGM: 15-05 says:

Zhu Zhenheng says: "Some do not know that the nature of mugwort is extremely hot. When it enters the patient through the fire of moxibustion, its qi moves downward. When it enters the patient through medicinals, its qi moves upward."[1]

This statement clearly shows that mugwort used for moxibustion has different effects than mugwort used internally. We cannot simply read the materia medica for mugwort and understand the mechanisms of moxibustion. It is also likely that the functions of other medicinals, such as ginger, garlic, and Fu Zi (Aconite) are somewhat changed when used as an isolating substance or when powdered medicinals are mixed in with the mugwort. We must regard the functions of moxibustion as somewhat different from the functions of the same substances when taken internally.

Going back to Zhu's statement that the qi of mugwort moves downward when used as moxibustion, we can conclude that this is one reason the ancients used moxibustion with confidence in heat conditions. The downward movement of the qi of mugwort fire helps counteract the upward movement of heat or fire evils within the body.

Certainly caution is needed when applying moxibustion. Many sources warn about its over-application to the upper body and head. **ZJDC: 9-27** discusses the number of cones: "Whenever applying moxibustion to the head and nape, stop at seven cones or stop when up to seven times seven cones are accumulated." **ZJDC: 9-25** says, "If you apply a lot of moxibustion to the head, it makes the person lose essence-spirit."

Perhaps we can use the image of the heating system in a house. If the heating vents are located near the ceiling, the air in that region becomes very hot, but it does not circulate. The feet of the occupants remain cold, yet if they raise their hands near the ceiling, they can feel the heat above them. When the vents are near the floor, the rising hot air will circulate and the whole room will have a more even

---

[1] This statement and the discrepancy between **BCGM: 15-05** and **ZJDC: 9-23** have been discussed in detail after **BCGM: 15-05** in the section on the translations of mugwort.

temperature through convection. Like this, we need the body's qi to circulate so we don't end up with a heat repletion above.

However, if we need to apply moxibustion to the upper body or head, there are ways to prevent this accumulation of heat from occurring. **ZJDC: 9-29** and **LJTY: 11-2-4** discuss the order of applying moxa cones. You always began at the top and work your way down, to help draw the fire qi down and make it circulate. In the discussion of Gao Huang Shu (UB 43), **ZJDC: 9-8** warns, "If the patient feels congestion and fullness after applying moxibustion, you can apply moxibustion to Qi Hai [Ren 6] and Zu San Li [ST 36] to drain down fire repletion." **LJTY: 4-27-4**, **6-3-36**, and **7-1-35** also mention the ability of moxibustion on Zu San Li (ST 36) to descend qi.

So it seems that Zhu's statement, "When the qi of mugwort enters the patient through the fire of moxibustion, its qi moves downward" is really for moxibustion applied to points of the lower body and legs.

Moxibustion attracts qi:

Moxibustion fire attracts qi, even hot qi. Applying moxibustion below draws fire repletion down from above as we have just seen.

Moxibustion can also raise falling qi by attracting it back up. **LJTY: 11-3-19-13** discusses prolapse of the rectum. It says Bai Hui (Du 20) "is like the drawstring of the yang vessels, uniting the body's yang qi. Whenever there is prolapse of the rectum, it is always because of the downward fall of yang qi. The *Classic* says, 'Raise what is descending.' That is why you should borrow the power of fire in order to lift the downward fall of qi." **LJTY: 11-3-14** also uses three cones of moxibustion on Bai Hui (Du 20) for enduring diarrhea from downward fall of qi.

Moxibustion scatters and vents evils and toxins:

Moxibustion can lure an evil out from inside the body. It scatters toxins, stagnation, and depressed evils, especially when these cause sores and abscesses. **LJTY: 10-1-7** explains the mechanism of the Bamboo Horse Point: "Abscesses are always toxins from retained and stagnant heart fire. When moxibustion is applied to this point, heart fire flows freely and the toxins scatter." **LJTY: 11-3-23** discusses eruptions on the back: "When not yet ulcerated, it must be that moxibustion is able to draw out and scatter the depressed toxins." **JYQS: 46-11** makes a similar statement: "If the sore has not ulcerated, steaming or moxibustion draws and leads out depressed toxins... Use mugwort cones for the power of fire which is able to thrust outward." **JYQS: 64-115** describes the treatment of pox, abscesses, and toxic sores: "The toxins follow the fire and scatter. This is a co-acting treatment method[2] of attacking and scattering depressed toxins. It has the great effect of returning the patient to life." **LJTY: 11-3-24** says, "Whenever there are snake, scorpion, or centipede bites... quickly apply moxibustion to the site of the bite using mugwort fire. This draws out and scatters the venom qi, promptly quieting the situation."

However, moxibustion does more than scatter evils in toxic sores. **JYQS: 23-1-5** says regarding accumulations and gatherings, "When the power of fire arrives, the qi of the hard gathering will naturally gradually resolve and scatter." Moxibustion on Bai Hui (Du 20) can even vent yang repletion. It is used in **LJTY: 11-3-1** for arched-back rigidity; **LJTY: 11-3-3** and **11-3-15** for mania or epilepsy; **LJTY: 11-3-18** for head wind; and **LJTY: 11-3-22** for fright wind. When draining moxibustion technique is applied, it can let the repletion vent out, like the valve on a pressure cooker.

---

[2]   A co-acting treatment method is using a like thing, instead of the opposite.

Special techniques and formulas were developed to help moxibustion scatter evils. **JYQS: 64-122** explains Zhang's *Formula of the Immortals for Fuming and Radiating*. Medicinals are ground up and mixed together, then rolled in paper and used like a moxa stick:

> Light it and burn it over the sores. It must be about a half *cun* away from the sores. From outside the sore's red halo, circle around slowly, slowly radiating [the heat and qi] in order to gradually take [this heat and qi] of the roll into the opening of the sore. This is what is called 'from the outside inward.' Further, you must suddenly lift the twisted section towards the outside in order to conduct the toxic qi out. This is the manipulation. The qi of the medicinals effuses upward from the fire end of the twist; when it penetrates into the sore, the toxins follow the qi and scatter, so they do not spontaneously invade the organs internally.

The twist is circled inwardly to help the qi penetrate into the sore and then suddenly lifted to grab the toxic qi and pull it out. This also illustrates the previous action of moxibustion attracting qi.

Moxibustion can make qi penetrate into the body or extend in all directions:

As we saw above, moxibustion can disperse evils, either by drawing them out or by scattering them. Scattering is one type of extending movement. The cones must be big enough to do this: **ZJDC: 9-25** says, "You should make the base of the cone three *fen* wide. If it is not three *fen*, the fire qi will not extend and you will not be able to cure the disease."

As for penetrating, if the evils are deep, the moxibustion must be able to reach in and grab them. **LJTY: 11-3-23** discusses eruptions on the back: "The person performing moxibustion must make the fire qi extend straight into the site of the toxins." In **BCGM: 06-07**, Li reveals his miraculous needle moxa roll. He said "Whenever there is dull pain in sinews and bones, use the miraculous needle on it. The fire qi

will directly extend into the diseased place." Later he added, "The hot qi enters directly into the diseased site." Medicinals such as musk were added into moxa rolls to help with this penetration. That is why Li claimed his miraculous needle could even treat pain in the bones. In fact, moxa rolls, peach twigs, and mulberry twigs were all called "needles" because they were used to make the effects penetrate more deeply, like an acupuncture needle.

Moxibustion can supplement or drain:

We are accustomed to the idea that moxibustion can be used to supplement, but it seems few modern practitioners remember the guidance of *Magic Pivot*, Chapter 51 which tells us that moxibustion can also be used to drain and gives techniques for both: "To use fire for supplementation, do not blow on the fire. You must wait for the fire to extinguish itself. Then press the point. To use fire to drain, quickly blow on the fire and leave the point open" (as stated in **ZJDC: 9-24**).

To supplement, let the cone burn itself out on the skin, but without making the fire overly bright and quick. You want the qi to penetrate, not to escape, so you close the hole. This will make a moxa sore as fire touches the flesh. But the flesh corresponds to spleen earth, and fire supplements earth. Spleen earth is also the root of post-heaven qi for the whole body. One of the most commonly-used points for supplementation is Zu San Li (ST 36), the earth point on the earth channel that shares the function of supplementing post-heaven qi. Supplementation using moxibustion is also common on points such as Guan Yuan (Ren 4) and Qi Hai (Ren 6), both associated with the lower *dan tian* and pre-heaven qi.

The directions from *Magic Pivot*, Chapter 51 were given in the context of the back-transport points, so this technique can also be used to target a specific organ through the 12 transport points.

In discussing the ability of moxibustion to scatter evils, we saw how it is used for eruptions on the back. However, sometimes eruptions do not heal and become chronic ulcers. This is usually due to insufficient qi and yang, which holds things closed (for example, the "pores" and the lower orifices). Moxibustion can also be used to supplement in this type of case. **LJTY: 11-3-23** says: "When sores have already ulcerated, moxibustion is able to supplement and receive yang qi; it easily promotes contraction." **JYQS: 46-11** has a similar statement: "When it has already ulcerated, steaming or moxibustion joins and supplements yang qi, and dispels and scatters cold evils. The opening of the sore will spontaneously close."

As for repletion, "To use fire to drain, quickly blow on the fire and leave the point open." This makes the mugwort fire burn more brightly so it can radiate outward, and the ensuing moxa sore is left open as an escape route for the evil. **JYQS: 46-11** says, "Moxibustion makes toxin qi discharge to the exterior. This is like a thief entering a household. You must open the gate to expel him. If not, he can enter the house and do harm."

This brings us to a discussion of moxa sores.

How do moxa sores benefit the body?

The most obvious answer is that when moxibustion causes a blister and a sore to develop, the intensity of treatment must be stronger than one that only leaves redness and a feeling of warmth. In addition, since a moxa sore can take a few weeks to a month to heal, one moxibustion treatment can give continuous stimulation to a point for an extended period of time. When we compare this to a patient that gets moxibustion once a week and only to the point of redness and warmth, we know there is a big difference in the "dosage."

It is apparent that ancient doctors felt moxa sores were necessary for effective treatment. Yang said, "When you are touched by mugwort, sores erupt. What the mugwort affects is promptly healed. If sores do not erupt, the disease does not recover" (**ZJDC: 9-31**). In fact, Yang thought the moxa sores

should suppurate and that this process is important for treating the root. "The ancients did not apply a medicinal paste to moxibustion sores. They thought it was important to get a lot of pus to come out in order to eliminate the disease… Modern people often … want quick recovery. This is not the idea of treating the root of the disease… If medicinal paste is applied, there is no decay… If the paste is quickly changed, there will be quick recovery of the moxa sores, and it is possible that the disease root is not entirely eliminated." **ZJDC: 9-32**

How can moxa sores eliminate a disease? In **ZJDC: 9-35**, Yang wrote, "Mugwort fire expels diseased qi." The sore is an exit route. The following has further insight in Yang's discussion of a medicinal ointment and a medicinal wash for moxa sores:

> This method uses a warm decoction of red-skinned scallions and Bo He [Herba Menthae Haplocalycis] to wash around the sores for about as long as a double-hour. It allows the expulsion of wind evils, exiting from the opening of the sore. In addition, it allows smooth going and coming inside the channels and vessels so recovery is naturally quick. **ZJDC: 9-34**

This decoction uses two medicinals that release the exterior and expel wind. Yang's image is of the wind actually being expelled through the opening of the sores. Since both medicinals are acrid, they also help to regulate qi-blood in the region. When qi and blood are regulated, wind evils cannot exist.

In **ZJDC: 9-33**, Yang gave a formula for an ointment, stating that it is the only one that can counteract the pathocondition. He repeated his earlier contention that "If perchance the moxa sore-opening closes easily, the disease qi is unable to exit." The moxa sores are a site where the disease qi can be expelled from the body. This action resembles expelling a wind evil by opening the 'pores' and inducing sweating. The difference is that moxa sores can be used for diseases that are deeper in the body since acu-moxa points connect to the interior through the channel system.

In this ointment, Yang also used medicinals that release the exterior, such as Bai Zhi (Radix Angelicae Dahuricae), Bo He (Herba Menthae Hapolcalycis), and Cong Bai (Bulbus Alli Fistulosi) along with medicinals to move the blood, such as Ru Xiang (Olibanum), Dang Gui (Radix Angelicae Sinensis), and Chuan Xiong (Rhizoma Chuanxiong). He also used a few cooling medicinals, including Dan Zhu Ye (Folium Bambusae) and Huang Lian (Rhizoma Coptidis). The moving medicinals are likely to have the dual purpose of regulating the blood so evils cannot linger and also to aid in healing the moxa sore without pain or permanent damage to the flesh.

If the body's defense qi is insufficient, it is unable to expel external evils through the "pores." In a similar way, "There is also the possibility that blood and qi are debilitated. Therefore, the sores do not erupt.

Take Si Wu Tang [Four Agents Decoction] to enrich and nourish blood and qi" (**ZJDC: 9-31**). The body must be strong enough to react to the moxibustion treatment for healing to occur. This is also why Yang gave many guidelines for self-care after moxibustion in **ZJDC: 9-35**. It becomes obvious that the body is not passively healed by moxibustion; moxibustion gives the body what it needs to heal itself.

Although I have not discussed every possible action of moxibustion, it is apparent that its mechanisms are complex and it can be used flexibly to bring healing to many types of conditions. Here is a summary of techniques to achieve various functions with moxibustion. They are taken both from the translations and the modern research. Keep in mind that all the techniques involve selecting appropriate acu-moxa points. (See the chart below.)

FUNCTION	TECHNIQUE
Supplement	direct moxibustion, let the cone burn down on its own, close the point
Drain	direct moxibustion, blow on the cone to increase the fire, do not close the point
Warm the interior (including sinews and bones)	use an isolating substance such as aconite, or use a moxa roll with penetrating medicinals (such as musk) and the sparrow pecking technique
Expel wind (including internal wind)	direct moxibustion to make an exit sore, use a wash of wind-expelling medicinals such as scallions and mint
Sores with heat and toxins	use an isolating substance such as garlic (if there is pain apply moxibustion until there is no pain; if there is no pain, apply moxibustion until there is pain), or use a moxa roll with a technique of circling inward to grab the evil qi and suddenly lifting up to extract it
Attract qi up	supplementation technique on Bai Hui (Du 20)
Attract qi down when there is repletion above	draining technique on appropriate points of the lower body, also on Fu Zi (Radix Lateralis Praeparata Aconiti) and isolated moxibustion or plasters on Yong Quan (KI 1)
Vent qi out when there is repletion above	draining technique on Bai Hui (Du 20)
Benefit the joints	warm needle on local points
Benefit pre-heaven qi in many diseases	plaster or moxibustion on Shen Que (Ren 8)
Prevent repletion when using moxibustion on the head or upper body	moxibustion on points on the lower body, such as Guan Yuan (Ren 4) or Zu San Li (ST 36), applied at the end of the treatment
Nourish life	frequent moxibustion with supplementation technique on points such as Qi Hai (Ren 6), Guan Yuan (Ren 4), or Zu San Li (ST 36)
Prevent disease	make a moxa sore on an appropriate point, *e.g.*, Zu San Li (ST 36), Jue Gu (GB 39), Feng Men (UB 12)

"When yang is generated, yin is also generated."

Moxibustion is used to treat or prevent disease and to nourish life. It is used to raise or lower qi, to drain or supplement, to penetrate inward or to draw out evils, to fortify yang or to nourish yin. What could the mechanism be? How can moxibustion be effective in treating so many types of disease patterns?

It seems obvious that yang is at the root of moxibustion. Its application uses fire, the nature of mugwort is warm, and it is picked on the fifth day of the fifth lunar month which is one of the most yang days of the year. It is used with other warming medicinals: ginger, *Fu Zi* (Radix Lateralis Praeparata Aconiti), garlic, *She Xiang* (Secretio Moschi), etc. Li Shizhen wrote that mugwort floss is pure yang (**BCGM: 15-05-1**). The mechanism of all its functions must be based on yang.

Since moxibustion is yang, it is easy to see how it can warm whatever is cold and move qi-blood. It makes sense that it can supplement yang and qi (which is a part of yang). But what about nourishing yin and blood?

We can discuss this from a macro level, the level of the big *tai ji* (heaven and earth). Moxa on the lower body (below the navel or on the legs) has the image of *tai gua* (gua 11 泰, peace) or *ji ji* (gua 63 既濟, already complete). *Tai* consists of earth (*kun*) over heaven (*qian*). *Ji ji* has water (*kan*) over fire (*li*). Both have the yang *gua* below and the yin *gua* above. In this way, yin descends to meet yang which is ascending. This is a relationship of interaction, of circulation. It brings to mind convection, or the evaporation of water from the ocean (due to the heat/yang

of the sun) so that clouds can form above, and rain can return the water to the ocean. Once heaven and earth communicate, how can any imbalance remain?

This concept has been applied on the level of the small *tai ji* (i.e., the human body) since the earliest times. Laozi wrote, "The sage keeps order by emptying his heart and filling his abdomen" *Dao De Jing*, Chapter 3.[3] The Mawangdui medical manuscripts state, "The sage cools his head and warms his feet" *Model of the Vessels*.[4]

The application of yang moxibustion below initiates circulation of qi: heat rises, beginning the communication between the upper and the lower. You can say that communication between yin and yang, above and below, is more important than the absolute levels of yin and yang. Once the *tai ji* moves, yin and yang regulate themselves.

Zhu Danxi, the master of nourishing yin, gave us a clue in his statement: "Great disease with vacuity desertion is rooted in yin vacuity. Use mugwort moxibustion on the *Dan Tian* (Cinnabar Field). This is done to supplement yang, because when yang is generated, yin is also generated."[5] The idea that "when yang is generated, yin is also generated" comes from *Elementary Questions*, Chapter 5.[6]

Other statements from *Elementary Questions*, Chapter 5 remind us that yin is treated through yang:

"Guide yin from yang" *Elementary Questions*, Chapter 5.[7]
"When yin is diseased, treat yang" *Elementary Questions*, Chapter 5.[8]

---

[3]   聖人之治：虛其心，實其腹。《老子·三章》
[4]   聖人寒頭而煖足。《脈法》
[5]   《金匱鉤玄·腳氣》 *Probing into the Subtleties of the Golden Cabinet* (Zhu 2000, 114).
[6]   《陰陽應象大論》 (Wu and Wu 1997, 31)
[7]   從陽引陰。《陰陽應象大論》 (Wu and Wu 1997, 42)
[8]   陰病治陽。《陰陽應象大論》 (Wu and Wu 1997, 43)

Besides the principle that yin and yang are interconnected and rely on each other, and that communication between the two is essential, some also champion the idea that yang is primary. While this concept is essential to the Ming dynasty school of warm supplementation, it can be traced back as far as *Huai Nan Zi*, Chapter 3, which says, "The bright emits qi and for this reason fire is the external brilliance of the sun; the obscure sucks qi in, and for this reason water is the internal luminosity of the moon. Emitted qi endows, retained qi is transformed. Thus yang endows and yin is transformed" (translated by Major 1993, 64-5).

Nature is our language. It is universally and eternally available to give us guidance. In a medical context, the relationship between the sun and yang is discussed in *Elementary Questions*, Chapter 3: "Yang qi is like sun in heaven. If it loses its proper place, longevity diminishes and does not manifest."[9] Wang Bing's notes say: "This passage compares people having yang to heaven having the sun. If heaven loses its proper place, the sun will not be bright; if man loses his proper place, yang is not firm. If the sun is not bright, heaven's region is dark; if yang is not firm, human lifespan is diminished. This says that for human life, it certainly is appropriate to borrow the sun's yang qi" (Wang, B. 1994, 15-16). Zhang Jiebin commented on the same passage in the *Categorized Classic*:

> When the sun is not bright, heaven is yin darkness. When yang is not firm, human life is cut short. Both are because yang qi loses its proper place. Heaven is not bright by itself. Its brightness is in the sun and moon. The moon's body is rooted in blackness. It is bright when it obtains the sun...

> Like this, when yang is located in *wu* (noon), it is daytime and the sun is connected to the center of heaven. It manifests with the image of spirit brightness and the yang lines of *li gua* located on the exterior. When yang is located in *zi* (midnight), it is

night and fire lies concealed in water. It is transformed into the formlessness of original qi, the yang line of kan located on the interior (Zhang, J.Y. 1965, 387-8).

Li gua	*Kan gua*
——— ———	——— ———
——— ———	——————
——— ———	——— ———

Zhang is pointing out the sun's correspondence with *li gua*. *Li gua* has two yang lines on the outside, resembling the sun's outward radiation of light and warmth. *Kan gua* corresponds to the moon, water, yin, and the kidneys. It has one yang line inside, the image of internal storage of yang; you can only see the reflection of yang. This yang should not radiate outwardly, but should be stored inside. While the moon, water, and the kidneys are yin, they are dead without the warmth and brightness of yang. Yang is what animates; yin without yang is form without function.

Zhang explains this idea further in *Appended Supplement of the Categorized Classic*:

> When discussing life and death, yang governs life while yin governs death... In the mechanism of life transformation, yang is first and yin comes after. Yang bestows while yin receives... The life of the ten-thousand things must be from yang; the death of the ten-thousand things is also from yang. It is not that yang is able to kill things. When yang comes, there is life; when yang goes, there is death... Although heaven and earth are great, if they did not have the sun, they would just be cold substance... The human body is a small *qian* and *kun*: when it obtains yang it is alive; when it loses yang it is dead... The great treasure in heaven is only the one ball of red sun. The great treasure in man is only the one breath of true yang (Zhang, J.Y. 1966, 395-8).[10]

---

[9] 陽氣者，若天與日，失其所，則折壽而不彰。《素問·生氣通天論篇第三》
[10] 《類經附翼·大寶論》

While these passages do not specifically discuss moxibustion, the ideas are relevant. It takes yang to transform yin. Yin can be acquired from food and drink if there is the yang qi to transform it. All of life's processes need yang. Moxibustion, especially below the umbilicus, is like the one yang line inside *kan gua*. It is used to animate the yin. It gives the body the ability to transform more yin from food and drink in order to restore balance.

It is also relevant that these passages compare yang to the sun. Mugwort is picked on the fifth day of the fifth lunar month to receive maximum yang from the sun. It is also dried in the sun. The best way to light mugwort, according to the old books, was with a "fire bead," "fire crystal," "yang speculum," or "fire mirror" (**ZJDC: 9-26, ZJDC: 9-18**, and **BCGM: 06-06**). These are all devices to light mugwort from the rays of the sun. So if the sun is necessary for life in the big *tai ji* of heaven and earth, then perhaps we can consider moxibustion an emissary of the sun that benefits life in the small *tai ji* of the human body.

According to Li Shizhen (**BCGM: 15-05**), one of the old names for mugwort is "ice platform" (冰台 *bing tai*). He points out that it is said that in ancient times, ice was cut into a lens and used to focus the sun's rays on mugwort. The mugwort would then catch on fire. While this may only be mythology, it provides an image of fire born from ice. The inseparable relationship of yin and yang, ice and fire are somehow inherent in this plant. It is a partial truth to say that mugwort is only yang or that the kidneys are essentially yin. *Li gua* contains a yin line in the center; *kan gua* contains a yang line in the center. The kidneys contain life gate fire. Mugwort contains the ability to bring benefit to yin or yang in the body. The key is knowing how to use it to achieve your intent.

What is clinically relevant today?

There are many deterrents to the fully-developed use of moxibustion in the modern Western clinic of Chinese medicine. These include the amount of time it takes to give a treatment, the ash, smoke alarms, worry about scarring or infection, possible harm by exposure to smoke, restrictions of malpractice insurance policies, the climate of bringing a lawsuit for even minor events perceived as adverse, and the ignorance of both the practitioner and the consumer towards the benefits of moxibustion.

Some of the old practices are clearly not sanitary; for example, mixing Fu Zi (Aconite) powder with spittle to make isolating cakes. Other techniques may be replaced by Western medicine; many patients might choose antibiotic therapy over hundreds of cones of moxibustion at the site of an abscess.

However, if an abscess does not close up and becomes chronic, perhaps moxibustion would be the treatment of choice. There are some diseases that may not readily recover with Western medicine or acupuncture but may respond well to moxibustion. *Magic Pivot*, Chapter 73 states, "Moxibustion is suitable for what the needle does not do." We have also seen the value Li, Yang, and Zhang put on the healing effects of moxa sores. The words of these great masters should be adequate to spark an investigation of their claims.

The Ming masters agree that moxa sores are necessary for treatment to be effective. Moxibustion as it is practiced today in the West is much weaker and treatments are less frequent. Therefore, results are not as good. To be able to practice blistering moxibustion in the West, we need to:

• Gather research from China on blistering moxibustion and sort through it to see if it appears effective, and for which conditions.[11]
• Develop clinical trials for the efficacy of blistering moxibustion in the U.S. or in the West, as Western doctors and scientists are reluctant to accept clinical studies from China.

---

[11] Examples: apoplexy (JTCM, June 1991); bronchial asthma (JCM 12, May 1983); recurrent herpes simplex (Zhongguo Zhen Jiu, 2005 April 25(4):255-6); knee pain (Zhongguo Zhen Jiu, 2007 July 27(7):513-5).

- Compare the risks and discomforts with those of Western medical procedures,[12] including voluntary ones such as cosmetic surgery. In reality, moxibustion must be relatively low risk compared to many accepted Western medical procedures.
- Lobby malpractice insurance and health insurance companies to cover direct moxibustion once we have "Western scientific" evidence of its efficacy and cost-effectiveness.
- Develop consent forms that adequately explain the risks and benefits.
- Practice and experiment on ourselves so we fully understand how the patient will experience it.[13]
- Educate practitioners and students of Chinese medicine.
- Educate the consumer.

We may also need to rely on technology and develop alternative methods of moxibustion. To reduce exposure to smoke, we can explore the use of air purifiers and other methods of increasing ventilation. Heavenly moxibustion, moxa patches, or liquid moxa also reduce smoke exposure.

The unavoidable truth of the 21st century is that time is at a premium and we prefer the most convenient methods. Therefore, stick-on and pre-manufactured cones are valued because they save time and make less mess. Perhaps we also need prepackaged isolating substances. Even stocking and slicing fresh ginger and garlic may be too much trouble for some practitioners.

Moxibustion seems to be valued less today than in the past. It is not taught as an equal partner of acupuncture in the schools and is less frequently included in the treatment of patients. Clinicians practice fewer moxibustion techniques and use it in more limited conditions than in the past. How to revive the practice of moxibustion is not within the scope of this book. However, this book may be able to contribute to such a revival.

What has been forgotten today? What have we lost? Or are we going in the right direction? Is it natural selection? Are we better off with more focus on acupuncture and less on moxibustion? Can we revive or adapt some of the older practices and make them relevant today? What practices must be eliminated because they are unsafe or ineffective? These questions cannot all be answered here, but asking them is a first step.

Since the most renowned of the ancient physicians, from Sun Simiao to Zhu Danxi to our three Ming masters, put such value on moxibustion, especially on blistering moxibustion, it must be worth our time to research this issue. As Zhang Jiebin wrote, "When the power of fire arrives, its merits are not insignificant"(**LJTY: 11-2-1**).

---

[12] For example, a search of the PubMed site (www.pubmed.com) on 6/16/06 received 31,793 hits for the phrase, 'nosocomial infection.'

[13] Self-experimentation has been a common research method in the West, used by medical students and doctors (Altman, 1986). In my experience with direct moxibustion resulting in moxa sores, the pain was much less than expected and the treatment was even pleasant at times. Usually blisters arise a few hours after treatment or the following day. No infections resulted and scarring has been minimal.

APPENDIX 1

SOURCES OF THE MING TEXTS AND BIBLIOGRAPHIES OF THEIR AUTHORS

The three giants of medicine during the late Ming dynasty cited in Part 2 of this book all published within 30 years of each other. Li Shizhen's *Great Pharmacopeia* was published in 1596, three years after his death. Yang Jizhou's *Great Compendium of Acupuncture and Moxibustion* was published five years later, in 1601. Zhang Jiebin's *Categorized Classic* and its *Supplements* were published in 1624. Each of these doctors had a different area of expertise:

Li Shizhen was a master of materia medica, although he also wrote about pulse diagnosis and the eight extraordinary vessels. Li some included information on acupuncture-moxibustion in his writings.

Yang Jizhou was a master of acupuncture-moxibustion. He passed on a family tradition in addition to gathering information and techniques from books and practitioners of his day.

Zhang Jiebin is celebrated today for his work on the theoretical aspects of Chinese medicine. He was one of the founders of the school of warm supplementa-

tion and he organized and codified the theories of medicine to a degree that had never been done before. Zhang is also renowned for his development and use of herbal formulas. He is less-well known in the field of acupuncture-moxibustion, although it is evident from his writings that he was a skilled practitioner of these modalities.

Fortunately, their writings originated during the Ming dynasty, a relatively recent time. Their texts were not copied repeatedly by hand, a process which brings about errors and variations. However, each of these texts had more than one early edition and these editions contained variations. Beyond this, modern editions also have typographical errors. Many of them have translated the traditional characters into simplified Chinese. This is another source of error or ambiguity. Some have "corrected" the texts in various ways. The main source texts used in this book are discussed after the biography of the author.

We now examine the lives and works of these three great physicians one by one:

LI SHIZHEN & THE *GREAT PHARMACOPEIA*

Li Shizhen (1518-1593) is among the most famous herbalists in the history of Chinese medicine. His *Great Pharmacopeia* is a major achievement, not only of Chinese medicine, but also of world-wide science. Li was born in 1518 just north of Qizhou,[1] Hubei province (Dharmananda 2001, 1). Coincidentally, Qizhou is the source of the best quality mugwort (Cheng 1987, 339). Li's grandfather had been a wandering doctor, considered to be a low position in society. His father, Li Yanwen,[2] raised the family position by becoming a scholar-doctor and obtaining an official rank. Li Yanwen authored the first treatise on ginseng, as well as books or papers on the four methods of diagnosis, pulse diagnosis, smallpox, and on the mugwort of his homeland (Dharmananda 2001, 1-2). Li Shizhen incorporated his father's treatise on ginseng in the *Great Pharmacopeia* and expanded his father's writings on pulse diagnosis in the *Lakeside [Master's] Study of the Pulse*,[3] but Li Yanwen's discussion of mugwort was not transmitted in the writings of his son and has since been lost.

Li Yanwen had three children, but not much is known about the other two. Young Shizhen was encouraged to study the classics and sit for the imperial exams. This would further raise the status of the family. However, Shizhen was frequently ill in his youth and so became interested in medicine. He helped his father collecting herbs, treating patients, and copying prescriptions. Li studied medicine and at the same time continued his studies of the non-medical classics. He passed the county level exams, but failed the national exams three times (Dharmananda 2001, 2).

At the age of 23, Shizhen was allowed to apprentice with his father. He studied the medical classics thoroughly and continued studying the classics in other fields. Li's recognition grew as he cured some important patients. He was eventually offered an official position, but Li did not feel suited for the job. So after a while he made excuses and returned home to private practice (Dharmananda 2001, 2).

Over a period of time, Li Shizhen realized that the pharmacopeias available had many errors and had been copied without revision for too many generations. At about 30 years of age, Li began his research for the *Great Pharmacopeia*. He traveled extensively, interviewing doctors, farmers, herb collectors, wood cutters, hunters, fishermen, and producers of medicinals. Li also collected and consulted 800 medical books (Dharmananda 2001, 3; Fu 1985, 43-44).

Li felt hands-on experience was as important as reading texts and interviewing people. He went out to observe pangolins himself to try to verify the old legend that pangolins opened their scales to attract their food, ants. He found that instead they use their tongues to tempt the ants. He also dissected them and saw that their stomachs were full of ants (Fu 1985, 44). Similarly, like a latter-day Shen Nong, Li Shizhen tried Man Tuo Luo (Datura) himself to see if it had the anesthetic effect that the ancient books described. In Volume 27 of the *Great Pharmacopeia*, Li also explained how to differentiate two similar looking herbs: Ji Chang Cao (Chicken Intestine Grass) and E Chang Cao (Goose Intestine Grass). He discovered that if the former is chewed, the mouth will salivate, but the latter does not have this effect. This is an indication that Li tasted many of the herbs about which he wrote (Fu 1985, 44-5).

Li Shizhen modeled his *Great Pharmacopeia* after a Song dynasty materia medica that appealed to him: the *Categorized Pharmacopeia for Emergencies* by Tang Shenwei.[4] This book included formulas under each medicinal to illustrate its usage (Dharmananda 2001, 3). The *Great Pharmacopeia* was completed in 1578

---

[1] 蘄州
[2] 李言聞
[3] 《濱湖脈學》, First published in 1564
[4] 唐慎微 《經史証類備急本草》 (c. 1090)

when Li was 60 years old, after about 30 years of work. It was revised a couple of times over the years. The final edition was illustrated and was completed with the assistance of Li's sons and grandsons. Li had the book printed himself and submitted a copy to the imperial court with the goal of having it officially published. It was delivered to the emperor after Li's death, and languished until the reign of the next emperor (Dharmananda 2001, 3).

The first two editions of the *Great Pharmacopeia* (1596 and 1603) were not widely distributed. The book was reorganized for the 1603 edition and the illustrations were re-drawn for a 1640 printing (with a total of 1,160 illustrations). Since the 1640 edition, the *Great Pharmacopeia* has been recognized as a classic and has been reprinted frequently. By the end of the 19th century, it had been translated into Japanese, Latin, French, English, Russian, and German (Dharmananda 2001, 3-4). Foreign Languages Press has recently released an English translation (Li 2004). It was not replaced as the most respected materia medica until 1959 (Dharmananda 2001, 4). In its present form, the *Great Pharmacopeia* lists 1,892 medicinals, including 374 that were not listed in previous materia medicas. Over 11,000 formulas were included, with more than 8,000 that Li collected from doctors or rare texts (Dharmananda 2001, 4).

Li also reorganized the medicinals into categories that are related to botany and zoology rather than by their usage in treatment. This arrangement is close to that of Carl Linnaeus, who developed the binomial system in the 18th century. It is said that the *Great Pharmacopeia* influenced Charles Darwin in his development of the theory of evolution (Dharmananda 2001, 5; Eckman 1996, 82). It is easy to observe why from the order of the contents. Li began with minerals, progressed to plants, and then to animals. Within each of the three kingdoms, he began with the less complex structures and moved toward the more complex, for example, from insects and worms to snakes and fish to birds to mammals to humans.

Throughout the history of Chinese medicine, most authors quoted liberally from earlier writings without citing the origin. Li Shizhen was one of the few doctors of his day who gave attributions for almost all of his sources. Li revised information about familiar medicinals. He corrected errors from previous pharmacopeias. For example, he wrote that the use of heavy metals in elixirs was toxic and harmed people rather than prolonging life (Dharmananda 2001, 4).

The name of Li's book is difficult to translate literally. *Ben Cao* 本草 is a materia medica or pharmacopeia. Like today's *Physicians Desk Reference*, it is an encyclopedia that lists the relevant information for each medicinal substance. Literally, *ben cao* means "roots and herbs." *Gang mu* 綱目 is a little more difficult. *Gang* refers to an outline, implying that individual items are arranged in a logical order. *Mu* means, among other things, a table of contents, a category (Zhang F.J. 1992, 934, 1059). Dharmananda (2001, 4) says that *gang* refers to each item or entry, while *mu* refers to the "technical criteria for arranging the herb descriptions."

The *Great Pharmacopeia* has 52 Volumes: (See chart on next page.)

Volumes 5 through 52 discuss medicinal substances, one by one. Each item includes some or all of the following: an illustration; a discussion of its name; explanation of its growth, production, harvest, preparation, etc.; its properties, functions, and indications along with explanations; and formulas illustrating its use. If more than one part of an item is used differently, each part received a separate discussion.

Li Shizhen wrote 11 other medical books, but only three have survived to the present (Dharmananda 2001, 6): two, *The Lakeside [Master's] Study of the Pulse*, mentioned above, and *Examination of the Eight Extraordinary Vessels*[5] are still important today. The

---

[5] 《奇經八脈考》

LI SHIZHEN'S *GREAT PHARMACOPEIA*	
VOLUME(S)	CONTENTS
1-2	general introduction, including historical information, basic theories of medicinals, etc.
3-4	prescribe treatments, arranged by disease
5	the properties and uses of various types of water
6	properties and uses of various types of fire
7	the properties and uses of various types of earth
8-11	the properties and uses of various types of metals, stones, and minerals
12-21	the properties and uses of various types of herbs
22-25	the properties and uses of various types of grains
26-28	the properties and uses of various types of vegetables
29-33	the properties and uses of various types of fruit
34-37	the properties and uses of various types of trees and wood
38	the properties and uses of various types of household or man-made objects, fabrics, and utensils
39-42	describes the properties and uses of various types products coming from insects, worms, and amphibians
43-44	the properties and uses of various types of products coming from animals with scales, like fish and snakes
45-46	the properties and uses of various types of products coming from animals with shells, like turtles and shellfish
47-49	the properties and uses of various types of products coming from birds
50-51	the properties and uses of various types of products coming from mammals
52	the properties and uses of various types of products from humans

third is *Pulse Formula Textual Research*,[6] which is only two pages in a modern printing (Li 1996, 1271-2).

The main source text used in this book is the 1996 Zhongguo Zhongyiyao edition,[7] edited by Hu Guochen[8] *et al.* The original manuscript used for the Zhongguo Zhongyiyao edition was the first edition engraving by Hu Chenglong.[9] The preface of the Zhongguo Zhongyiyao edition says the original was printed in 1590[10] (page 1). However, most other sources say this edition was published in 1596[11] (for example, Unschuld 1986a, 148; Chen and Luo 1995, 104). The reason for this confusion is probably that a preface was written for this first edition, signed and dated by Wang Shizhen[12] in 1590, even though

the book itself was not published until six years later. The editors of the modern edition have cut out the pictures (a common practice) and removed any lemmas that had only a heading but no content.

Li did not write a section on moxibustion. He focused more often on the internal application of medicinals, or even external ointments and washes. However, Li scattered references to moxibustion throughout the book. For example, in Volumes 3 and 4, moxibustion is discussed in the treatment of various diseases. Volume 6 describes the properties of the fire from mugwort and the fire from a moxa stick called the "thunder-fire miraculous needle." Throughout the rest of the book, moxibustion is dis-

---

[6] 《脈訣考證》
[7] Chinese Medicine and Herbal Publishers 中國中醫藥出版社 (Li, 1996).
[8] 胡國臣
[9] 胡承龍
[10] The 18th year of Ming emperor 萬曆 Wan Li
[11] The 24th year of Ming emperor 萬曆 Wan Li
[12] 王世貞

cussed under mugwort and other medicinals, such as those used as isolating substances.

Moxibustion was only a small part of the discussion of any medicinal. Because of this, only exerpts of the relevant lemmas are translated for this book. For example, under garlic (Suan), the sections about its properties, indications, and its use in moxibustion are relevant, but its use in internal formulas is irrelevant. Therefore, Li's contribution to this book is in smaller, edited clips.

YANG JIZHOU & THE GREAT COMPENDIUM OF ACUPUNCTURE AND MOXIBUSTION

Yang Jizhou (1522-1620, Zhejiang province) was born into a family of scholar-physicians. His grandfather was an imperial physician. Yang, like Li Shizhen, first studied the classics in order to sit for the exams and become an official. However, it is said that because a local examiner disliked him, he failed to pass the examinations. After this, Yang turned to his family's profession of medicine. The Yang family had all the necessary resources for becoming a good doctor: a big library and lots of experience. Yang Jizhou soon developed a reputation and he was asked several times to treat members of the royal family. He served as an imperial physician in Beijing for many years (Yang and Liu 1994, vi-vii). Yang traveled extensively to treat various patients and collect techniques from local doctors (Huard and Wong 1968, 51).

Yang Jizhou had a dream of collecting all the important writings on acupuncture-moxibustion and publishing them. This was a difficult task as there was no commercial press at the time. He needed to come up with a significant sum of money to finance his project (Yang and Liu 1994, vii). Fortunately for Yang, the governor of Shanxi, Zhao Wenbing,[13] was suffering from a serious chronic disease that other doctors were

unable to treat successfully. Zhao consulted with Yang, who was able to cure him after only three treatments. The governor was grateful and impressed with Yang's skill; so he offered to give Yang assistance in publishing (Yang and Liu 1994, vii-viii).

As for the title of this book, *zhen jiu* 針灸 means "acupuncture-moxibustion." *Da cheng* 大成 literally means something like "great achievement." *Da* can be translated as big or great. *Cheng* is an accomplishment, achievement, or something that is fully developed. The phrase *da cheng* is used to indicate the "ultimate completion of a great work, the consummate understanding of all relevant branches of a science, and an all-embracing collection" (Yang and Liu 1994, x). The sources for the *Great Compendium* include the Yang family experience and the writings of many previous authors, including Gao Wu, Xu Chunfu, Wang Ji, Li Chan, the *Inner Canon*, and the *Classic of Difficulties*.[14] The engraving was begun in 1579 and the book was finally published in 1601 (Huard and Wong 1968, 51).

The *Great Compendium of Acupuncture and Moxibustion* consists of 10 volumes shown in the chart on the next page.

Yang Shouzhong said, "Ever since its birth, this work has been universally acknowledged as the most authoritative and mature in the pre-modern literature of acupuncture and moxibustion. Even until now, no other work can be said to truly challenge either its theoretical or practical value" (Yang and Liu 1994, x).

Yang Jizhou emphasized the integrated use of acupuncture, moxibustion, medicinals, and massage. Yang wrote a rather large section on moxibustion; he felt moxibustion was as important as acupuncture (Wei 1987, 82). Yang included the writings of many previous authors on moxibustion in Volumes 3 and 9. Volume 9 is especially useful as a clinical guideline,

---

[13] 趙文炳
[14] 高武，徐春甫，汪機，李梴，《内經》，《難經》

YANG JIZHOU'S *GREAT COMPENDIUM OF ACUPUNCTURE AND MOXIBUSTION*	
VOLUME(S)	**CONTENTS**
1	Theories of acupuncture and moxibustion from the *Inner Canon* and the *Classic of Difficulties*.
2-3	Memorization poems
4	Discussion of acupuncture and moxibustion techniques, especially supplementation and draining, by famous doctors, including the Yang family. This also includes a list of points forbidden for moxibustion.
5	Discussion of various methods of chrono-acupuncture.
6-7	Discussion of the organs, channels, network vessels, and points.
8	A treatment formulary for various diseases, already translated into English as the *Divinely Responding Classic* (Yang & Liu, 1994).
9	Specific acupuncture and moxibustion techniques from various doctors. This volume includes a large section on moxibustion. At the end, it also has a number of case histories.
10	Treatment of children, especially pediatric massage.

discussing the materials used in moxibustion, methods of lighting a fire, the number of cones, care before and after moxibustion, the eruption of moxibustion sores, a formula for an ointment to be used on moxibustion sores, etc. Yang covered everything a practitioner would need to know about moxibustion, although unlike Zhang Jiebin, he did not give a moxibustion treatment formulary for every disease. This is because Yang's treatment with moxibustion was integrated with other modalities, while Zhang favored moxibustion over acupuncture and massage.

Many passages of the *Great Compendium* reveal Yang's treatment philosophy: acupuncture and moxibustion should be used together as equals. For example, the *Song of Victorious Jade*[15] says, "This is the Yang family's true secret transmission: sometimes acupuncture and sometimes moxibustion is used based on the venerable teachings…" Another example comes after his discussion of the confluence points of the eight extraordinary vessels, "Some use mugwort for moxibustion. You also can do this… You cannot focus on and constrain yourself with the needle."[16] It is clear that Yang did not hold a bias towards acupuncture.

In clinical practice, Yang combined acupuncture and moxibustion. For example, 15 of his 31 case studies use acupuncture and moxibustion together. There are some that only use acupuncture, but there are also a few that only use moxibustion. Yang was able to select the appropriate modality based on the merits of each method and the requirements of the case: "Sometimes you can use the needle and so you needle. Sometimes, you can use moxibustion and so you apply moxibustion… Sometimes acupuncture and moxibustion can be chosen together, so you choose them together."[17]

The main source used for the translations was the *Grand Compendium of Famous Works on Acupuncture and Moxibustion*,[18] published in 2000 by Cathay Publishers.[19] This is a collection of many important works on acupuncture-moxibustion, including the *Great Compendium*. The editor, Huang Longxiang,[20] says that there is no existing copy of the original 1601 edition of the *Great Compendium*. There are some old editions that state they are from the Ming dynasty, and later publishers have taken that claim at face value. However, the truth is that the "Ming editions" were actually printed during the

---

[15] 《針灸大成·卷三·勝玉歌》 (Huang 1996, 837)
[16] 《針灸大成·卷五·八脈圖並治症穴》 (Huang 1996, 895)
[17] 《針灸大成·卷三·穴有奇正策》 (Huang 1996, 847)
[18] 《針灸名著集成》
[19] 華夏出版社 (Huang, 2000)
[20] 黃龍祥

Qing dynasty by Li Yuegui[21] who published two editions: one in 1656[22] and the other in 1698.[23] The 1656 edition was also reprinted in 1680.[24] These editions had a number of corrections from the original printing, and even some new plates. Therefore, they cannot be called Ming editions. The main manuscript used for *Grand Compendium of Famous Works on Acupuncture and Moxibustion* was the 1656 edition with the 1680 reprinting as a second reference (page 786).

In Volume 9, Yang wrote one long section on moxibustion. This is translated in its entirety. Throughout the rest of the *Great Compendium*, moxibustion is mentioned in many places. A few selected passages are also translated in this book.

ZHANG JIEBIN, THE CATEGORIZED CLASSIC, ITS SUPPLEMENTS, AND [ZHANG] JINGYUE'S COMPLETE BOOK[25]

Zhang Jiebin (1563-1640), also known as Zhang Jingyue, was an author and famous physician during the late Ming dynasty. He was also one of the founders of the school of warm supplementation (Chen and Luo 1995, 126). Zhang grew up in Shaoxing,[26] Zhejiang province, not too far from Hangzhou, and across the bay from Shanghai. During his youth, Zhang showed that he was naturally gifted and clever. He studied with his father, who was proficient in medical theory, until he was 14 years old (Chen and Luo 1995, 126). Zhang studied the usual subjects of an aspiring Confucian scholar and especially liked *Sunzi's Art of War* and the *Yellow Emperor's Inner Canon* (Zhang 1999, 1863). Later, Zhang traveled to Beijing with his father. There, he made friends with many scholars, and studied medicine for 10 years with a famous doctor, Jin Ying[27] (Li 1995, 837). Zhang also researched astronomy, astrology, mathematics, numerology, *kan yu* (*feng shui*), music, military arts, and *Yi Jing* theory (Hong 2000, 146; Ren 1986, 126; Zhang J.Y. 1995, 1830; and Zhang 1999, 1863).

In his adult years, Zhang "threw away his pen and joined the military." He was sent to the far north: Liaoning and Heilongjiang provinces, and what is now North Korea (Chen and Luo 1995, 126). The Ming period lay between two dynasties that were ruled by Northern foreigners (Yuan and Qing). There were many incursions from the Northern tribes into China during the Ming dynasty. Even its capital, Beijing, was attacked a few times. The Ming government put its military might into defending the Northern border and a concerted effort was made to reinforce the Great Wall (Yan 1998). Zhang's military service must have been a part of this effort. Zhang passed some years in the military but without recognition. In addition, his parents were old and his family poor. Around 1620, when Zhang was almost 60 years old, he returned home (Zhang 1999, 1863). There, Zhang focused on his interest in medicine. His fame spread and patients flocked to his door (Chen and Luo 1995, 126).

Zhang Jiebin wrote diligently his whole life. He left us many large books, such as the *Categorized Classic*, and its appended texts: the *Illustrated Supplement* and the *Appended Supplement*. These were published together in 1624, when Zhang was 61 years old (Li 1995, 837). The 32 volumes of the *Categorized Classic* contain Zhang's research into the *Inner Canon*. Zhang worked on this book for 30 years, rewriting the manuscript four times before completing it. In it, Zhang combined and reorganized *Elementary Questions* (*Su Wen*) and *Magic Pivot* (*Ling Shu*) into 12 categories and 390 sections, adding comprehensive annotations and

---

21 李月桂
22 Qing dynasty emperor 順治 Shun Zhi's 14*th* year
23 康熙 Kang Xi's 37*th* year
24 康熙 Kang Xi's 19*th* year
25 《類經》, 《類經圖翼》, 《類經附翼》, 《景岳全書》, hereafter called the *Categorized Classic*, the *Illustrated Supplement*, the *Appended Supplement*, and *Zhang's Complete Works*, respectively.
26 紹興
27 金英 (also known as Jin Mengshi 金夢石)

ZHANG JIEBIN'S *ILLUSTRATED SUPPLEMENT*		
VOLUME(S)	**CONTENTS**	
1-2	The five transports and the six qi.[28] This is the theory of predictive epidemiology discussed in *Elementary Questions*, Chapters 66 through 71, and Chapter 74.	
3-10	The channels and network vessels	
	Volume 4	Includes a memorization poem listing points that are contraindicated for moxibustion, and another section that lists guidelines for acupuncture and moxibustion, but is focused on moxibustion. These sections are translated above.
	Volume 10	Lists extraordinary points, many of them used for moxibustion. Portions of this are also translated above.
11	Entitled *Essential Reading on Acupuncture and Moxibustion*.[29] After a short section on points, there is a lengthy treatment formulary almost exclusively prescribing moxibustion. This is also translated above.	

explanations (Zhang J.Y. 1995, 1811). This book transformed the disorganization of the *Inner Cannon* into an orderly text, convenient for searching, reading, and studying (Chen and Luo 1995, 126).

The two *Supplements* (literally "wings") are additional explanations on various topics to help the main text "fly." One of them, the *Illustrated Supplement*, contains a detailed discussion of moxibustion. This book has 11 volumes (see chart above).

In addition, Zhang finished the *Complete Works* in his later years, around 1636 or 1637. This monumental book compiled his theories and clinical experience. It is organized by specialty (internal medicine, external medicine, gynecology, pediatrics, etc.) and begins with some volumes on medical theory. It is a complete handbook on the theory and practice of medicine during the late Ming dynasty. This book emphasizes Zhang's warm supplementation theory (Chen and Luo 1995, 126). Zhang's *Complete Works* has 64 volumes:

ZHANG JIEBIN'S *COMPLETE WORKS*	
VOLUME(S)	**CONTENTS**
1-3	Medical theory
4-6	Pulse diagnosis
7-8	Cold damage
9-37	Various internal disease patterns and their treatments
38-39	Gynecology
40-41	Pediatrics
42-45	Pox and rashes
46-47	External diseases
48-49	A materia medica
50-64	Medicinal formulas. This section includes formulas for moxa sticks as well as ointments for moxibustion sores.

---

[28] 五運六氣
[29] 《類經圖翼·針灸要覽》

Volumes 7 through 47 contain a number of acupuncture-moxibustion protocols, although the vast majority of treatments use medicinals. Zhang wrote one other small book in his later years, *Calling the Record into Question*.[30] It has 45 short sections on various topics (Zhang J.Y. 1995, 1812).

Much of Volume 11 and sections of Volume 4 of the *Illustrated Supplement* are primary sources for the translations in this book. Occasional selections from Zhang's *Complete Works* are also translated. The main source for the *Illustrated Supplement* is an edition of the *Categorized Classic* (including its two *Supplements*), published in 1991 by Shanghai Ancient Text Publishers.[31] This is the *Four Treasuries* edition, a facsimile of a Qing dynasty Qian Long[32] period (1736-1795) edition that was completed in 1783. It is part of a series of books called the *Four Treasuries Medical Collection of Books*,[33] which is part of the encyclopedic *Four Treasuries Complete Book*.[34] Only seven copies were made for the emperor's collection, all hand written. Currently there are four surviving sets (Liu 1985, 92-3).

An edition of Zhang's *Complete Works* that was published in 1995 by Renmin Weisheng Chubanshe[35] and edited by Zhao Lixun[36] was also used as a source text. In its introduction, Zhao states that Zhang's *Complete Works* had three editions published within a 13-year period, beginning in 1700:

Published by Lu Chao in 1700[37]
Published by Jia Tang in 1710[38]
Published by Zha Li'nan in 1713[39]

From these three, at least 40 other editions were published. Zhao choose the second edition as his chief source as he felt it had fewer mistakes than the first edition. The third edition copied the second edition, without correcting any errors and adding more. Zhao compared the second edition to the other two for reference (page 4).

---

[30] 《質疑錄》
[31] 上海古籍出版社 (Zhang, 1991)
[32] 乾隆
[33] 《四庫醫學叢書》
[34] 《四庫全書》
[35] 人民衛生出版社 (Zhang, 1999)
[36] 趙立勛
[37] 魯超, 康熙, Kang Xi's 39th year
[38] 賈棠, Kang Xi's 49th year
[39] 俀禮南, Kang Xi's 52nd year

APPENDIX 2

TIMELINE OF MEDICAL BOOKS ON MOXIBUSTION

Below is an outline of important Chinese-language books in the development of moxibustion theory and practice. Most of these are also mentioned in Chapter 3: The History of Moxibustion.

Early

- 馬王堆 Mawangdui silk books (found in 1973) Hunan province, sometime before 168 B.C.E. The earliest recorded literature on moxibustion received at the present.
  - 《陰陽十一脈灸經》 *Moxibustion Canon of the Eleven Yin and Yang Vessels*
  - 《足臂十一脈灸經》 *Moxibustion Canon of the Eleven Vessels of the Foot and Forearm*
  - 《五十二病方》 *Formulas for Fifty-two Diseases*
- The *Yellow Emperor's Inner Classic*, the Warring States Period and Spring and Autumn Period (Unschuld: 400 BCE to 260 CE; Eastern Han according to Kaptchuk). The earliest book that has been continuously used for acupuncture, moxibustion, and medical theory.
  - 《素問》 *Elementary Questions*, 81 chapters
  - 《靈樞》 *Magic Pivot*, 81 chapters

Han dynasty (206 B.C.E.-220 C.E.)

- 張仲景 Zhang Zhongjing (159-219), today's Henan province. Influential books, the basis of the idea that yang patterns are appropriate for acupuncture and yin patterns are appropriate for moxibustion, and that in critical patterns, only moxibustion can quickly extract a deep illness.
  - 《傷寒論》 *Treatise On Cold Damage*
  - 《金匱要略》 *Essential Prescriptions of the Golden Cabinet*
- 曹翁 Cao Weng, 《曹氏灸經》 *Master Cao's Moxibustion Classic*. 7 volumes (lost). The earliest moxibustion therapy treatise.

Jin晉, Southern and Northern, and Sui dynasties (265-618)

- 皇甫謐 Huangfu Mi (214-282), today's Gansu province, compiled 《針灸甲己經》 the *Systematic Classic of Acupuncture and Moxibustion*, 12 volumes, published in 282 C.E. Gives number of cones for each point and

points that are contraindicated for moxibustion. First to mention suppurative moxibustion. Compiled from:
- *Elementary Questions*
- *Magic Pivot*
- 《明堂孔穴針灸治要》 *Acupuncture and Moxibustion Treatment Essentials from the Bright Hall of Points*, c. 100 B.C.E. (lost)
- 王叔和 Wang Shuhe (dates unknown, Wei and/or Jin dynasty), today's Shandong province, 《脈經》 the *Pulse Classic*, 10 volumes, published in 280. Summarized Zhang Zhongjing's statements on which conditions are appropriate for moxibustion.
- 葛洪 Ge Hong (c. 261-341), today's Jiangsu province, 《肘後備急方》 *Emergency Prescriptions to Keep Up Your Sleeve*, 8 volumes, published c. 341 C.E. Emphasized moxibustion for emergency patterns and was the first to use moxibustion on isolating substances.
- 陳延之 Chen Yanzhi (dates unknown), 《小品方》 *Short Sketches of Formulas*. The original is lost. Its contents were copied and scattered in other books, such as *Secret Necessities of a Frontier Official*. He wrote about practical issues regarding moxibustion, such as how many cones were appropriate for the different regions of the body. Advocated suppurative moxibustion.
- Gong Qingxuan, (c. 495) 《劉涓子鬼遺方》 *Formulas Left Behind by Liu Juanzi's Ghost*, 10 volumes, on external medicine, based on Liu Juanzi (c. 370-450), from Zhenjiang.

Tang dynasty (618-907)

- 孫思邈 Sun Simiao (581-682), today's Shaanxi province. He treated moxibustion as equal to acupuncture and medicinal formulas, used it in heat conditions, used large numbers of cones, used isolating substances and other variations in applications.
  - 《千金要方》 *Essential Prescriptions Worth a Thousand Pieces of Gold*, 30 volumes, published in 652.
  - 《千金翼方》 *Supplement to Prescriptions Worth a Thousand Pieces of Gold*, 30 volumes, published in 682.
- 王燾 Wang Tao (670-755), today's Shaanxi province, 《外台秘要》 *Secret Necessities of a Frontier Official*, 40 volumes, published in 752, wrote about medicinal formulas and moxibustion but felt acupuncture could easily cause injury.
- Archeological finds at Dunhuang, including Moxibustion Diagrams and 《灸經明堂》 the *Moxibustion Classic of the Bright Hall*

Song dynasty (960-1279) and Jin dynasty 金 (1115-1234)

- 王懷隱 Wang Huaiyin, Henan province, 《太平聖惠方》 *Sage-like Prescriptions of the Taiping Era*, 100 volumes, published in 992, ordered by the Song emperor Taizong. Gave moxibustion formulas for many diseases. Advocated suppurative moxibustion.
- 王惟一 Wang Weiyi (c. 987-1067), 《銅人腧穴針灸圖經》 the *Illustrated Classic of Acupuncture Points as Found on the Bronze Man*, 3 volumes, published 1026. This book standardized point location. It also gave the number of cones for each point and named the points contraindicated for moxibustion.
- Imperial Medical College compilation, 《聖濟總錄》 *General Record of Sage-like Benefit*, 200 volumes, published in 1117. Gave moxibustion formulas for many diseases.
- 許叔微 Xu Shuwei (1080-1154), Jiangsu province, 《普濟本事方》 *Prescriptions of Universal Benefit from My Own Practice*, 10 volumes, published in 1132. Gave moxbustion formulas for many diseases.
- 竇材 Dou Cai (1100-1164), Hebei province, 《扁鵲心書》 *Book of Bian Que's Heart*, 3 volumes, published in 1146. Gave moxibustion formulas for many diseases. Used moxibustion for warm supplementation. Used moxibustion preventatively and for achieving longevity. Recommended large numbers of cones. First to

recommend anesthesia for applying
moxibustion.

- 劉完素 Liu Wansu (c. 1110-1200), Hebei
province, books like 《素問病機氣宜保命集》
*Collection of Writings on the Mechanisms of Illness,
Suitability of Qi, and the Safeguarding of Life as
Discussed in the Su Wen*, 3 volumes, published in
1186. Used moxibustion in heat diseases.
- 莊綽 Zhuang Chuo (12th c.), Shanxi
province, 《灸膏肓俞穴法》*Moxibustion on
Gaohuangshu UB 43*, 1 volume, published in
1127. Treating consumption with moxibustion.
- 東軒居士 Dongxuan Jushi or Scholar who
Resides on the Eastern Veranda (12th c.,
Song), 《衛濟寶書》*Precious Book of Protecting
and Aiding*, 1 volume. The earliest mention of
Riding the Bamboo Horse moxibustion.
- 許洪 Xu Hong (Southern Song) wrote the three
volumes 《指南總論》*Guidebook Overall
Discussion* as an appendix to 《太平惠民和
劑局方》*Professional and Popular Prescriptions
from the Taiping Era*, published in 1208.
Opposed moxibustion in heat conditions.
- 王執中 Wang Zhizhong (dates unknown),
Zhejiang province, 《針灸資生經》*Classic of
Nourishing Life with Acupuncture and Moxibustion*,
7 volumes, published in 1220. Gave
moxibustion formulas for many diseases. Used
few cones and few points. Used acupuncture,
moxibustion (including heavenly moxibustion),
and medicinal decoctions together.
- 聞人耆年 Wenren Qi'nian (Knowledgeable Aged
Person) (dates unknown), Zhejiang province,
《備急灸法》*Moxibustion for Emergencies*, one
volume, published in 1226. Favored moxibustion for acute diseases. Used Ride the
Bamboo Horse moxibustion. Advocated
suppurative moxibustion.
- 張從正 Zhang Congzheng, also known as
Zhang Zihe 張子和 (c. 1156-1228), Henan
province, books like 《儒門事親》*Confucians'
Duties to their Parents*, 15 volumes, published in
1228. Urged caution and moderation in
moxibustion.
- 李東垣 Li Dongyuan (1180-1251), Hebei

province, books like 《脾胃論》*Discussion of the
Spleen and Stomach*, published in 1249.
Moxibustion can be used in heat conditions.
- 西方子 The Western Master (dates unknown),
《西方子明堂灸經》the *Western Master's
Moxibustion Classic from the Bright Hall*, 8
volumes. Followed Wang Tao in emphasizing
moxibustion over acupuncture.

Yuan dynasty (1271-1368)

- 羅天益 Luo Tianyi (1220-1290), Hebei province,
《衛生寶鑒》*Precious Mirror of Protecting Life*, 24
volumes. Advocated warm supplementation
and treatment of windstroke using
moxibustion.
- 危亦林 Wei Yilin (1277-1347), Jiangxi province,
《世醫得效方》*Effective Formulas Obtained from
Generations of Doctors*, 19 volumes, published in
1345. Collected many moxibustion formulas.
- 朱丹溪 Zhu Danxi (1281-1358), Zhejiang
province, books like 《丹溪心法》*Heart Methods
of [Zhu] Danxi*, 5 volumes, published in 1347.
Used moxibustion for heat conditions. Used
isolating substance moxibustion.

Ming dynasty (1368-1644)

- 朱橚 Zhu Xiao (died 1425), *et. al.*,《普濟方》
Prescriptions of Universal Benefit, 168 volumes,
published in 1406. Gave moxibustion formulas
for many diseases.
- 徐鳳 Xu Feng (14th c.), Jiangxi province,
《針灸大全》*Great Completion of Acupuncture
and Moxibustion*, 6 volumes, published in 1439.
Gave moxibustion formulas for many diseases.
- 朱權 Zhu Quan, 《壽域神方》*Miraculous
Formulas from Longevity Land*. First moxa roll.
- 虞摶 Yu Tuan (1438-1517), Zhejiang province,
《醫學正傳》*True Transmission of Medicine*, 8
volumes, published in 1515. Moxibustion can
be used in all conditions, including heat.
- 汪機 Wang Ji (1463-1539), Anhui province,
《針灸問對》 *Questions and Answers on
Acupuncture and Moxibustion*, 3 volumes,

published in 1532. Gave moxibustion formulas for many diseases. Moxibustion can be used in all conditions, including heat.

- 高武 Gao Wu (16th c.), Zhejiang province, 《針灸聚英》*Gatherings from Eminent Acupuncturists*, 4 volumes, published in 1529. Gave moxibustion formulas for many diseases. Felt doctors should integrate acupuncture, moxibustion, and medicinal formulas.

- 薛立齋 Xue Lizhai, also known as 薛己 Xue Ji (c. 1486-1558), Suzhou province. Used isolating substance moxibustion.

- 李梴 Li Chan (16th c.), Jiangxi province, 《醫學入門》*Entering the Gate of Medicine*, 7 volumes, published in 1575. Moxibustion can be used in all conditions, including heat.

- 李時珍 Li Shizhen (1518-1593), Hubei province, 《本草綱目》the *Great Pharmacopoeia*, 52 volumes, completed in 1578, first published (posthumously) in 1596. First recorded '雷火神針 Thunder Fire Miraculous Needle in Volume 9.

- 龔信 Gong Xin, Jiangxi province, father of Gong Yanxian, 《古今醫鑒》*Ancient and Modern Mirror of Medicine*, 16 volumes.

- 龔延賢 Gong Yanxian (16th c.), Jiangxi province, son of Gong Xin, 《壽世保元》*Long Life and Protecting the Origin*, 10 volumes. Has a chapter on moxibustion, including practical advice, points to be used, and treatments for many diseases. Advocated suppurating moxibustion, but suggested tapping around the burning cone to diffuse the pain.

- 楊繼洲 Yang Jizhou (1522-1620), Zhejiang province, 《針灸大成》*Great Compendium of Acupuncture and Moxibustion*, 10 volumes, published in 1601. Felt doctors should integrate acupuncture, moxibustion, and medicinal formulas. Summarized the achievements of moxibustion during the Ming dynasty and before.

- 吳崑 Wu Kun (1551-1620), Anhui province, 《針方六集》*Six Collections of Acupuncture Formulas*, 6 volumes, published in 1618. Felt doctors should integrate acupuncture,

moxibustion, and medicinal formulas.

- 張介賓 Zhang Jiebin, also known as Zhang Jingyue 張景岳 (1563-1640), Zhejiang province. Gave moxibustion formulas for many diseases. Used moxibustion for warm supplementation. Opposed moxibustion in heat conditions. Used isolating substance moxibustion.
  - *Illustrated Supplement to the Categorized Classic*, 11 volumes, published in 1624.
  - 《景岳全書》*[Zhang] Jingyue's Complete Works*, 64 volumes, completed in 1636 and published in 1700.

- 龔居中 Gong Juzhong, Zhejiang province, 《紅爐點雪》*A Spot of Snow on a Red [Hot] Stove*, 4 volumes, published in 1630. Moxibustion can be used in all conditions, including heat.

Qing dynasty (1644-1911)

- Anonymous, 《采艾編翼》*Organized Supplement of Gathering Mugwort*, 3 volumes, published in 1711. Moxibustion treatise, covering each specialty.

- 吳謙 Wu Qian, Anhui province, *et. al.*, 《醫宗金鑒》*Golden Mirror of Medicine*, 90 volumes, published in 1742. Gave moxibustion formulas for many diseases, as well as many memorization poems.

- 葉桂 Ye Gui also known as 葉天士 Ye Tianshi (1667-1746), Jiangsu province, 《种福堂公選良方》*Collectively Selected Good Formulas from the Hall of Planting Happiness*, 1 volume. Used moxa rolls.

- 陳延銓 Chen Yanquan, Hunan province, 《羅遺篇》*Collecting Missing Writings*, 3 volumes, published in 1763. Moxibustion on non-channel points.

- 魏之琇 Wei Zhixiu (1722-1772), 《續名醫類案》*Additional Categorized Cases of Famous Doctors*, 36 volumes, published in 1770. Many case studies involving moxibustion, including using moxibustion on heat diseases.

- 李守先 Li Shouxian (1736-?), Henan province, 《針灸易學》*Easy Studies in Acupuncture and*

Moxibustion, 2 volumes, published in 1798. Advocated suppurative moxibustion.

- 趙學敏 Zhao Xuemin (c. 1730-1805), Zhejiang province, 《串雅全書》 *Chuanya Complete Book*, written in 1759, two sections with a total of 8 volumes, published in 1851. Collected folk medicine, including many moxibustion techniques.
- 李學川 Li Xuechuan, 《針灸逢源》 *Meeting the Source of Acupuncture and Moxibustion*, 6 volumes, published in 1817. Used moxibustion on external diseases.
- 陳修園 Chen Xiuyuan (1753-1823), Fujian province. Used moxa rolls.
- 周雍和 Zhou Yonghe, 《太乙神針附方》 *Miraculous Needle Appended Formulas*, the introduction was by 郭寅皐 Guo Yingao, published in 1823. This book passed on the teachings of 範毓奇 Fan Yuqi (dates unknown). Described a type of moxa roll.
- 吳亦鼎 Wu Yiding or 吳倪丞 Wu Yancheng (19th c.), Anhui province, compiled 《神灸經綸》 *Principles of Miraculous Moxibustion*, 4 volumes, published in 1853. Summarizes the major developments of moxibustion from the Qing dynasty and earlier. Used moxibustion in urgent patterns.
- 王孟英 Wang Mengying or王士雄 Wang Shixiong (1808-1866), Zhejiang province.

Opposed moxibustion in yin vacuity.

- 孔廣培 Kong Guangpei (dates unknown), 《太乙神針集解》 *Taiyi Miraculous Needle Collection and Explanation*, published in 1872. Described a type of moxa roll.
- 廖潤鴻 Liao Runhong (born c. 1834), Hunan province, 《針灸集成》 *Collected Works of Acupuncture and Moxibustion*, 4 volumes, published in 1874.
- 雷少逸 Lei Shaoyi (1833-1888), Zhejiang province, 《雷火針法》 *Thunder Fire Needle Method*. He also wrote 《灸法秘傳》 *Secret Transmission of Moxibustion*, 1 volume, published in 1883, from information passed down by 金冶田 Jin Yetian. Used moxa rolls.
- 韓貽豐 Han Yifeng (18th c.), 《太乙神針心法》 *Taiyi Miraculous Needle Heart Method*, 2 volumes, introduction by Qiu Shimin 邱時敏. Used moxa rolls.
- 陳惠疇 Chen Huichou, Hunan province, 《太乙神針方》 *Taiyi Miraculous Needle Formulas*. Used moxa rolls.

Compiled from: (Kaptchuk 2000), (He 2003), (Wei 1987), (Deadman 1998), (O'Conner & Bensky 1981), (Chen & Luo 1995), (Li 1995), (Zhang 1994), (Unschuld 1985), etc. The number of volumes may vary depending on the edition. Also occasionally the dates vary from source to source.

APPENDIX 3
INDEX OF TRANSLATED ENTRIES

Below is an index of all the entries that have been translated from the books of Yang Jizhou, Zhang Jiebin, and Li Shizhen. The column on the far right shows the Chapter in this book in which the entry is found.

Chapter Contents

	BCGM 李時珍《本草綱目》 (Ben Cao Gang Mu) LI SHIZHEN'S *GREAT PHARMACOPEIA*		
VOLUMES	**ENTRY**		**CHAPTER**
3 & 4	Various Selections on Indications		11
06-03	Fire from Mulberry Twigs	桑柴火 *sang chai huo*	20
06-06	Fire from Mugwort	艾火 *ai huo*	5
06-07	Fire from a Miraculous Needle	神針火 *shen zhen huo*	9
06-09	Fire from Lamps	燈火 *deng huo*	9
11-01	Salt	食鹽 *shi yan*	8
15-05	Mugwort	艾葉 *ai ye*	8
17-17-1	Radix Lateralis Praeparata Aconiti	附子 *fu zi*, 大附子 *da fu zi*	8
17-21-1	Radix Aconiti	烏頭 *wu tou*	8
17-22	Radix Typhonii	白附子 *bai fu zi*	8
22-08	Buckwheat	蕎麥 *qiao mai*	8
25-01	Semen Praeparatum Sojae	大豆豉 *da dou chi*, 淡豆豉 *dan dou chi*	8
26-03	Bulbus Allii Fistulosi	蔥白頭 *cong bai tou*	8
26-09	Bulbus Allii Sativi	葫 *hu*, 大蒜 *da suan*	8
26-17	uncooked Rhizoma Zingiberis	生薑 *sheng jiang*	8
27-07	Chinese Chives	小蒜 *xiao suan*	8
29-06-08	Stems and White Bark of Peach Tree	桃樹莖及白皮 *tao shu jing ji bai pi*	8
35-21	Fructus Gleditsiae	皂莢 *zao jiao*	8
35-47	Semen Crotonis	巴豆 *ba dou*	8
38-42	Arrow Shaft and Head	箭（竹+可）及鏃 *jian ke ji cu*	8
38-58	Axle Grease of Carts and Wagons	車脂 *che zhi*	8
40-05	Jujube Cat	棗貓 *zao mao*	8

	JYQS 張介賓《景岳全書》(*Jing Yue Quan Shu*) Zhang Jiebin's *[Zhang] Jingyue's Complete Works*		
	ENTRY		**CHAPTER**
11-1-15	Windstroke, Moxibustion	《非風・灸法》	11
19-3-7	Hiccoughs, Moxibustion	《呃逆・灸法》	11
22-1-8	Swelling and Distention, Acupuncture and Moxibustion	《腫脹・針灸法》	11
23-1-5	Accumulations and Gatherings, Acupuncture and Moxibustion	《積聚・針灸法》	11
25-2-4	Pain of the Rib-sides, Moxibustion	《脅痛・灸法》	11
27-1-5	Eyes, Acupuncture and Moxibustion	《眼目・針灸法》	11
28-3-6	Teeth, Acupuncture and Moxibustion	《齒牙・針灸法》	11
32-1-8	Leg Qi, Acupuncture and Moxibustion	《腳氣・針灸》	11
35-2-15	Moxibustion for Gu Toxins	《諸毒・灸蠱毒法》	11
46-11	External Medicine, Discussion on Moxibustion	《外科・論灸法》	11
48-71	Mugwort [*Ai*]	《艾》	8
49-229	Garlic [*Suan*]	《蒜》	8
51-54	Thunder Fire Needle	《雷火鍼》	9
58-115	Decoction to Support Yang and Reinforce the Stomach	《扶陽助胃湯》	12
60-63	Moxibustion for Sudden Deafness	《暴聾灸法》	9
60-237	Snake Venom	《蛇毒》	11
60-239	Rabid Dog Bite	《瘋犬傷人》	11
60-243	Moxibustion for all Dog and Insect Bites	《諸犬咬蟲傷灸法》	11
60-266	Smoke Tube for Coughing	《嗽煙筒》	9
60-267	Magic Gem Smoke Tube	《靈寶煙筒》	9
60-278	Formula for Cold Stroke Abdominal Pain after Sexual Activity	《事後中寒腹痛方》	11
60-279	Damp Mounting [*Shan*] Testicular Pain	《濕疝陰丸作痛》	11
61-66	Moxibustion to Terminate Childbirth	《斷產灸法》	11
63-117	Miraculously Effective Moxibustion on Garlic	《神效隔蒜灸法》	8
64-115	Method of the Immortals for Moxibustion on Garlic	《神仙隔蒜灸法》	8
64-116	*Fu Zi* [Aconite] Cakes	《附子餅》	8
64-117	*Dou Chi* [Fermented soybean] cakes	《豆豉餅》	8
64-118	*Mu Xiang* [Auklandia] Cakes	《木香餅》	9
64-119	*Xiang Fu* [Cyperus] Cakes	《香附餅》	9
64-120	Miraculously Effective Mulberry Twig Moxibustion	《神效桑枝灸》	9
64-121	Miraculously Effective Ironing with Scallions	《神效蔥熨法》	8
64-122	Formula of the Immortals for Fuming and Radiating	《神仙熏照方》	9
64-265	Moxibustion for Lockjaw	《破傷風灸法》	11
64-324	Jasper [Colored] Oil Ointment	《碧油膏》	5

	LJTY 張介賓 《類經圖翼》 (Lei Jing Tu Yi) Zhang Jiebin's *Illustrated Supplement to the Categorized Classic*		
	ENTRY		CHAPTER
4-17	Blood Avoidance Song	《血忌歌》	13
4-26	Song of Contraindicated Moxibustion Points	《禁灸穴歌》	7
4-27	Various Rules of Acupuncture and Moxibustion	《針灸諸則》	5
Volumes 6-8	Various Points of the Fourteen Channels		6, 7
Volume 10	Various Extraordinary Points		6, 7
11-2	Important Points Used for Applying Moxibustion to All Patterns	《諸證灸法要穴》	5
11-3	Moxibustion Treatments for Various Diseases		10

	ZJDC 楊繼洲 《針灸大成》 (Zhen Jiu Da Cheng) Yang Jizhou's *Great Compendium of Acupuncture and Moxibustion*		
	ENTRY		CHAPTER
4-27	Contraindicated Moxibustion Points Song	《禁灸穴歌》	7
4-31	Various Entries on Day Selection		13
9-6	Quick Essentials of Moxibustion	《捷要灸法》	6
9-7	Master Cui's Method of Applying Treatment to the Four Flowers	《崔氏取四花穴法》	6
9-8	Method for Applying Treatment to Gao Huang [UB 43]	《取膏肓穴法》	6
9-9	Ride the Bamboo Horse Moxibustion Point Method	《騎竹馬灸穴法》	6
9-10	Applying Moxibustion to the Taxation Point	《灸勞穴法》	6
9-11	Method to Apply Treatment to Shen Shu [UB 23]	《取腎俞穴法》	6
9-12	Method to Apply Moxibustion for Heart Qi	《取灸心氣法》	11
9-13	Method to Apply Moxibustion for Hemorrhoids and Fistulas	《取灸痔漏法》	11
9-14	Method to Apply Moxibustion to the Small Intestine Shan [Mounting] Qi Point	《灸小腸疝氣穴法》	11
9-15	Method to Apply Moxibustion for Intestinal Wind and Bloody Diarrhea	《灸腸風下血法》	11
9-16	Moxibustion for Bound Chest and Cold Damage	《灸結胸傷寒法》	11
9-17	Moxibustion for Yin Toxins Binding the Chest	《灸陰毒結胸》	11
9-18	Thunder Fire Needle Method	《雷火針法》	9
9-19	Method of Steaming the Umbilicus to Treat Disease	《蒸臍治病》	9
9-20	Reading the Weather and Time	《相天時》	13
9-21	Moxibustion from A Thousand Pieces of Gold	《《千金》灸法》	11
9-22	Method to Make Moxa Sores Erupt from the Precious Mirror	《《寶鑑》發灸法》	13
9-23	Mugwort Leaf	《艾葉》	8
9-24	Supplementation and Draining with Mugwort Moxibustion	《艾灸補瀉》	5
9-25	The Size of Mugwort Cones	《艾炷大小》	5
9-26	Lighting Mugwort Fire	《點艾火》	5
9-27	Number of Cones	《壯數多少》	5
9-28	Moxibustion	《灸法》	5
9-29	Order of Burning the Cones	《炷火先後》	5
9-30	Moxibustion for Chills and Fever	《灸寒熱》	11
9-31	Important Method for Moxibustion Sores	《灸瘡要法》	5
9-32	Applying Medicinal Paste to Moxibustion Sores	《貼灸瘡》	5
9-33	Moxibustion Sores Ointment Method	《灸瘡膏法》	5
9-34	Washing Moxibustion Sores	《洗灸瘡》	5
9-35	Nursing Health after Moxibustion	《灸後調攝法》	5
9-36	Appended Case Studies of Master Yang	《附楊氏醫案》	12

GLOSSARY

1. SYMPTOM, DISEASE, OR CONDITION TERMINOLOGY

Below is a list of more unusual terms found in the translations for symptoms, diseases, or conditions. Besides a definition, there is a listing of one or more entries where it is found. The entries listed are not comprehensive.

abstraction (恍惚 *huang hu*): "Inattention to present objects or surroundings, or low powers of mental concentration." (Wiseman 1998, 3) **ZJDC: 9-6**

bone-clinging flat-abscess (附骨疽 *fu gu ju*): "A headless flat-abscess located on a bony and sinewy part of the body." (Wiseman 1998, 44) **LJTY: 11-3-23**

bulging mounting ([疒 + 頹] *tui*): A type of mounting [*shan*] where a bulge is visible on the body. "A general name for diseases of the anterior yin, including in males, swelling of the testicles and sagging of one testicle etc; and in females, vaginal protrusion, etc." (Wiseman 1998, 51) **LJTY: 10-1-4-33**

clove sore (疔瘡 *ding chuang*): "A small, hard sore with a deep root like a clove or a nail, appearing most commonly on the face and the ends of the fingers." (Wiseman 1998, 75) **LJTY: 11-3-23**

dysphagia-occlusion (膈噎 *ye ge*): "A disease charac-terized by sensation of blockage on swallowing, difficulty in getting food and drink down, and, in some cases, immediate vomiting of ingested food." (Wiseman 1998, 163) **ZJDC: 9-8**

eruptions on the back (發背 *fa bei*): Wiseman translates this as "effusion of the back" and writes that the term means, "A headed flat-abscess of the back, usually on the governing vessel or bladder channel and attributable to stagnation in the channels and blockage of qi and blood stemming either from fire toxin brewing internally or exuberant yin vacuity fire." (Wiseman 1998, 168-9) **LJTY: 11-3-23**

flat-abscess (疽 *ju*): "1. Headless flat-abscess. A deep malign suppuration in the flesh, sinew, and even the bone, attributed to toxic evil obstructing qi and the blood. 2. Headed flat-abscess. Prior to the Song dynasty, the term *ju* meant only headless flat-abscess. From the Song dynasty, it came to be used to denote certain su-perficial sores." (Wiseman 1998, 209) **LJTY: 11-3-23**

ghost strike (鬼擊 *gui ji*): Sudden gripping pain of the chest and abdomen or bleeding (vomiting blood, nosebleed, bleeding from the lower orifices) (Li 1995, 1110). It seems like injuries received from an attack, yet there was no visible attack. **LJTY: 11-3-20**

glomus lump (痞塊 *pi kuai*): Any type of palpable abdominal mass. (Wiseman 1998, 242) **LJTY: 11-3-7**

goose foot wind (鵝掌風 *e zhang feng*): "A skin disease of the hand characterized by vesicles, itching, and thickening of the skin." (Wiseman 1998, 244) **BCGM: 04-22-8, BCGM: 15-05-40**

gu toxins (蠱毒 *gu du*): In ancient times it was believed that people could make a poison from insects and use it to harm others. Later it was associated with drum distention because it has a similar pronunciation. It is still thought to be caused by toxins from poisonous insects or reptiles. (Wiseman 1998, 249) **LJTY: 11-3-24**

hostility (忤 *wu*): Hostility is short for visiting hostility (客忤 *ke wu*). Wiseman (1998) says it is "crying, fright, disquietude, or even changes in complexion in infants brought on by seeing a stranger or a strange sight, or being exposed to unfamiliar surroundings or circumstances" (p. 60). **ZJDC: 9-6-7**

hu huo (狐惑 *hu huo*): *Hu huo* is a type of worm disease. Erosion due to worms in the genitals and anus is *hu*. Erosion due to worms in the throat is *huo* (Li 1995, 967). This syndrome is discussed in Chapter 3 of the *Golden Cabinet* 《金貴要略》. The *Golden Cabinet* says to treat erosion in the anus by fuming with *Xiong Huang* (Realgar). **BCGM: 15-05-13, ZJDC: 9-6**

infixation (疰 or *zhu*): Wiseman (1998) says that 疰 *zhu* infixation is related to 蛀 *zhu*, which means to be eroded by worms. 疰 *Zhu* infixation means an evil lodges permanently, causing disease (Li 1995, 1291). Cadaverous infixation denotes pulmonary consumption. (Wiseman 1998, 300) **ZJDC: 9-6-7**

invisible-worm (虫+匿 *ni4*): Worm-erosion disease (Wiseman 1998, 319). These worms often target the nose or teeth. (Li 1995, 1711) **BCGM: 26-09, BCGM: 04-23-7**

malign stroke (中惡 *zhong e*): A disease attributed to

demons, contracted after the victim went into a temple or graveyard, or attended a funeral. (Wiseman 1998, 384) **BCGM: 29-06-08**

occlusion qi (氣膈 *qi ge*): Blockage of the throat with chest and rib-side counterflow fullness and putrid belching. (Wiseman 1998, 481) **LJTY: 11-3-8**

oppressive ghost dreams (魘 *yan*): Also called 夢魘 *meng yan* or 鬼魘 *gui yan*. Malign bizarre dreams, perhaps with a feeling of something heavy pressing on the body, often with sudden fright. Although this phrase can be translated as nightmares, it is different than ordinary bad dreams; it suggests ghosts or spirits (whether real or imagined) as etiology. (Li 1995, 1686) **ZJDC: 9-6-2, LJTY: 10-1-4-33, LJTY: 11-3-20**

outcropping ((弩+肉) *nu3*): This is an improperly written character commonly substituted for 胬 *nu*. Malign flesh, putrid flesh. It can also grow over an eye like a membrane. An abscess can also have an outcropping. (Li 2001, 59; Wiseman 1998, 181 & 422) **BCGM: 17-17-1-114**

patch wind (癜風 *dian feng*): Also known as purple and white patch wind (紫白癜風 *zi bai dian feng*) or sweat macules (汗斑 *han ban*). A skin condition with shiny purplish and whitish patches that may scale and itch. It begins with small patches that grow and merge. The edges are clear. (Li 1995, 1494; Wiseman 1998, 473) **ZJDC: 9-6-12**

reachable sore (搭手 *da shou*): Eruptions on the back that the patient can reach with his own hand. They can be on the upper, middle, or lower back. (Wiseman 1998, 168-9 & 492) **LJTY: 11-3-23**

reverse flow (厥逆 *jue ni*): 1. From the *Discussion on Cold Damage*, reversal cold of the extremities. 2. From *Magic Pivot*, Chapter 22, acute chest pain with sudden cold of the extremities. 3. From *Elementary Questions*, Chapter 47, a kind of enduring headache. (Wiseman 1998, 505) **LJTY: 11-3-2**

shank sores (臁瘡 *lian chuang*): "A sore on the shin,

characterized by redness, swelling, and itching." (Wiseman 1998, 528) **BCGM: 15-05-44**

she gong (射工 *she gong*): Li Shizhen (1995, 1265) says *she gong* is some kind of toxic insect. It is discussed in **BCGM: 42-15**, where it is also called "ravine ghost insect" (溪鬼蟲). This passage says its feet are angled like a crossbow and it uses qi as "arrows." It shoots people's shadows and they become ill. **BCGM: 27-07, BCGM: 26-09**

she wang (射罔 *she wang*): A poison from *Fu Zi* (Aconite) used to coat weapons like arrow tips. (Harper 1998, 238) **BCGM: 17-21-1**

streaming sores (流注 *liu zhu*): "A sore deep in the body, so called because of the tendency of its toxin to move from one place to another, as if flowing through the flesh." (Wiseman 1998, 584) **JYQS: 64-119**

summer influx (注夏 *zhu xia*): (Also called summer infixation) a condition that recurs each summer, with poor appetite, fatigue, weakness, low fever, and gradual recovery in the autumn. It is a type of damp obstruction. (Wiseman 1998, 592) **LJTY: 11-3-4**

thoroughflux diarrhea (洞泄 *dong xie*): Diarrhea with untransformed food in the stool that comes after eating. (Wiseman 1998, 612) **LJTY: 11-3-14, 11-3-19-13**

twisted intestines with internal hooking (盤腸內釣 *pan chang nei diao*): This is spasmodic abdominal pain that feels like the intestines are being twisted or pulled with a hook. (Li 1995, 1404-5) **BCGM: 26-03**

ulcerate (潰 *kui*) The opening up of a sore. (See also the section below on *Moxibustion Treatment Terminology*.) **LJTY: 11-3-23**

welling-abscess (癰 *yong*): "A large suppuration in the flesh characterized by a painful swelling and redness that is clearly circumscribed, and that before rupturing is soft and characterized by thin, shiny skin. Be-

fore suppuration begins, it can be easily dispersed; when pus has formed, it easily ruptures; after rupture, it easily closes and heals. It may be associated with generalized heat, thirst, yellow tongue fur and a rapid pulse." (Wiseman 1998, 670) **LJTY: 11-3-23**

white turbidity (白濁 *bai zhuo*): Cloudy white urine. It can also mean a white discharge from the urethra. (Wiseman 1998, 677) **LJTY: 11-3-19-3, LJTY: 11-3-21**

2. MOXIBUSTION & TREATMENT TERMINOLOGY

apply medicinals externally (貼 *tie*)

blistering moxibustion (發泡灸 *fa pao jiu*)

cone (炷 *zhu* or 壯 *zhuang*)

direct moxibustion (直接灸 *zhi jie jiu* or *ming jiu* 明灸 or *zhu fu jiu* 著膚灸)

heavenly moxibustion (天灸法 *tian jiu fa*)

indirect moxibustion (間接灸 *jin jie jiu* or 間隔灸 *jian ge jiu*)

moxa floss (熟艾 *shu ai*)

moxa pole (艾條灸 *ai tiao jiu*)

moxa punk (熟艾 *shu ai*)

moxa roll (艾卷灸 *ai juan jiu*)

moxa sore (灸瘡 *jiu chuang*)

moxa stick (艾條灸 *ai tiao jiu*)

moxa wool (熟艾 *shu ai*)

moxibustion (灸法 *jiu fa*)

moxibustion using isolating substances (間接灸 *jian jie jiu* or 間物灸 *jian wu jiu* or 間艾 *jian ai*)

mugwort from Qizhou (蘄艾 *qi ai*)

non-scarring moxibustion (無瘢痕灸 *wu ban hen jiu*)

number of cones based on years of age (隨年壯灸之 *sui nian zhuang jiu zhi*)

scarring moxibustion (瘢痕灸 *ban hen jiu*)

session (報 *bao*): A technical term used in moxibustion. It indicates separate times to repeat application of a moxibustion formula. It was used as far back as Sun's *Prescriptions*, "Do not surpass 30 cones of moxibustion, one session every three days."

suppurative moxibustion (化膿灸 *hua nong jiu*)

take medicinals internally (服 *fu*)

ulcerate (潰 *kui*): The opening up of a moxa sore

(See also the section above on *Symptom, Disease, or Condition Terminology*.)

3. SOME REGIONS OF THE BODY

heart region and abdomen (心腹 *xin fu*): "The pit of the stomach and the abdomen as a whole." (Wiseman 1998, 271)

lesser abdomen (少腹 *shao fu*): The lateral lower abdomen, although sometimes it is used as a synonym for the smaller abdomen. (Wiseman 1998, 343)

smaller abdomen (小腹 *xiao fu*): The lower abdomen, the area below the umbilicus. (Wiseman 1998, 541)

stomach duct (胃脘 *wei wan*): More commonly translated as the epigastrium. (Deng 1999, 82)

REFERENCES

Anonymous. 1999. 《詩經》 *The book of songs*. Shandong: Shandong Friendship Press.

Bai, H.M. 白鶴鳴. 1996. 《術數精要》 *Essentials of calculation skills*. Hong Kong: Juxian Guan Ltd.

Baldwin, G.C. 1970. *Schemers, dreamers, and medicine men*. New York: Four Winds Press.

Bensky, D. and Gamble, A. 1993. *Chinese herbal medicine: Materia medica*. Seattle: Eastland Press.

Chao, Y.F. 巢元方. 1992. 《諸病源候論校註》 *Proofread and annotated discussion on the origins of symptoms in illness*. Beijing: People's Health Publishing House.

Chen, R.L. 陳瑞隆, 1993. *Secret canon of day selection knowledge*. 《擇日學秘典》 Tainan: Shifeng Publishing.

Chen, F.H. 陳復華, ed. 1998. 《古代漢語詞典》 *Ancient Chinese dictionary*. Beijing: Commercial Printing Shop.

Chen, W.J. 陳文杰 and Luo, D.H. 羅得懷. 1995. *Drawings of 100 famous Chinese doctors*. Guangdong: New Century Publishers.

Chen, Y.B. and Deng, L.Y., eds. 1989. *Essentials of contemporary Chinese acupuncturists' clinical experiences*. Beijing: Foreign Languages Press.

Chen, Y.Z. 陳延之. 1993. 《小品方新輯》 *New compilation of short sketches of formulas*. Ed. by Zhu, X.N. 祝新年. Shanghai: Shanghai Chinese Medicine College Publishing House.

Cheng, X.N. 程莘農. 1964. 《中國針灸學》 *Chinese acupuncture and moxibustion*. Beijing: People's Health Publishing House.
———. 1987. *Chinese acupuncture and moxibustion*. Beijing: Foreign Languages Press.

Deadman, P., *et al.* 1998. *A manual of acupuncture*. Hove, East Sussex, England: JCM Publications.

Deng, T.T. 1999. *Practical diagnosis in traditional Chinese medicine*. Edinburgh: Churchill Livingstone.

Dharmananda, S. 1998. *Borneal, artemisia, and moxa*. Portland: ITM's START Group.
———. 2001. *Li Shizhen: Scholar worthy of emulation*. Portland: ITM's START Group.
———. 2004. *Moxibustion: Practical considerations for modern use of an ancient technique*. Portland: ITM's START Group.

Dongxuan Jushi 東軒居士. 1989. 《衛濟寶書》 *Precious book of protecting and aiding*. Beijing: People's Health Publishing House.

Dou, C. 竇材. 1991. 《扁鵲心書 · 神方》 *Book of Bian Que's heart*. Seoul: All China Publishers.

———. 2000.《扁鵲心書》*Book of Bian Que's heart.* Beijing: Chinese Medicine Ancient Book Publishing House.

Duan, Y.S. 段逸山, ed. 1984.《醫古文》*Ancient medical texts.* Shanghai: Shanghai Science and Technology Publishing House.

Eberhard, W. 1986. *A dictionary of Chinese symbols.* London: Routledge.

Eckman, P. 1996. *In the footsteps of the Yellow Emperor.* San Francisco: Cypress Book Company.

Ellis, A., Wiseman, N., and Boss, K. 1989. *Grasping the wind.* Brookline: Paradigm Press.
———. 1991. *Fundamentals of Chinese acupuncture.* Brookline: Paradigm Press.

Flaws, B., trans. 1998. *The Lakeside Master's study of the pulse.* Boulder: Blue Poppy Press.
———. 2003. *Liquid moxa as a species of applied moxibustion.* Boulder, CO: Blue Poppy Enterprises: www.bluepoppy.com/press/down load/articles/liquidmoxa_sp

Fruehauf, H. 1998. Driving out demons and snakes: *gu* syndrome. *Journal of Chinese Medicine* 57:10-17.
———. 1999. Chinese medicine in crisis. *Journal of Chinese Medicine* 61:6-14.

Fu, W.K. 1985. *Traditional Chinese medicine and pharmacology.* Beijing: Foreign Languages Press.

Gao W. 高武. 1999.《針灸聚英》*Gatherings from eminent acupuncturists.* Beijing: Chinese Medicine Ancient Book Publishing House.

Ge H. 葛洪. 1996.《葛洪肘後備急方》*Ge Hong's emergency prescriptions to keep up your sleeve.* Beijing: People's Health Publishing House.

Gong Y.X. 龔延賢. 1999.《龔延賢醫學全書》*Gong Yanxian's complete medical works.* Beijing: China Chinese Medicine Herbal Publishing House.
———. 2001.《壽世保元》*Long life and protecting the origin.* Beijing: People's Health Publishing House.

Gu, C.S. 賈春生 and Zhao, J.X. 趙建新. 1994.
《特種灸法臨床精要・保健灸法史略》*Essentials of special types of clinical moxibustion: A brief history of preventive moxibustion.* Beijing: Chinese Medicine Herbal Science and Technology Publishing House.

Gu, Y.S. 顧悦善 and Hao, X.J. 郝學君. 1996.
《灸法養生》*Moxibustion to nourish life.* Liaoning: Liaoning Science and Technology Publishing House.

Guo, L.W. 1991. The proper application of herb stick moxibustion. *Journal of Chinese Medicine* 37:15-16.

Han, Y. 韓愈. 2002.《韓愈全集》*Complete collection of Han Yu.* http://www.yasue888.net/hon_yue.html.

Harper, D. 1998. *Early Chinese medical literature: The Mawangdui Medical Manuscripts.* London: Kegan Paul International.

He, P.R. 賀普仁. 2003.《灸具灸法》*Utensils and methods of moxibustion.* Beijing: Scientific and Technical Documents Publishing House.

Hong, D.G. 洪敦耕. 2000.《醫易入門》*Introduction to medical yi.* Hong Kong: Heaven and Earth Book Limited Company.

Hu, Y.S. 胡裕樹, ed. 1997.
《新編古今漢語大詞典》*New edition of the great ancient and modern Chinese dictionary.* Shanghai: Shanghai Lexicography Publishing House.

Huang, L.X. 黃龍祥, ed. 1996.《針灸名著集成》*Grand compendium of famous works on acupuncture and moxibustion.* Beijing: Cathay Publishing House.
———, ed. 2003.《中國針灸史圖鑒》*Illustrated handbook of the history of Chinese acupuncture and moxibustion.* Qingdao: Qingdao Publishing House.

Huang, Z.J. 黃志杰, ed. 1973.
《黄帝内經, 神農本草, 中藏經, 脈經, 男精精譯》*Essential interpretation of Yellow Emperor's inner canon, the Divine Peasant's materia medica, classic of the central viscera, pulse classic, and classic of difficulties.* Beijing: Sci-

entific and Technical Documents Publishing House.

Huangfu, M. 皇甫謐. 1993. *The systematic classic of acupuncture and moxibustion*. Trans. by Yang, S.Z. and Chace, C. Boulder, CO: Blue Poppy Press.

———. 1997.《針灸甲乙經》*The systematic classic of acupuncture and moxibustion*. Liaoning: Liaoning Science and Technology Publishing House.

Huard, P. and Wong, M. 1968. *Chinese medicine*. New York: World University Library.

Ji, D.Z. 齊德之. 1990. *The profound significance of external medicine*. 《外科精義》 Beijing: People's Health Publishing House.

Ji, W.H. 吉文輝. 2000. *A study of editions of ancient Chinese medical books*.《中醫古籍版本學》 Shanghai: Shanghai Science and Technology Publishing House.

Kaptchuk, T. 2000. *The web that has no weaver*. Chicago: Contemporary Books.

Lhasa OMS. 2003-2004. Medical supplies catalogue. Weymouth, MA.

Li, C. 李梴. 1999.《醫學入門》*Entering the gate of medicine*. Tianjin: Tianjin Science and Technology Publishing House.

Li, D.Y. 李東垣 1993.《東垣醫集》*Li Dongyuan's medical collection*. Beijing: People's Health Publishing House.

Li, J. W. 李經緯. 1995.《中國大辭典》*Great dictionary of Chinese medicine*. Beijing: People's Health Publishing House.

Li, S.B. 李順保. 2001.《中醫中藥醫古文難字字典》*Dictionary of difficult characters from ancient Chinese medicine and Chinese herbal texts*. Beijing: Xueyuan Publishing.

Li, S.Z. 李時珍. 1962. *Illustrated great pharmacopeia*. 《圖解本草綱目》Seoul: High Culture Publishing.

———. 1996. *Li Shizhen's complete medical works*.

《李時珍醫學全書》 Ed. by Hu, G.C. 胡國臣, *et al.* Beijing: China Chinese Medicine Herbal Publishing House.

———. 1999.《濱湖脈學》*The Lakeside [Master's] study of the pulse*. Tianjin: Tianjin Science and Technology Publishing House.

———. 2004. *Compendium of materia medica (Bencao Gangmu)*. Trans. by Luo, X.W. Beijing: Foreign Languages Press.

Li, Z.D. 1989. *Chinese traditional auspicious patterns*. Shanghai: Shanghai Popular Science Press.

Liao, R.H. 廖潤鴻. 1986.《針灸集成》*Collected works of acupuncture and moxibustion*. Seoul: All China Publishers.

Liu, G.J. 劉冠軍. 1991.《中醫灸療集要》*Collected essentials of Chinese moxibustion*. Nanchang: Jiangxi Science and Technology Publishing House.

Liu, W.D. 劉文典. 1980.《莊子補正》*Zhuangzi additions and corrections*. Kunming: Yunnan People's Publishing House.

Liu, W.S. 劉完素. 1998.《素問病機宜氣保命集》*Collection of writings on the mechanisms of illnesses, suitability of qi, and the safeguarding of life as discussed in the Su Wen*. Beijing: Chinese Medicine Ancient Book Publishing House.

Liu, Z.C. 劉正才. 1999. *A study of Daoist acupuncture*. Boulder, CO: Blue Poppy Press.

Lo, V. and Cullen, C. 2005. *Medieval Chinese medicine: The Dunhuang medical manuscripts*. London: Routledge Curzon.

Lu, G.D. and Needham, J. 1980. *Celestial lancets: A history and rationale of acupuncture and moxa*. Cambridge: Cambridge University Press.

Lu, T.L. 魯兆麟, *et al.*, eds. 1996.《二續名醫類案》*Two additional categorized cases of famous doctors*. Liaoning: Liaoning Science and Technology Publishing House.

Ma, S. 馬蒔, 1999. 《黃帝內經素問注証發微》*Yellow Emperor's inner canon elementary questions, annotated, validated, and its subtleties elucidated*. Beijing: Science and Technical Documents Publishing House.

Mair, V. H., trans. 1994. *Wandering on the way: Early Taoist tales and parables of Chuang Tzu*. Honolulu: University of Hawaii Press.

Major, J.S. 1993. *Heaven and earth in early Han thought*. Albany: State University of New York Press.

Mathews, R.H. 1943. *Mathews' Chinese-English dictionary*. Cambridge: Harvard University Press.

Mengzi, Yi, F. 易夫, ed. 1997.《孟子》*Mengzi*. Beijing: Religion and Culture Publishing House.

Menzies, G. 2002. *1421: The year China discovered America*. New York: Perennial Books.

O'Connor, J. and Bensky, D. 1981. *Acupuncture: A comprehensive text*. Seattle: Eastland Press.

Qi, H. 漆浩, *et al.* 1995.《艾灸養生祛病法》*Methods of nourishing life and dispelling disease with mugwort moxibustion*. Beijing: Beijing Physical Culture University Publishing House.

Ren, Y.Q. 任應秋, *et al.* 1986.《中醫各家學說》*The theories of each school of Chinese medicine*. Shanghai: Shanghai Science and Technology Publishing House.

So, J.T.Y. 1987. *Treatment of disease with acupuncture*. Brookline, MA: Paradigm Publications.

Sun, S.M. 孫思邈. 1994.《千金方》*Prescriptions worth a thousand pieces of gold*. Beijing: Cathay Publishing House.
———. 1996.《千孫真人千金方》*True Person Sun's prescriptions worth a thousand pieces of gold*. Beijing: People's Health Publishing House.
———. 1997a.《千金翼方》*Supplement to prescriptions worth a thousand pieces of gold*. Liaoning: Liaoning Science and Technology Publishing House.
———. 1997b.《備急千金要方校釋》*Essential prescriptions for emergencies worth a thousand pieces of gold, corrected and explained*. Beijing: People's Health Publishing House.

Tamba, Y. 丹波康賴. 1993.《醫心方》*Medical heart formulas*. Beijing: People's Health Publishing House.

Unschuld, P.U. 1985. *Medicine in China: A history of ideas*. Berkeley: University of California Press.
———. 1986a. *Medicine in China: A history of pharmaceuticals*. Berkeley: University of California Press.
———. 1986b. *Nan-ching: The classic of difficult issues*. Berkeley: University of California Press.
———. 2000. *Medicine in China: Historical artifacts and images*. Munich: Prestel.
———. 2003. *Huang di nei jing su wen: Nature, knowledge, imagery in an ancient Chinese medical text*. Berkeley: University of California Press.

Walters, D. 1992. *Chinese astrology*. Northampton England: Aquarian/Thorsons.

Wang, B. 王冰, ed. 1994.《黃帝內經素問》*The Yellow Emperor's inner canon: elementary questions*. Beijing: People's Health Publishing House.

Wang, S.H. 王叔和. 1996.《脈經》*The pulse classic*. Beijing: Science and Technology Literature Publishing House.
———. 1997. *The pulse classic*. Trans. by Yang S.Z. Boulder, CO: Blue Poppy Press.

Wang, T. 王燾. 1955.《外台秘要》*Secret necessities of a frontier official*. Beijing: People's Health Publishing House.

Wang, X.T. 王雪苔. 1984. Research into the methods of classical moxibustion. Trans. by Moffett, J. *Journal of Chinese Medicine* 15:1-9.
———, ed. 1994.《特種灸法臨床精要》*Essentials of special types of clinical moxibustion*. Beijing: Chinese Medicine Herbal Science and Technology Publishing House.

Wei, J. 魏稼 ed. 1987.《各家針灸學說》*The theories of each school of acupuncture and moxibustion*. Shanghai: Shanghai Science and Technology Publishing House.

Wei, Y.L. 危亦林 1964.《世醫得效方》*Effective formulas obtained from generations of doctors*.

Shanghai: Shanghai Science and Technology Publishing House.

Wilcox, L. 2007. *Moxibustion in the Ming dynasty* (dissertation). Los Angeles American University of Complementary Medicine.

Wiseman, N. 1995. *English-Chinese Chinese-English dictionary of Chinese medicine*. Changsha: Hunan Science and Technology Publishing House.

Wiseman, N. and Ye, F. 1998. *A practical dictionary of Chinese medicine*. Brookline MA: Paradigm Publications.

Wolfe, H.L. 2003. *Pushing the envelope of moxibustion*. Boulder, CO: Blue Poppy Enterprises. www.bluepoppy.com/press/journal/issues/articles/apr03/apr

Wright, A.F. and Twitchett, D., eds. 1973. *Perspectives on the T'ang*. New Haven: Yale University Press.

Wu, L.S. and Wu, A.Q. 1997. *Yellow Emperor's canon internal medicine*. Beijing: China Science and Technology Press.

Xu, C.F. 徐春甫 1991.《古今醫統大全》*Great completion of unified ancient and modern medicine*. Beijing: People's Health Publishing House.

Xu, H. 許洪 1997.《指南總論》*Guidebook overall discussion* (appendix to《太平惠民和劑局方》*Professional and popular prescriptions from the Taiping era*). Liaoning: Liaoning Science and Technology Publishing House.

Xu, S. 許慎. 1997.《說文解字今釋》*Modern explanation of the analytical dictionary of Chinese characters*. Changsha: Yuelu Publishers.

Yan, X.Q. 1998. *The great wall*. Trans. by Zhang, S.N. *Chinese Literature Magazine* (#3).

Yang, J.Z. 楊繼洲. 1908.《繪圖針灸大成》*Illustrated great compendium of acupuncture and moxibustion*. Shanghai: Shanghai Zhang Fu Ji Shi Yin.
———. 1998.《針灸大成》*Great compendium of acupuncture and moxibustion*. Beijing: Chi-

nese Medicine Ancient Book Publishing House.

Yang, S.Z., trans. 1993. *Master Hua's classic of the central viscera*. Boulder, CO: Blue Poppy Press.

Yang, S.Z. and Liu, F.T., trans. 1994. *The divinely responding classic*. Boulder, CO: Blue Poppy Press.

Yang, Z.M. 楊兆民. 1996.《刺法灸法學》*Needling and moxibustion studies*. Shanghai: Shanghai Science and Technology Publishing House.

Ye, T.S. 葉天士. 1999.《葉天士醫學全書》*Ye Tianshi's complete medical works*. Beijing: China Chinese Medicine Herbal Publishing House.

Zhang, F.J. 張芳杰. 1992. *Far East Chinese-English dictionary*. Taibei: The Far East Book Company, LTD.

Zhang, J. 張吉. 1994.《各家針灸醫籍選》*Selections from medical texts of each school of acupuncture and moxibustion*. Beijing: China Chinese Medicine Herbal Publishing House.

Zhang, J.Y. 張景岳. 1965.《類經》*Categorized classic*. Beijing: People's Health Publishing House.
———. 1966.《類經圖翼·類經附翼 評注》*Illustrated supplement to the categorized classic and appended supplement of the categorized classic with annotations*. Eds. Wang, Y.S. 王玉生 *et al*. Xi'an: Shanxi Science and Technology Publishing House.
———. 1982.《類經圖翼，附：類經附翼》*Illustrated supplement of the categorized classic; Appended: Appended supplement of the categorized classic*. Seoul: Great Star Culture Society.
———. 1991.《類經》*Categorized classic*. Shanghai: Shanghai Ancient Text Publishing House.
———. 1995.《景岳全書》*Jingyue's complete works*. Ed. by Zhao, L.X. 趙立勛. Beijing: People's Health Publishing House.
———. 1999.《醫學全書》*Complete medical works*. Ed. Li, Z. Y. 李志庸. Beijing: China Chinese Medicine Herbal Publishing House.

Zhang, Q.W. 張奇文. 1992.《中國灸法大成》*Great compendium of Chinese moxibustion*. Tianjin:

Tianjin Science and Technology Publishing House.

Zhang, R. 張仁 and Liu, J. 劉堅. 2004. 《中國民間奇特灸法》*Unusual Chinese folk moxibustion*. Shanghai: Shanghai Science and Technology Publishing House.

Zhang, Z.H. 張子和. 1996. 《子和醫集》*[Zhang] Zihe's medical collection*. Beijing: People's Health Publishing House.

Zhang, Z.J. 張仲景. 1992. 《金匱要略按案》*Essential prescriptions of the golden cabinet annotations and cases*. Hong Kong: Juxian Guan Ltd.

———. 1995. *Cold damage fascicle.* 《傷寒分冊》Ed. Cheng, Z.H. 程昭寰. Beijing: China Science and Technology Publishing House.

Zhao, X.M. 趙學敏 1998. 《串雅全書》*Complete writings of stringing together the refined*. Beijing: China Chinese Medicine Herbal Publishing House.

Zhu, D.X. 朱丹溪. 2000. 《丹溪醫集》*[Zhu] Danxi's medical collection*. Beijing: People's Health Publishing House.

AUTHOR/BOOK INDEX

SUBSTANCES INDEX

GENERAL INDEX

withdrawal, 77, 80, 155, 168
worms, 68, 78, 103, 121, 122,
  124, 125, 144, 145, 186, 195,
  208, 220, 221, 239, 240, 258

Y
yang speculum, 62, 206, 234
Yao Yan (M-BW-24), 26, 68, 78,
  83, 145, 215, 220

Z
zi wu liu zhu, 206, 210
Zhou Jian (M-UE-46), 69
Zu San Li (ST 36), 4, 25, 30, 32,
  58, 64, 72, 74, 75, 81, 83, 86,
  88, 89, 107, 108, 141-146, 148-
  153, 155-157, 159, 160, 171,
  172, 178, 183, 184, 191, 226,
  228, 229, 231

OTHER BOOKS ON CHINESE MEDICINE AVAILABLE FROM:

BLUE POPPY PRESS

1990 57th Court North, Unit A, Boulder, CO 80301
For ordering 1-800-487-9296 PH. 303\447-8372   FAX 303\245-8362
Email: info@bluepoppy.com Website: www.bluepoppy.com

ACUPOINT POCKET REFERENCE
by Bob Flaws
ISBN 0-936185-93-7
ISBN 978-0-936185-93-4

ACUPUNCTURE & IVF
by Lifang Liang
ISBN 0-891845-24-1
ISBN 978-0-891845-24-6

ACUPUNCTURE FOR STROKE REHABILITATION
Three Decades of Information from China
by Hoy Ping Yee Chan, *et al.*
ISBN 1-891845-35-7
ISBN 978-1-891845-35-2

ACUPUNCTURE PHYSICAL MEDICINE:
An Acupuncture Touchpoint Approach to the Treatment of
Chronic Pain, Fatigue, and Stress Disorders
by Mark Seem
ISBN 1-891845-13-6
ISBN 978-1-891845-13-0

AGING & BLOOD STASIS:
A New Approach to TCM Geriatrics
by Yan De-xin
ISBN 0-936185-63-6
ISBN 978-0-936185-63-7

BETTER BREAST HEALTH NATURALLY
with CHINESE MEDICINE
by Honora Lee Wolfe & Bob Flaws
ISBN 0-936185-90-2
ISBN 978-0-936185-90-3

BIOMEDICINE: A TEXTBOOK FOR PRACTITIONERS OF
ACUPUNCTURE AND ORIENTAL MEDICINE
by Bruce H. Robinson, MD
ISBN 1-891845-38-1
ISBN 978-1-891845-38-3

THE BOOK OF JOOK:
Chinese Medicinal Porridges
by Bob Flaws
ISBN 0-936185-60-6
ISBN 978-0-936185-60-0

CHANNEL DIVERGENCES
Deeper Pathways of the Web
by Miki Shima and Charles Chase
ISBN 1-891845-15-2
ISBN 978-1-891845-15-4

CHINESE MEDICAL OBSTETRICS
by Bob Flaws
ISBN 1-891845-30-6
ISBN 978-1-891845-30-7

CHINESE MEDICAL PALMISTRY:
Your Health in Your Hand
by Zong Xiao-fan & Gary Liscum
ISBN 0-936185-64-3
ISBN 978-0-936185-64-4

CHINESE MEDICAL PSYCHIATRY
A Textbook and Clinical Manual
by Bob Flaws and James Lake, MD
ISBN 1-845891-17-9
ISBN 978-1-845891-17-8

CHINESE MEDICINAL TEAS: Simple, Proven, Folk
Formulas for Common Diseases & Promoting Health
by Zong Xiao-fan & Gary Liscum
ISBN 0-936185-76-7
ISBN 978-0-936185-76-7

CHINESE MEDICINAL WINES & ELIXIRS
by Bob Flaws   Revised Edition
ISBN 0-936185-58-9
ISBN 978-0-936185-58-3

CHINESE MEDICINE & HEALTHY WEIGHT
MANAGEMENT
An Evidence-based Integrated Approach
by Juliette Aiyana, L. Ac.
ISBN 1-891845-44-6
ISBN 978-1-891845-44-4

CHINESE PEDIATRIC MASSAGE THERAPY: A Parent's &
Practitioner's Guide to the Prevention & Treatment of
Childhood Illness
by Fan Ya-li
ISBN 0-936185-54-6
ISBN 978-0-936185-54-5

CHINESE SELF-MASSAGE THERAPY:
The Easy Way to Health
by Fan Ya-li
ISBN 0-936185-74-0
ISBN 978-0-936185-74-3

THE CLASSIC OF DIFFICULTIES:
A Translation of the *Nan Jing*
translation by Bob Flaws
ISBN 1-891845-07-1
ISBN 978-1-891845-07-9

A CLINICIAN'S GUIDE TO USING GRANULE
EXTRACTS
by Eric Brand
ISBN 1-891845-51-9
ISBN 978-1-891845-51-2

A COMPENDIUM OF CHINESE MEDICAL
MENSTRUAL DISEASES
by Bob Flaws
ISBN 1-891845-31-4
ISBN 978-1-891845-31-4

CONCISE CHINESE MATERIA MEDICA
by Eric Brand and Nigel Wiseman
ISBN 0-912111-82-8
ISBN 978-0-912111-82-7

CONTEMPORARY GYNECOLOGY: An Integrated
Chinese-Western Approach
by Lifang Liang
ISBN 1-891845-50-0
ISBN 978-1-891845-50-5

IMPERIAL SECRETS OF HEALTH & LONGEVITY
by Bob Flaws
ISBN 0-936185-51-1
ISBN 978-0-936185-51-4

INSIGHTS OF A SENIOR ACUPUNCTURIST
by Miriam Lee
ISBN 0-936185-33-3
ISBN 978-0-936185-33-0

INTEGRATED PHARMACOLOGY: Combining Modern Pharmacology with Chinese Medicine
by Dr. Greg Sperber with Bob Flaws
ISBN 1-891845-41-1
ISBN 978-0-936185-41-3

INTRODUCTION TO THE USE OF
PROCESSED CHINESE MEDICINALS
by Philippe Sionneau
ISBN 0-936185-62-7
ISBN 978-0-936185-62-0

KEEPING YOUR CHILD HEALTHY WITH
CHINESE MEDICINE
by Bob Flaws
ISBN 0-936185-71-6
ISBN 978-0-936185-71-2

THE LAKESIDE MASTER'S STUDY OF THE PULSE
by Li Shi-zhen, trans. by Bob Flaws
ISBN 1-891845-01-2
ISBN 978-1-891845-01-7

MANAGING MENOPAUSE NATURALLY WITH
CHINESE MEDICINE
by Honora Lee Wolfe
ISBN 0-936185-98-8
ISBN 978-0-936185-98-9

MASTER HUA'S CLASSIC OF THE CENTRAL VISCERA
by Hua Tuo, trans. by Yang Shou-zhong
ISBN 0-936185-43-0
ISBN 978-0-936185-43-9

THE MEDICAL I CHING: Oracle of the Healer Within
by Miki Shima
ISBN 0-936185-38-4
ISBN 978-0-936185-38-5

MENOPAIUSE & CHINESE MEDICINE
by Bob Flaws
ISBN 1-891845-40-3
ISBN 978-1-891845-40-6

MOXIBUSTION: A MODERN CLINICAL HANDBOOK
by Lorraine Wilcox
ISBN 1-891845-49-7
ISBN 978-1-891845-49-9

MOXIBUSTION: THE POWER OF MUGWORT FIRE
by Lorraine Wilcox
ISBN 1-891845-46-2
ISBN 978-1-891845-46-8

A NEW AMERICAN ACUPUNTURE By Mark Seem
ISBN 0-936185-44-9
ISBN 978-0-936185-44-6

POCKET ATLAS OF CHINESE MEDICINE
Edited by Marne and Kevin Ergil
ISBN 3-131416-11-7
ISBN 978-3-131416-11-7

POINTS FOR PROFIT: The Essential Guide to Practice
Success for Acupuncturists 4rd Edition
by Honora Wolfe, Eric Strand & Marilyn Allen
ISBN 1-891845-25-X
ISBN 978-1-891845-25-3

PRINCIPLES OF CHINESE MEDICAL ANDROLOGY: An
Integrated Approach to Male Reproductive and Urological
Health by Bob Damone
ISBN 1-891845-45-4
ISBN 978-1-891845-45-1

PRINCE WEN HUI's COOK: Chinese Dietary Therapy
By Bob Flaws & Honora Wolfe
ISBN 0-912111-05-4
ISBN 978-0-912111-05-6

THE PULSE CLASSIC:
A Translation of the Mai Jing
by Wang Shu-he, trans. by Yang Shou-zhong
ISBN 0-936185-75-9
ISBN 978-0-936185-75-0

THE SECRET OF CHINESE PULSE DIAGNOSIS
by Bob Flaws
ISBN 0-936185-67-8
ISBN 978-0-936185-67-5

SECRET SHAOLIN FORMULAS FOR THE TREATMENT
OF EXTERNAL INJURY
by De Chan, trans. by Zhang Ting-liang & Bob Flaws
ISBN 0-936185-08-2
ISBN 978-0-936185-08-8

STATEMENTS OF FACT IN TRADITIONAL
CHINESE MEDICINE   Revised & Expanded
by Bob Flaws
ISBN 0-936185-52-X
ISBN 978-0-936185-52-1

STICKING TO THE POINT: A Step-by-Step Approach to
TCM Acupuncture Therapy
by Bob Flaws & Honora Wolfe   2 Condensed Books
ISBN 1-891845-47-0
ISBN 978-1-891845-47-5

A STUDY OF DAOIST ACUPUNCTURE
by Liu Zheng-cai
ISBN 1-891845-08-X
ISBN 978-1-891845-08-6

THE SUCCESSFUL CHINESE HERBALIST
by Bob Flaws and Honora Lee Wolfe
ISBN 1-891845-29-2
ISBN 978-1-891845-29-1

THE SYSTEMATIC CLASSIC OF ACUPUNCTURE &
MOXIBUSTION
A translation of the Jia Yi Jing
by Huang-fu Mi, trans. by Yang Shou-zhong & Charles Chace
ISBN 0-936185-29-5
ISBN 978-0-936185-29-3

THE TAO OF HEALTHY EATING: DIETARY
WISDOM ACCORDING TO CHINESE MEDICINE
by Bob Flaws   Second Edition
ISBN 0-936185-92-9
ISBN 978-0-936185-92-7

TEACH YOURSELF TO READ MODERN
MEDICAL CHINESE
by Bob Flaws
ISBN 0-936185-99-6
ISBN 978-0-936185-99-6

TEST PREP WORKBOOK FOR BASIC TCM THEORY
by Zhong Bai-song
ISBN 1-891845-43-8
ISBN 978-1-891845-43-7

TEST PREP WORKBOOK FOR THE NCCAOM BIO-
MEDICINE MODULE: Exam Preparation & Study Guide
by Zhong Bai-song
ISBN 1-891845-34-9
ISBN 978-1-891845-34-5

TREATING PEDIATRIC BED-WETTING WITH
ACUPUNCTURE & CHINESE MEDICINE
by Robert Helmer
ISBN 1-891845-33-0
ISBN 978-1-891845-33-8

TREATISE on the SPLEEN & STOMACH: A Translation
and annotation of Li Dong-yuan's
Pi Wei Lun
by Bob Flaws
ISBN 0-936185-41-4
ISBN 978-0-936185-41-5

THE TREATMENT OF CARDIOVASCULAR DISEASES
WITH CHINESE MEDICINE
by Simon Becker, Bob Flaws &
Robert Casañas, MD
ISBN 1-891845-27-6
ISBN 978-1-891845-27-7

THE TREATMENT OF DIABETES MELLITUS WITH
CHINESE MEDICINE
by Bob Flaws, Lynn Kuchinski &
Robert Casañas, M.D.
ISBN 1-891845-21-7
ISBN 978-1-891845-21-5

THE TREATMENT OF DISEASE IN TCM, Vol. 1:
Diseases of the Head & Face, Including Mental &
Emotional Disorders   New Edition
by Philippe Sionneau & Lü Gang
ISBN 0-936185-69-4
ISBN 978-0-936185-69-9

THE TREATMENT OF DISEASE IN TCM, Vol. II:
Diseases of the Eyes, Ears, Nose, & Throat
by Sionneau & Lü
ISBN 0-936185-73-2
ISBN 978-0-936185-73-6

THE TREATMENT OF DISEASE IN TCM, Vol. III:
Diseases of the Mouth, Lips, Tongue, Teeth & Gums
by Sionneau & Lü
ISBN 0-936185-79-1
ISBN 978-0-936185-79-8

THE TREATMENT OF DISEASE IN TCM, Vol IV:
Diseases of the Neck, Shoulders, Back, & Limbs
by Philippe Sionneau & Lü Gang
ISBN 0-936185-89-9
ISBN 978-0-936185-89-7

THE TREATMENT OF DISEASE IN TCM, Vol V: Diseases
of the Chest & Abdomen
by Philippe Sionneau & Lü Gang
ISBN 1-891845-02-0
ISBN 978-1-891845-02-4

THE TREATMENT OF DISEASE IN TCM, Vol VI:
Diseases of the Urogential System & Proctology
by Philippe Sionneau & Lü Gang
ISBN 1-891845-05-5
ISBN 978-1-891845-05-5

THE TREATMENT OF DISEASE IN TCM, Vol VII:
General Symptoms
by Philippe Sionneau & Lü Gang
ISBN 1-891845-14-4
ISBN 978-1-891845-14-7

THE TREATMENT OF EXTERNAL DISEASES WITH
ACUPUNCTURE & MOXIBUSTION
by Yan Cui-lan and Zhu Yun-long, trans. by Yang Shou-zhong
ISBN 0-936185-80-5
ISBN 978-0-936185-80-4

THE TREATMENT OF MODERN WESTERN
MEDICAL DISEASES WITH CHINESE MEDICINE
by Bob Flaws & Philippe Sionneau
ISBN 1-891845-20-9
ISBN 978-1-891845-20-8

UNDERSTANDING THE DIFFICULT PATIENT: A Guide
for Practitioners of Oriental Medicine
by Nancy Bilello, RN, L.ac.
ISBN 1-891845-32-2
ISBN 978-1-891845-32-1

WESTERN PHYSICAL EXAM SKILLS FOR
PRACTITIONERS OF ASIAN MEDICINE
by Bruce H. Robinson & Honora Lee Wolfe
ISBN 1-891845-48-9
ISBN 978-1-891845-48-2

YI LIN GAI CUO (Correcting the Errors in the Forest of
Medicine)
by Wang Qing-ren
ISBN 1-891845-39-X
ISBN 978-1-891845-39-0

70 ESSENTIAL CHINESE HERBAL FORMULAS
by Bob Flaws
ISBN 0-936185-59-7
ISBN 978-0-936185-59-0

160 ESSENTIAL CHINESE READY-MADE MEDICINES
by Bob Flaws
ISBN 1-891945-12-8
ISBN 978-1-891945-12-3

630 QUESTIONS & ANSWERS ABOUT CHINESE
HERBAL MEDICINE:
A Workbook & Study Guide
by Bob Flaws
ISBN 1-891845-04-7
ISBN 978-1-891845-04-8

260 ESSENTIAL CHINESE MEDICINALS
by Bob Flaws
ISBN 1-891845-03-9
ISBN 978-1-891845-03-1

750 QUESTIONS & ANSWERS ABOUT ACUPUNCTURE
Exam Preparation & Study Guide
by Fred Jennes
ISBN 1-891845-22-5
ISBN 978-1-891845-22-2